I hope that what people might say about this book is "Hey, these guys have really listened to Ann & Rud Turnbull in thinking about families". That's the best compliment I can imagine.

I miss you.

George Singer

With highest respect & deepest appreciation to you, Ann & Rud, for your nurturing & mentorship to make who I am now.

Mian

SUPPORTING FAMILIES OF CHILDREN WITH DEVELOPMENTAL DISABILITIES

EVIDENCE-BASED PRACTICES

SERIES EDITORS:

David E. Biegel, PhD
Elizabeth M. Tracy, PhD
Jack, Joseph and Morton Mandel
School of Applied Social Sciences,
Case Western Reserve University

Family Psychoeducation for Serious Mental Illness
Harriet P. Lefley

School Social Work
An Evidence-Informed Framework for Practice
Michael S. Kelly, James C. Raines, Susan Stone, and Andy Frey

Mental Health Treatment for Children and Adolescents
Jacqueline Corcoran

Individual Placement and Support
An Evidence-Based Approach to Supported Employment
Robert E. Drake, Gary R. Bond, and Deborah R. Becker

Preventing Child and Adolescent Problem Behavior
Evidence-Based Strategies in Schools, Families, and Communities
Jeffrey M. Jenson and Kimberly A. Bender

Supporting Families of Children with Developmental Disabilities
Evidence-Based and Emerging Practices
Mian Wang and George H. S. Singer

The Evidence-Based Practices series is published in collaboration with the Jack, Joseph and Morton Mandel School of Applied Social Sciences at Case Western Reserve University.

SUPPORTING FAMILIES OF CHILDREN WITH DEVELOPMENTAL DISABILITIES

EVIDENCE-BASED AND EMERGING PRACTICES

Mian Wang and George H. S. Singer
University of California, Santa Barbara

OXFORD
UNIVERSITY PRESS

OXFORD
UNIVERSITY PRESS

Oxford University Press is a department of the University of Oxford. It furthers the University's objective of excellence in research, scholarship, and education by publishing worldwide. Oxford is a registered trade mark of Oxford University Press in the UK and certain other countries.

Published in the United States of America by Oxford University Press
198 Madison Avenue, New York, NY 10016, United States of America.

First Edition published in 2016

Library of Congress Cataloging-in-Publication Data
Wang, Mian, 1964– author.
Supporting families of children with developmental disabilities :evidence-based and emerging practices/ by Mian Wang & George H.S. Singer; with contribution by Yeana W. Lam, Jiyeon Kim, Kelsey Oliver, Whitney Detar-Smith, Robin Dodds, Angela Ente and Louisa Wood.
pages cm. — (Evidence-based practices)
Includes bibliographical references and index.
ISBN 978–0–19–974307–0 (alk. paper)
1. Developmentally disabled—Family relationships—United States. 2. Social work with people with disabilities—United States. 3. Parents of developmentally disabled children—United States. 4. Caregivers—Services for—United States. 5. Family services—United States. 6. Family social work—United States. I. Singer, George H. S.,author. II. Title.
HV1570.5.U6W35 2016
362.1968—dc23
2015032484

1 3 5 7 9 8 6 4 2

Printed by Sheridan, USA.

We dedicate this book to Ann and Rud Turnbull, friends, mentors, and our role models as creative scholars and engaged public intellectuals.

CONTENTS

PREFACE

This book brings together the work of hundreds of researchers, many of whom were and are parents or siblings of individuals with developmental disabilities. They work in the academic wings of many disciplines that feed knowledge to the social sciences involved in helping families who have members with developmental disabilities. There are many helping professions that impact the lives of families of children, youth, and adults with intellectual disabilities or autism. A partial list includes pediatrics, general and special education, clinical and counseling psychology, school psychology, occupational and physical therapy, speech and language therapy, social work, school administration, and early intervention, to name some but by no means all of them. All of these professions require extensive training to enter and implement, training that is a combination of authoritative knowledge, craft knowledge, and situated praxis. This book is about the accumulation and comprehension of cumulative research aimed at yielding the authoritative knowledge that can help professionals effectuate the changes that families seek when they ask for help.

In the social sciences affiliated with the helping professions, it has long been a central aim to ground professional practice in scientific research. The evidence from research studies is meant to be like a building in which one brick is placed on top of a another that was previously mortared in place; it is meant to be a cumulative enterprise. The metaphor of incremental development and construction of a solid structure has not always fit the reality of social science research. Following the construction analogy, there are many walls that have been started and abandoned and there have been disagreements over what building should be built in the first place, so that sometimes there are several separate structures partly built. Some bricks that were at first ignored later become foundational, whereas others that may be of equal value are left in a stack to the side. Many of the builders have not been content to add another brick in a long-term construction process but instead have aimed to start their own wall. Some bricks, even foundational ones, are sometimes found to be faulty and risk bringing down a whole structure. Nonetheless, much applied knowledge has been developed by interlayered studies that have constructed sound and useful edifices. Simply put, after 50 years of research in the social sciences involved with helping families, we have learned a thing or two. This book is about several of those things and the evidence that convinces us they are indeed useful.

Traditional and relatively new ways of collating research now permit meaningful summarization of large bodies of research literatures in the helping-related social sciences. Procedures for reviewing and synthesizing the results of experimental studies have brought to light the extent to which research can and sometimes does build incrementally on itself so that helping practices are developed, refined through successive iterations, and repeatedly evaluated to establish confidence in the data that support them. This book is a gathering of studies about social and psychological interventions for families of children, youth, and adults with intellectual disability or autism. We have used tools that have evolved over time for making sense of a large amount of scientific data. The first major tool is the literature review, which uses brief verbal descriptions to summarize the key features of research studies and comment on their quality, importance, and implications. This kind of writing follows a set of genre rules that have been agreed on for accomplishing the work of giving an overall picture of a research topic in a relatively small amount of space. The second major tool is research synthesis, often referred to as meta-analysis. It is relatively newer and is still being developed, with the aim of using statistics to add together and characterize the outcomes of experiments in such a way as to create a common metric that applies across studies even though they may use very different ways of measuring outcomes. This approach relies on thorough, usually computer-aided, searches for studies, culling huge data bases where social science studies are cataloged. It makes use of a set of statistics that have been in existence for many years but that were only used to synthesize the numerical results of experimental research first in the 1970s. These statistical ideas and procedures are still being refined and extended. A meta-analysis standardizes very different kinds of results from studies about a given practice and reports on them in terms of one statistic that gives an indication of the strength of that practice when tested via controlled experiments. Meta-analyses are increasingly considered the gold standard for evaluating the effect of medical and psychological treatments. They frequently make the news about science and medicine because of their breadth and elegant simplicity by generating a number, an effect size, which gives a reading of the efficacy of whole groups of repeated studies. A meta-analysis can help answer three interrelated questions—"Is this practice efficacious when evaluated repeatedly with high-quality group experiments?," "To what extent does this practice change an outcome in a desirable way?," and "How robust is this finding?" When literature reviews and meta-analyses are combined, it is possible to develop fleeting but incisive overviews of large intellectual territories. At the same time, the specificity of the literature reviews and syntheses can help point out to practitioners and consumers specific practices for helping or being helped. They can also reveal to scholars and applied researchers where more work needs to be done. They typically do not provide enough information to serve as a working guide on how to implement practices, but instead they indicate which practices are likely to be effective and thus are worth acquiring more detailed knowledge about implementation.

The general public is most familiar with meta-analyses and the idea of science-based practices from the way new drugs are tested prior to their release. It is taken for granted that drugs that have been approved by the Food and Drug Administration have been evaluated by well-designed, rigorous experiments. Though the analogy is far from exact, the basic notion that interventions should be well defined, measurable, and repeatedly tested out via controlled experiments prior to adopting them pertains to psychosocial practices as diverse as support groups for parents of children with disabilities, Parent to Parent self-help programs, behavioral parent training, management of educational planning meetings, and coaching parents in advocacy skills.

The Oxford University Press series that includes this volume is predicated on a movement in the medical and social sciences centered on determining which practices have been reliably effective and deserve particular attention from practitioners and which ones have yet to be developed to this level. The movement is alternatively called the evidence-based practice or science-based practice movement. Professional organizations representing researchers in several fields have promulgated standards for determining what is required from research to determine that a practice can be reliably depended on.

The idea that what a practitioner does in the field should be guided by published research has not been without its critics. Some believe that professional practice is an art that must be guided by intuitive situated understanding of specific cases rather than a more formally structured endeavor based on generalizable data from experimental studies. Our sense is that the human arts requiring engaged emotional intelligence and the products of scientific research are not mutually exclusive and that the most effective practitioners combine both in a symbiotic way.

There are some important aspects of research on helping practices for families that a reader will not find in this volume. The reader will not meet the people who carried out the many studies reviewed in this book nor more importantly the participants and their children. We have not included biographical portraits of families or their loved ones who have disabilities, nor have we given a flavor of the kind of interpersonal caring and sometimes wrenching changes the intervention practices have sometimes required of parents. We do not include the testimonies of family members who were helped or not helped by the practices under review. Space and the conventions of scientific review have also not allowed us to detail the many ways that researchers have been the learners under parents' informal tutelage and the powerful ways that the needs and strengths of their children have motivated the research. This knowledge published here has been acquired because of the generosity of the many hundreds of people who voluntarily participated in the studies. Often this participation entailed allowing researchers to enroll them in extensive programs where they were required to make substantial commitments of time and energy. The many parent-training programs reviewed in this book often involved repeatedly allowing researchers into families' homes and intervening in the ways parents and children related to one another. We hope the reader will keep in mind that the formal summaries and statistical syntheses reported here represent important human endeavors for all concerned, ones that sometimes have had enormous impacts on the lives of the researchers and above all their subjects. Despite the formality of the genre and the abstract nature of the statistics, these studies are fundamentally works of the human heart aimed at doing the ongoing work of caring for one another in the face of difficult circumstances. And often in practice the people doing the research have been supported and uplifted by the resilience, relentless commitment, humor, and hope of the parents and their children with disabilities. They have often developed their interventions based on listening and learning from parents and siblings who have learned through lived experience ways of solving problems posed by caregiving. Further, the individuals with intellectual disability and autism who are the reason for the studies have often been the best guides to the kind of parenting and support they most need. This research represents human work in which researchers and the people who participate in their studies have educated one another in the practice of mutual caring. We hope that it will be useful for fellow scholars, practitioners, and above all to the families and their children.

ACKNOWLEDGMENTS

We thank the families who have shared their experiences, opened their homes, and risked implementing new ways of parenting in order that others in the future can benefit from practices based on science. They have been our inspiration and tutors.

Mian also wants to thank his mom, Xiangyu He, for her inspiration and constant confidence on him and is grateful to his wife, Xiaohong Li, and daughter Yidi Wang for their steadfast love and support during the period of writing this book and beyond.

LIST OF CONTRIBUTORS

Whitney Detar-Smith

Robin Dodds

Jiyeon Kim

Yeana W. Lam

Kelsey Oliver

SUPPORTING FAMILIES OF CHILDREN WITH DEVELOPMENTAL DISABILITIES

1

INTRODUCTION

George H. S. Singer and Mian Wang

Many citizens of the United States experience lifelong cognitive disabilities and require various degrees of assistance in daily living throughout the life course. Estimates of the prevalence of children and adults with intellectual disability (ID) or autism in the United States range widely from 3.8 to 7.7 million (Boyle et al., 2011; Larson et al., 2001). Over 75% of adults either live with their families of origin or rely on them for support well into middle age and their parents' elder years (Seltzer, Begun, Mailick Seltzer, & Krauss, 1991). Despite the centrality of families in assisting individuals with disabilities, only 4% of public funds for developmental disability (DD) services are allocated for family support (Braddock et al., 2015). Caregiving families have substantial needs for services aimed at bolstering their capacity to provide support and to achieve a high quality of life. There is a compelling need for evidence-based practices (EBPs) for providing such support.

Many individuals with DDs, specifically ID and autism, require some form of lifelong assistance that goes beyond what is normally required for nondisabled citizens to live independently, work in the community, have friends, enjoy leisure activities, and determine their own goals and preferences in small and large life decisions. Families provide the majority of this assistance over the life course. Family assistance may include relatively minor intermittent help with independent living, such as accompanying an adult with ID to baseball games with a favorite home team. It may also include ongoing and extensive help with activities of daily living, such as providing physical assistance to help a son or daughter scoop food with a spoon to eat healthy meals at the dinner table with the family.

Most families willingly take on the responsibility of caring for family members who need assistance with the demands of daily living. Many report that giving support to family members with disabilities is a source of satisfaction that enhances their quality of life

(Hastings, Beck, & Hill, 2005; Hastings & Taunt, 2002). For many people caregiving is central to their sense of what it means to be a good person and to live a good life. Under the right conditions, raising a child with ID or autism also brings with it opportunities for perceived benefits in the form of improved family cohesion, a sense of meaning and empowerment, and pride in the child's achievements, to name but a few of the many benefits that family members report (Hastings, Kovshoff, et al., 2005). In the right ecology of supports, families perceive and enjoy reciprocal benefits from caregiving. This book is about some of the many forms of community support that can contribute to these positive outcomes.

Family caregiving is also beneficial to society as a whole. Mahoney (1976) described it as a national treasure. If it were necessary for the government to provide for all of the care given by families to all relatives requiring 8 hours per week or more of support, the costs would be in the hundreds of billions of dollars (Arno, Levine, & Memmott, 1999); when converted to 2014 dollars, the national costs would range from $221.8 billion to $376 billion, depending on the estimated wage level of paid caregivers. Caregiving families make an enormous public contribution to US society by providing essential assistance that otherwise is very expensive, monetary costs that go well beyond the general safety net programs available in the United States. Further, it is care provided by loved ones and thus more likely to be personalized in a way that is difficult for paid providers to match. When families have sufficient internal resources and external support they report mutual benefits from caregiving (Hastings & Taunt, 2002; Stainton & Besser, 1998). Under the right conditions, a majority of these families adapt to their long-term assistance roles (Seltzer, Greenberg, Floyd, Pettee, & Hong, 2001).

The reason that families require access to generic community services and to government-sponsored forms of support is that raising children with disabilities through adulthood at home often entails unusual costs. These costs are captured by the term "caregiving stress" and include psychological, social, physical, and financial strains. In the absence of community supports, families are at risk of long-term caregiving stress, which can lead to fatigue, physical illnesses, and mental health problems, particularly in mothers (Witt, Riley, & Coiro, 2003). Evidence has been emerging for the past four decades suggesting strongly that caregiver stress can be prevented or reduced by providing family-centered services through the lifespan (Dunst, 2002). The stress response can be prevented or reduced by solving problems in caregiving, providing opportunities for rest and recreation, establishing social support, and using several forms of active coping skills. Furthermore, there is far more than stress to family adjustment in living with and loving a family member with a DD (Bernheimer & Weisner, 2007).

THE EVIDENCE-BASED PRACTICE MOVEMENT

The EBP movement offers the hope of some quality control in the services that are provided to families. The field of disability has been prone to treatment fads and to outright quackery in practices and services. A community-based support system risks failure if the quality of the services is not high. There are many factors that contribute to the quality of a social service, whether it is a private behavior analysis practice or a public school classroom. These include the training, expertise, and average performance level of the practitioners who staff these services. They also include the sufficiency of resources available to the service. For example, in-home training for helping a parent whose child has a severe behavior problem is likely to take several sessions and may require periodic booster sessions as the children and their problem behaviors change with age. For individuals with the most challenging and long-standing behavior problems, effective treatment may require months or even years of frequent home visits by therapists who coach caregivers. An insurance allocation to pay for 10 days of treatment may well be insufficient, and access to this service may mean little. The cultural fit of practitioners with the culture of families in their community is also likely to be a contributor to the effectiveness of a service system, as are many key structural variables.

One important contributor to the ultimate success of the service system is that its various services use programs that have a reasonable chance of success and that are not based on discredited theories or techniques. There needs to be a level of quality control on the content and delivery of support practices. The EBP movement is one important effort to increase the likelihood of effective and scientifically valid forms of supports. We do not believe that it is sufficient of itself, and there are some very real limitations to the move from judging the efficacy of a treatment under experimental conditions to establishing its effectiveness when delivered by ordinary practitioners in the context of community services. We discuss some of these limitations in chapter 7. Nonetheless we believe that the EBP movement is an important step in the evolution of a larger family support movement, a development that is ethically compelling and entirely necessary.

The idea of EBPs began as a movement within academic medicine, gaining momentum over the last quarter of the 20th century. Currently, several professions with a scientific knowledge base have taken up the idea. The ideal of professions that practice their work based on high-quality scientific evidence dates at least to the Enlightenment era. In the ideal, research scientists conduct rigorous experiments to establish procedures that can precisely target groups of people with specific characteristics. Evidence for initial efficacy is usually disseminated at first through scientific journals and at professional meetings, and subsequently through pre-service and in-service education. Evidence that the program is effective under real-world circumstances and at a large scale evolves more slowly. Ideally, pre-service professionals are educated to implement both basic and specific interventions to alleviate suffering. Scientifically analyzed interventions ideally become standard practice on a large scale, and these in turn are sustained and improved over time. In this ideal sequence, moving from problem identification to testing practices and finally informing services, a key early stage is determining that a practice is efficacious.

CLASSIFICATION OF EVIDENCE-BASED PRACTICES

The EBP movement has affected the helping professions concerned with individuals with DDs and their families. Several professional organizations serve these families and have provided standards for establishing that a practice is effective. These organizations include Division 12, the Division for Child and Adolescent Therapy of the American Psychology Association; the Division of Research for the Council for Exceptional Children (CEC); the US Department of Education's What Works Clearing House; the American Association of School Psychologists; and the National Autism Center. For example, the National Autism Center (2009) has provided standards for evaluating how efficacious and effective practices are likely to be on the basis of quantity and quality of research evidence supporting them. In this book, evidence-based and promising practices fall into two major groups. The first consists of those interventions that directly serve the parent or other family members other than the individual with a DD. For the most part, these interventions are drawn from a treatment tradition consisting of cognitive-behavioral interventions, mindfulness-based practices, and coping skills instruction. A second major group of interventions aims to reduce parental stress associated with children's problem behaviors and skill deficits by providing parent training and education so that parents can act as therapists. To be considered family support methods in this book, studies of this second group of practices must evaluate not only impacts on children with developmental disabilities but also impacts on parents and/or other family members. That is, behavioral parent-training studies must provide evidence of benefit to family members in addition to the child with a disability to be considered family support practices and to be included here.

The influence of social and medical research on the helping professions predates the current expansive trend toward identifying and disseminating EBPs. Graduate schools educating helping professionals have long drawn on research in training their students, although the quality and quantity of the research and the weight given to empiricism has varied greatly. There are four long-standing trends that have accelerated the adoption of EBPs and increased their importance. First, consumers as well as funders, including government and insurance agencies, have insisted on more accountability and have increasingly required empirical support for the potential benefits of interventions as a warrant to expend public funds. Congress routinely asks the Congressional Research Service for syntheses and reviews of outcome research when deliberating over legislation to fund programs. In addition, the quality of practice and intervention research has gradually improved over the past half-century so that its validity and trustworthiness has overcome some of the earlier skepticism about the relevance of research to professional practice. As part of this developing trust, the growing acceptance of meta-analysis since its inception in the 1970s has provided practitioners with a succinct way to identify distinctive practices and quantify their efficacy and effectiveness. It has also allowed researchers to come to conclusions about a group of studies other than the formerly common finding that studies were inconclusive and more research was needed. Finally, many of the helping professions have had to cope with practice fads, which have often been unscientific but nonetheless have gathered large followings. Unfortunately, fads based on unscientific beliefs have often offered false promises while consuming limited resources that otherwise might be allocated for better substantiated practices (Offit, 2008). In response to such wasteful and sometimes tragic trends, professional organizations and family advocates have pushed for better ways to safeguard vulnerable families from false or unsubstantiated claims. We are not so naïve as to believe that unscientific practices will vanish from the scene, but it is our hope, shared with many other researchers and practitioners, that scientific evidence informing professional standards of practice can help prevent or mitigate the worst of these fads.

PROCEDURES OF STUDY SELECTION, CATEGORIZATION, REVIEW, AND SYNTHESIS

We conducted extensive searches of the research literature over a period of 3 years to find published studies that met our criteria for evidence of how effective support programs can be in helping families adapt. We defined family support practices in the following way: Family support practices are planned interventions designed to support the caregiving capacity and enhance the quality of life of families of individuals with ID (formerly mental retardation) or autism through the lifespan. Practices can be categorized as: (1) techniques (e.g., contingent parental praise), (2) programs consisting of multiple techniques (e.g., stress management training [SMT], behavioral parent training [BPT], Parent to Parent programs), (3) interventions consisting of two or more major programs, and (4) planned processes of organizational or systems change (e.g., cash and counseling programs, public school full inclusion) or a social policy at the regional, state, or national levels (e.g., closing state hospitals, diverting Medicaid funds to establish family support services, providing families with subsidies). Practices are designed for use by families, individuals with disabilities, and the organizations and systems that serve them, with the express expectation that implementation will result in measurable quality-of-life benefits for the individuals and families who are the ultimate recipients of the practice (Horner, Carr, Halle, McGee, Odom, & Wolery, 2005).

We conducted repeated searches of the major social science publication databases. When we found studies that appeared to fit well with this broad definition we then screened them to make sure that their subjects were family members of children or siblings with either autism or ID ages 4 through adulthood. The studies had to be experiments that used either randomized clinical trial (RCT) designs, quasi-experimental designs (QEDs), or single-subject designs (SSDs) to evaluate the interventions.

We conducted searches in commonly used databases such as Article First, BlackWell Synergy, ERIC, Google Scholars, JSTOR, Medline Plus, Pro-Quest Nursing and Allied

Health, PsycINFO, PubMed, Sage Journals On-Line, Science Direct, Social Service Abstracts, Social Work Abstracts, and WilsonWeb. A great number of search terms used as either a single term or a combination of terms were adopted in the search process, including "developmental disabilities," "autism," "intellectual disabilities," "retardation," "handicap," "autism spectrum disorders," "Asperger syndrome," and "pervasive developmental disorders," and various combinations of keywords related to parents (e.g., "parents," "mothers," "caregivers," "fathers," "home-based") and family-based and parent-implemented interventions. We focused preliminary screening on reading the titles and abstracts of all identified articles, book chapters, and books generated from the search. From myriads of publications that survived the preliminary screening, empirical studies that fell into the categorization of RCT, QED, and SSD were further reviewed in full text.

Once we determined that a study met our inclusion criteria, we extracted key information and summarized the studies with their outcomes. For the group comparison studies we also synthesized the findings using meta-analysis to determine the effect size of the interventions (Cooper, Hedges, & Valentine, 2009). Finally, we made an evaluative decision classifying an intervention as established, promising, or unproven.

In this book we focus on those interventions that have been published regarding families of individuals with DDs beginning at age 4 and up. We have excluded ages birth to 3, because there is a large differentiated literature that is of sufficient quantity and quality to require its own separate analyses. Our review examines studies of families in which the family member with ID or autism resides with at least one other family member who is the primary caregiver.

EVALUATING AND CATEGORIZING THE EVIDENCE

We followed a two-stage process for evaluating the quality of the research on family support practices. The first level was a set of inclusion criteria that a study had to meet in order to be considered for review: First, it had to be available in a published peer-reviewed journal. Further, to be included, a study must have a standard experimental design from either the group comparison tradition or the SSD approach. This means that we have not included correlational evidence or practices that have only been described but not tested experimentally.

These studies had to meet the criteria for quality research as described in the CEC's Standards for Evidence-Based Practices in Special Education (Council for Exceptional Children [CEC], 2014). We reviewed standards developed for evaluating evidence from other professional and government organizations including the American Psychological Association Division 12 standards, the US Department of Education What Works Clearinghouse standards, the Cochrane Collaborative, and others. We settled on the CEC standards because they address with precision the features of research that are commonly the focus of other sets of standards in the social sciences and helping professions. Although they are derived from research on children with disabilities usually in school settings, the characteristics of high-quality research are sufficiently consistent across the helping professions and social sciences that we determined the CEC standards are robust when applied to research on family support and sufficient for consumers to have confidence in the quality of evidence reviewed with these criteria. The CEC standards are comprehensive, specifying necessary characteristics of reported evidence regarding the subjects, settings, dependent measures, intervention procedures, qualifications of interventionists, research designs, necessary numbers of studies and subjects, and criteria for determining the valence of outcomes based on effect sizes.

Different terminology has been used across various professional groups to categorize practices according to the extent to which they are supported by empirical evidence. We adopted three categories to summarize the evidence regarding the effectiveness of a treatment and the confidence that can be placed in the evaluation research: (1) established practices, (2) promising practices, and (3) unproven practices. In our terminology an *established practice* is equivalent to the CEC standards category *evidence-based practice,* a *promising practice* is the same as CEC's *potentially evidence-based practice,* and an *unproven practice* is equivalent to the CEC *insufficient evidence category.* We did not use categories for *mixed evidence* or *negative effects* because we did not find sufficient examples in the family support literature to warrant their use. For studies evaluated with group comparison design experiments, we evaluated a practice as established if supported by two high-quality RCTs. Established practices had to have no record of published studies with overall negative effects or a ratio of at least 3:1 studies with positive effects to those with neutral or mixed effects. We modified the CEC standards in some cases based on our editorial judgement of the overall quality of the evidence regarding a practice. The authors of the CEC standards argue that studies used to evaluate EBPs must meet to the letter all of the standards they have promulgated. We believe that this requirement in some instances is excessive and results in erring on the side of ruling out groups of high-quality studies and, as a consequence, unnecessarily reducing the interventions recommended for adoption by practitioners. As stated in the CEC standards, this kind of editorial judgement is allowed regarding fidelity of implementation data. In some cases we inferred fidelity of implementation when the authors were the originators of a program and it was either carefully described in the methods section or a manual.

A second area in which we did not always strictly adhere to the CEC standards concerned the total number of subjects needed to categorize a practice as established. Here too we exercised editorial judgement. We did not require the 60 total number of subjects included in the CEC standards. These standards are oriented toward studies of groups of children in public school classrooms, in which larger numbers are available, whereas many of the studies in this book focus on parents of children with low-incidence disabilities. Instead we required that each study have sufficient numbers of subjects so that the statistical analyses were sound as judged by common published requirements for meeting analytic assumptions. In most cases this meant studies of established practices had a minimum of 48 subjects in the requisite two RCT studies. In a few high-quality cases we determined a practice to be established with fewer subjects when the studies had relatively high effect sizes, met statistical assumptions, and were otherwise sound.

We evaluated a practice as promising if it was supported by one well-designed RCT or two well-designed QED studies. The studies in this category must not include any with negative effects or must have at least a 2:1 ratio of studies with positive effects to those with neutral or substantially mixed effects. The total number of subjects for the one required RCT study for a promising practice usually was a minimum of 24, or 48 when the evidence consisted of two QED studies.

Many research studies that are reviewed in this book have been evaluated through an alternative research methodology to group comparison studies. Rather than RCT or QED designs, most of the research concerning the education and treatment of individuals with DDs and their families has used SSDs. This methodology has been successful in demonstrating the efficacy of many behavioral interventions through the intensive study of their functional effects on observable behavior. An SSD is particularly suited for research with participants who may have a limited ability to report their well-being before and after treatment and for research with low-incidence populations, where large samples are difficult to obtain. Single-subject research designs are also particularly effective for demonstrating a functional relationship between a treatment and changes in the subject's behavior; that is, internal validity. Because of the small number of subjects involved, this tradition requires a larger number of studies in order to be confident of the external validity, that is, the extent to which the treatment can be generalized.

Following CEC standards, we considered a practice investigated with SSD methods to be established when (1) a minimum of five SSD studies that meet acceptable methodological criteria and document experimental control have been published in peer-reviewed journals; (2) the studies have been conducted by at least two different researchers, one of whom was not an originator of the treatment; (3) the five or more studies included a total of at least 20 participants; and (4) there was no evidence of negative effects in these studies. The second criterion is one we added to the CEC standards based on recommendations by Horner et al. (2005). In keeping with the CEC standards, a practice was designated as promising if supported by at least two to four high-quality SSD studies with no evidence of negative effects.

Unproven practices received this label under three conditions. First, the practice, although used in the field, has not been studied with controlled research. Second, if a practice has been studied with experiments but the research evidence is sufficiently compromised by problems in the design and/or implementation of the evaluation, or lack of crucial information, we considered it to be unproven. Third, the intervention has been studied in well-designed evaluations but it has failed to achieve positive statistically significant differences between treatment and no-treatment comparison groups or has not achieved substantial changes compared with baseline in SSD studies.

The centrality of replication in determining how to categorize a practice requires a clear definition of the extent to which the practices that were evaluated were the same.

We judged that a study had been replicated if the independent variables used in the original study were used in the subsequent evaluations based either on descriptions in the procedures sections of published research reports or those in publicly available treatment manuals. We allowed in some instances for some minor differences in procedures in deciding that a practice had been evaluated in a replication study. In some cases, studies shared the same basic approaches and foundational theories but varied in one or more of the key specific techniques making up the practice. For example, in chapter 2 we review psychoeducational programs that centered on training for parents of various coping skills. These studies were similar in that interventionists used meetings with groups of parents to teach clearly defined skills such as problem-solving, self-monitoring of physical stress responses, and interpersonal communication skills. The programs taught several skills, often one new coping skill a week for each of 8 to 10 meetings. Several studies took this basic skills-training approach consistent with a behavioral theoretical orientation, and all reported some positive outcomes. However, most of the coping skills programs did not use the same combination of skills. In this case and others like it we judged that the practices had not been copied with sufficient sameness of content to judge them as fully replicated, a requirement for a practice to be categorized as established. In this and other instances we comment that the general approach as a family of practices appears likely to be promising based on similar but not identical studies, but no specific combination of practices could be said to be established. By contrast, two of the stress management studies we reviewed listed the same set of independent variables that were derived from the same published manual (e.g., Benn, Akiva, Arel, & Roeser, 2012; Dykens, Fisher, Taylor, Lambert, & Miodrag, 2014). In this instance we were able to categorize mindfulness-based stress management (Kabot-Zinn & Hahn, 2009) as established. The distinction is between evaluating a relatively homogeneous but by no means identical family of studies versus evaluating one specific intervention with close replication. We confined ratings of "established" to the latter, and when the evidence warranted, we commented on the overall family as likely to be useful but did not formally rate it.

To our knowledge, there are no EBPs that have been evaluated with a large and diverse enough sample to claim they will be generally effective on average for most parents of children with DDs. However, the better-designed studies provide enough descriptive data so that it is possible to indicate the group of parents who participated in the evaluation research. All treatment generalization is constrained in some way in this field of research. Judgment will be required for a practitioner to decide whether a specific EBP has a high probability of success in a particular set of circumstances with a particular family.

SYNTHESIZING GROUP COMPARISON STUDIES: META-ANALYSIS

Meta-analysis is a statistical approach to synthesizing the findings from a group of related research studies. It aims to provide an overall characterization of these findings both through an indicator of central tendency, confidence intervals, and through identification of sources of heterogeneity in groups of studies. Since it was introduced in the 1980s, meta-analysis has been adopted across the social sciences and medicine. A search of the database PsychInfo in October of 2012 generated 2,504 articles from a search using the term as a descriptor word for publications in psychology and education. Databases have been established for both the fields of education and medicine, and standards set for filing meta-analyses in them. Further, meta-analysis has become a prominent feature of policy analysis including decisions by the Food and Drug Administration (FDA) regarding the safety of medications. The methodology for synthesizing research based on group comparison design studies is well established and has been used to summarize the results of research about families of children with ID and children with autism (Risdal & Singer, 2004; Singer, 2006; Singer, Ethridge, & Aldana, 2007). In this book we use meta-analysis to evaluate the average effectiveness of interventions. Effect sizes have little meaning out of context and are most useful when compared with other research studies. When possible we present effect sizes with comparative findings from other related research syntheses. We use Cohen's effect size, d, to characterize groups of studies. It is a standardized measure of the differences between two group means (Cohen, 1987). In keeping with current best practice when studies are analyzed as a group, we first tested for homogeneity of variance with the Q statistic. A significant Q indicates that there are variances between some of the studies such that they should not be analyzed in the aggregate. In these instances we conducted subsequent analyses to establish subgroups with homogeneity of variance. For simplicity we report the overall Q statistic and then present effect sizes for the subgroupings of studies that emerged from subsequent analyses of homogeneity of variance (Borenstein, Hedges, Higgins, & Rothstein, 2009).

The methodology for group comparison design studies is sufficiently well established that a small set of effect sizes are commonly presented in the literature of meta-analysis and are viewed as valid (Cooper et al., 2009). This is not the case, however, concerning syntheses of SSD studies. There is considerable controversy about whether or not meta-analysis is appropriate for combining and characterizing studies with small numbers of subjects. Several different ways of synthesizing studies using this methodology have been presented, but as of yet there is not a consensus on the best statistic for presenting a summary of groups of these studies. We chose not to synthesize the SSD studies in this book, given the unsettled state of the field. However, if there are at least five high-quality published studies with a total of at least 20 subjects, and if at least one of the studies has been performed by a group other than the originators, we scored it as established. With two or more studies we labeled the method as promising. To be included in this review, SSD studies had to conform to several quality indicators. We drew these from the recommendations of the CEC standards.

BACKGROUND OF THE EVIDENCE-BASED PRACTICE MOVEMENT IN FAMILY SUPPORT

The programs we reviewed belong to a historical and cultural context that has evolved since they were first developed. There are three strands that form this backdrop: (1) a changing view of the impact of children with DDs on families, (2) the creation and evolution of a family support movement, and (3) the EBP movement in the helping professions.

THE CHANGING VIEW OF IMPACTS ON FAMILIES

There is an important question about first premises when discussing support for caregiving families. It concerns how best to characterize the impact of children with ID and autism on the family and how families adapt over time to their caregiving role. Glidden and Schoolcraft (2003) point out how essential these views are in designing family supports.

> An almost monolithic conception of the inevitability of distress, crisis, and pathology has been replaced by recognition of extreme variability of family response and an understanding of the importance of identifying the antecedent causes of that variability. (Glidden, 2003, p. 3)

Francis Galton, the intellectual patriarch of the eugenics movement, published his first observations on heredity and its influence on society in 1865. For the next 90 years this line of thought dominated public policy and attitudes about people with ID and, later, autism. Under its influence, people with ID were viewed, at best, as potentially detrimental to the national gene pool and, at worst, as dangerous potential criminals. At its high-water mark the movement led to the forced sterilization of an estimated 60,000 people believed to be feebleminded and the institutionalization of thousands. These practices were legitimized by state laws and even the US Supreme Court in 1926 in *Buck v. Bell,* a case that gave states a green light to perform involuntary sterilizations. For a century, eugenics was endorsed by the best and the brightest until the horrors of the Nazi's atrocities in the name of racial purity became widely known in the last years of World War II. During this long period, family support consisted of the kindness of relatives and neighbors. The only service offered by the government was institutionalization. Until 1960 the standard desk reference book for physicians recommended institutionalization of children with moderate and severe ID at any time, as it was assumed to be the most humane course of action for the family. Institutionalization represented the dominant pubic commitment to this group of Americans for over a century. To a lesser extent, schools offered limited services to some children with ID. At the turn of the 20th century, a few of the large cities in the United States began offering special classes for children with ID. Autism was not defined until Kanner described the condition in 1943 (Kanner, 1943). For most of its history, services for people with autism were one and the same as those for people with ID. Individuals who would currently be said to have autism would instead be given a diagnosis of mental retardation.

At its peak, no more than 5% of people with mental retardation resided in state-run facilities; most of the other 95% lived in family homes (Landesman & Butterfield, 1987). Institutions, however, represented the sole governmental response to family needs, and so they had a disproportionate influence on how ID was understood and how people with this label were devalued (Trent, 1994). Under the influence of eugenics ideology, children and adults with ID were considered to be highly detrimental to families. In 1948 Deutsch, arguing for more hospital beds for children with disabilities, wrote that the birth of a child with mental retardation was one of the "great tragedies of American life" (Risdal & Singer, 2004). A decade later Farber and Kirk (1959) reviewed the literature on the impact of a child with severe mental retardation (*sic*) on parents:

> Various other studies report on the feelings of frustration, projection, doubts, fears, guilt feelings, and other behavior indicating personal maladjustment of the parents of mentally retarded children. (Farber & Kirk, 1959, p. 23)

The blanket assumptions were that the birth or diagnosis of a child with ID or autism constituted a long-term tragedy and source of shame for families. There were a few dissenting voices, but they remained in the background until the mid-1980s. As early as 1964, direct observers of families of children with ID found adjustment rather than dysfunction as the rule (Barsch, 1961). This view remained an anomaly until two decades later, when researchers began to identify strengths in families (Wikler, Wasow, & Hatfield, 1981) and call attention to the positive contributions of children with disabilities to their families (Turnbull, Blue-Banning, Behr, & Kerns, 1986). A revision in the characterization of the impact of family caregiving has evolved slowly and is still underway.

The dominant worldview regarding families and DDs had a profound impact on the kinds of psychological and social supports that were designed to help families beginning in the early 1970s. Raised in this cultural milieu, it was perhaps inevitable that early researchers on families adopted eugenics-tinged assumptions without question. The interventions were often termed "therapies," and techniques were transferred from treatments for people with a defined mental illness to parents of these individuals. In this book, whenever possible, we have referred to support programs as "interventions," or more generically as "structured supports" rather than therapies; perhaps a subtle but, we hope, a meaningful difference. We urge the people who use this book to ask themselves whether any given intervention can be offered to family members without needing to draw on an assumption of pathology and without the language of therapy. We believe that most of the interventions can be helpful without needing the language of medical or psychological therapy based on the assumption that families are invariably disturbed. We discuss this issue in more detail in chapter 7.

The contemporary view of families of children with disabilities reflects major changes in US society on behalf of its citizens with disabilities. Parents and people with ID and autism have become effective advocates. Institutions are considered outmoded at best and cruel at the worst. A community system for adults with DDs has been established in most states so that living, working, and recreating with disabled peers has become familiar to younger citizens, increasing numbers of whom are growing up in inclusive public schools where they learn side by side with peers with disabilities. Many helping professions now serve individuals with DDs and their families. Families are currently viewed as allied with professionals. A small but growing body of research indicates that many, perhaps most, families of children with disabilities adapt well and view their family members with disabilities as contributors to the families' positive quality of life. Contemporary research indicates that many families adapt, find benefits in caregiving, and hold their children with DDs dear (e.g., Hastings, Beck, et al., 2005; Seltzer et al., 2001). As Glidden and Schoolcraft (2003) have pointed out, it matters how family experience in this respect is characterized.

> If families with children who have mental retardation continue to be seen as victims, and their positive outcomes viewed with skepticism, services and interventions will be inappropriate. Providing supports for families to help them make accommodations to their children is a very different enterprise from helping them deal only with their pain and tragedy. (Glidden & Schoolcraft, p. 251)

Our aim in this book is to contribute to helping families make accommodations by identifying ones that have evidence supporting their probable efficacy. A corollary of a more positive characterization of the impact of caregiving on families is that families' knowledge and skills should be viewed as funds of knowledge, which are potentially very useful for professionals. In order to understand how best to assist families in accommodating the needs of their children with disabilities, it is important to have a clear view of what stands in the way of this adaptation in some families. Our purpose here is not to review the large body of research on the challenges they face. Rather we highlight a few of the most important stressors. Our assumption is that these can be effectively addressed so that families can adapt positively.

Economic Stress

The families we focus on in this book on average have an elevated risk of economic hardship compared with families of nondisabled children. Fujiara and Yamaki (2000) reported that 28% of children with disabilities lived below the poverty level, compared with 16% of children without disabilities. To begin with, the children born to families with low incomes have a higher risk of DDs for a variety of reasons, including less access to prenatal care, inadequate nutrition, maternal stress during pregnancy, increased levels of maternal depression, and increased exposure to environmental toxins. Financial hardship is also more commonplace because children and adults with DDs, on average, require more specialized therapies and have a greater need for supervision, and because of the higher costs of providing for adult children; that is, the expenses of raising children last much longer than for families of nondisabled individuals, who often leave home in late adolescence and become self-supporting in early adulthood, unlike the majority of adults with DD. Further, many parents find they need to give up or cut back on work outside the home to address the needs of their children with disabilities, a decision that reduces family income.

A recent study compared several kinds of economic hardship in families with and without children with disabilities (Parish, Rose, Grinstein-Weiss, & Andrews, 2008). They reported findings as odds ratios in which any number over 1 meant increased risk whereas any number less than 1 meant less risk compared with the general population. They found that in families of children with ID, the odds ratio of worrying that food would run out was 1.78; the odds that food would not last through the month, 1.52; that they would be unable to pay rent, 1.72; that they would have to move in with others, 1.24; and that they had no telephone for a day in the past month, 1.81. These hardships remained high even in families with incomes 300% higher than the federal poverty level. This last point is notable because it indicates that unlike families without long-term caregiving demands, increases in income up to three times the poverty level do not translate into reductions in hardships as they do for other low-income families moving up the economic ladder (Parish et al., 2008).

There is a large body of evidence that on average, parents (usually mothers in the research), experience higher levels of stress and associated depressive symptoms and more frequent physical illness than matched parents of nondisabled children (Hastings & Beck, 2004; Witt et al., 2003). The extent of these problems does not inevitably rise to the level of family tragedy as was formerly believed, but there are real challenges that can overtax the resources of families (Hastings & Beck, 2004; Singer, 2006).

Problem Behaviors

Although there are many causes of caregiver stress, one that repeatedly surfaces in research is elevated prevalence of problem behaviors in family members with ID or autism (e.g., Bailey, Golden, Roberts, & Ford, 2007). Rates of problem behaviors in both populations are much higher than in typically developing children, and these challenging behaviors persist into adulthood without effective treatment. A recent longitudinal study of children with ID in Australia found that by adulthood over 40% were diagnosed as having a mental disorder in addition to ID. Dekker, Koot, Ende, and Verhulst (2002) in the Netherlands compared a sample of over 1,000 children with ID with a large, random population sample and found that odds ratios for incidence of problem behaviors indicated elevated risk. The odds ratio for children with moderate/severe ID was 3.7 for aggressive behaviors, 2.4 for anxious and depressed symptoms, and 4.0 on the total problem behavior score on a commonly used measure of the overall aberrant behavior, the Child Behavior Checklist (CBCL; Dekker et al., 2002). Other sources of stress have been conceptualized as interactions between children's characteristics and adversity in the family such as economic pressure, marital discord, troubles with siblings, and a child's caregiving demands (Quine & Pahl, 1985). It appears to be the concurrence of family adversity and challenging features of DD that are most likely to give rise to distress in families.

Adaptation is complicated both within the individuals who make up families and across diverse families so that they defy easy categorization in simple dichotomous terms. Within families the balance of positive and negative attributions may vary over time both with stages in the family lifecycle and changing family conditions (divorce, birth of siblings, unemployment, job promotion, etc.). Some family members may have a positive outlook, whereas others may "see the glass as half empty." Additionally families vary on many dimensions including their structure (two parent married, one parent, same sex partners), socioeconomic status (SES), ethnicity, and family cohesion. Intellectual disabilities and autism also encompass a wide range of variability from relatively mild cognitive disability to severe limitations in several domains including communication and comprehension of language. In a recent study, Bayat (2007) surveyed parents of children with autism about caregiving impact on their families. Approximately one-third described parenting their child with autism as primarily beneficial, one-third as both positive and negative, and the remaining one-third as primarily negative in impact.

Availability of Supports

The kinds of supports necessary to help more families make progress are not yet widely available in many parts of the United States. The proportion of funds for DD services that has gone to family support systems has not exceeded 4% since the 1980s, and it simply has not been enough to build comprehensive systems of family support. The shortfall can be seen in data from a 2011 national survey of over 2,500 parents of individuals with ID from all 50 states (L. Anderson, Larson, & Wuorio, 2011). They were given a list of common family needs and asked to rate whether meeting them was no problem, some problem, or a major problem. On all items, over 50% of the families reported major problems. Table 1.1 presents the findings in part.

The table shows that much of what caregiving families need is not yet available. It also indicates that the research on practices reported in this book could address some of these needs, some very important ones, but they are only part of the system that is called for.

TABLE 1.1 CHALLENGES THAT POSED MAJOR PROBLEMS FOR OVER 50% OF CAREGIVERS SURVEYED

Having enough retirement savings.
Finding noninstitutional, community-based care.
Finding trained and reliable home care providers.
Finding after school care/summer care.
Finding affordable residential care.
Overall economic security.
Being able to go on regular vacations.
Meeting my personal needs such as personal time, exercise, etc.
Having enough money to pay for care.
Balancing other family responsibilities, e.g., children, marriage, housework
Respite care to have time to take care of my own needs.
Building inclusive friendships for my family member.
Getting enough rest.
Adjusting my work schedule, meeting my work responsibilities.
Find out about legal options.
Understanding government programs such as Medicare or SSI.
Trying to provide care when I have my own health issues.
Emergency care when I need to care for another family member (i.e., sandwich generation issues).
Dealing with breakdowns in caregiving arrangements.
Dealing with dangerous, unwanted, or difficult behaviors of the person I care for.
Day care so I can work.
Having someone to talk to who understands what I deal with.
Doing end of life planning.
Getting cooperation and assistance from other family members.
Support for siblings of the individual with a disability.
Ensuring the safety of the person I am caring for.
Identifying available transportation options.

Source: L. Anderson et al. (2011)

SUPPORTING FAMILY ACCOMMODATION

Family support services have evolved along with changing views on family impact. The history of the family support movement is another important part of the historical backdrop to the EBP movement. Until relatively recently there was not a system of support for families in the community, and in many states it is still in a nascent stage. With the exception of federal Social Security benefits, family support programs are entirely under the jurisdiction of state governments, and they differ dramatically according to policies at the state level. The variability can be seen in 2011 data on average annual state spending per family with a child or adult with ID/autism, which ranged from $508 in Alabama to $33,400 in Louisiana (Braddock et al., 2011). Early family support efforts were small, aimed only at families with the highest risk of institutionalizing their family members with ID/autism. By 1990, 129,000 families in the United States received some form of formal support, constituting only about 3% of total funding on people with DDs (Braddock et al., 2011).

A watershed year for the beginning of widespread change from segregated state hospitals and segregated services was 1981, the year that Congress established the Medicaid Home and Community Waiver Program, which for the first time since Medicaid was established in the 1960s permitted allocation of small proportions of state and federal Medicaid funds for services for families of people with ID who resided in their family homes. The Medicaid Waiver program in 1981 is a prime example of a change in national policy that has impacted the lives of many families. These policy changes were driven by criticism of Medicaid from leaders of the disability rights movement and by parents of children with DDs. They managed to call national attention to a powerful critique of the dominant philosophy of minimal community services for people with DD and of the virtual nonexistence of services for families. In response to this critique, Congress granted states the right to negotiate with the federal Health Services Administration to divert to the community some Medicaid funds earmarked for paying for the care of people in large state hospitals.

Originally these funds had to be used to prevent or delay institutionalization of people with disabilities living with their family of origin. As a result, only a relatively small number of families of individuals with the most severe disabilities received support. Soon after Congress created the waiver program, several states began using these funds to help families maintain children with ID in their own homes, provided that administrators could make the case that the recipients were destined for the state hospital if their families did not receive assistance.

The first efforts to create family support services involved agencies that purchased or directly provided a limited range of services, which constituted a fixed menu of choices for families. Several forms of support were made available in some locales and few, if any, in others. The larger systems paid for services to families for several needs. Services offered in some states included respite care, family counseling, architectural adaptation of homes, parent training, assistance for siblings, education and behavior management services, and provision of specialized equipment, among many others (Braddock et al., 2011). The control of these resources became a source of controversy as parents gained more experience with these early support systems.

Parents who led advocacy groups were usually from middle-class families and did not settle for the traditional ways of providing state aid to families in poverty. In this older social welfare model, the power relationship between professionals and parents was hierarchical; it was assumed the recipient needed help that only professionals as experts could select because they held specialized knowledge that could relieve or prevent inevitable family pathology if only parents chose to comply with the prescribed program. As described earlier, it was often assumed that having a child with ID or autism was a family tragedy. In social services for families the model was largely based on welfare practices, which were designed to sort the worthy and deserving poor from the unworthy and prevent fraud and abuse. These services were professionally driven, because it was assumed that poor people needed professional control and oversight or they would use resources wastefully, or even immorally. The paradigmatic image of the welfare recipient as an untrustworthy, passive taker was the "welfare queen." She was described as a swindler or a wastrel, or both, who mooched off taxpayers' resources and had illegitimate and/or misbehaving children. The assumption of family tragedy was wedded to taken-for-granted assumptions that families who had fallen in such straights as to need support were feckless and that agencies were easy targets for welfare queens in the guise of parents of children with disabilities. These two assumptions in more traditional services were a heady mix, one that many parents found stifling and disempowering.

Many traditional practices were meant to be helpful, but helpfulness was defined by the governing agency rather than the people receiving assistance. The traditional service model was built under the influence of residualism (Mahoney, 1976). In residual welfare service models, public assistance was meant to be provided only to a small residual population of people in extremis after they had already failed to support their families independently. When early family support services were started for parents of children with disabilities they took up several of the assumptions built into the residual welfare model: an assumption that families were unformed and not altogether trustworthy, power-over relationships, and assistance only for families likely to institutionalize their children. In the most recent stage of family support program development, the emphasis moved from broadening the kinds of supports available to reforming the fundamental design and operation of the programs. Much of the thinking that guided this shift came from contemporary design of early intervention services and from a movement within pediatric medicine to create a model of family-centered services (Brewer, McPherson, Magrab, & Hutchins, 1989; Dunst, Trivette, & Deal, 1988; Turnbull et al., 2007). It was a deliberate attempt to break out of the older residualist model of state-supported assistance to families.

Family-Centered Support

Dunst, Trivette, Gordon, and Starnes (1993) operationalized family-centered support by identifying key characteristics. Family support in this paradigm aims to enhance a sense of community and the interdependence of the community members with the family. A key to this approach is that whenever possible, supports and services should be provided by generic organizations that help families of typically developing children as well as families of children with special needs. This emphasis in turn brings to light the need for capacity-building in the community so that, for example, churches, public schools, day care centers, and amateur sports teams can be welcoming and provide accommodations as needed. Dunst et al. argued that mobilizing resources and supports was a key function of family support programs. In this paradigm the informal social supports are recognized as among the most important sources of assistance; extended family, friends, neighbors, other parents of children with disabilities, and coworkers are able to provide kinds of social support not available from most professionals.

These family-centered programs share responsibility and collaboration. Dunst et al. (1993) explained, "ideas and skills [are shared] in ways that build collaborative arrangements" (p. 91). The relationship between professionals and parents has received considerable attention in the emergence of the family-centered service discourse. Summers et al. (2005) have defined and investigated the value of parent–professional partnerships in which both parties share their respective knowledge and skills to jointly achieve outcomes chosen by the family. When services are respectful of a family's culture and value system they are more likely to build mutual trust and shared effort in achieving goals chosen by the family. In an empirical study of the impact of parent–professional partnership, Summers et al. (2005) found that parent/professional partnerships mediated families' perceived adequacy of early intervention programs with their perceived quality of family life. A key element of this kind of service design and delivery is the way power is allocated. "Interventions should be made available to families in ways that maximize the family's control over and decision making power regarding services they receive" (Dunst et al., 1993). Finally, interventionists should aim to promote positive family outcomes rather than solely focusing on amelioration of suffering.

By the 1990s, parents' organizations in several states advocated for shifting the control of service selection and resource allocation from state agencies directly to families. They sought control for designing their family support plans and choosing the kinds of supports, selecting who or what organization provided the assistance, when, and for how long. Rather than confining the options available to a checklist of programs approved by the DD agencies, activist parents demanded and gained the right to receive an allocation of funds and to directly decide along with a case manager how the funds would be spent to best help the family. Caregiving families have many different needs that vary by the family's life stage, depending on factors such as the health and capabilities of caregivers, ethnicity, SES, employment status, and the changing needs of the family member with a disability over time. Rather than trying to create a "one size fits all" program, families in some of the most innovative states are given funds and some counseling to enable them to choose and purchase the services they need. These are called "cash and counseling" programs.

This shift in control of public funds and services represents a dynamic experiment in the human services. The evolution of respite care services in some states illustrates the change from top-down service models to family-centered services. In the mid-1980s some regional DD agencies began offering respite care, brief behavioral parent training, and case management. The services were purchased by the regional center from approved professionals and from respite care providers who were given some training and granted authority to bill the centers for their work. Parents were given a list of approved respite providers and a limited number of hours for someone to look after their children. The problem for families was that respite providers were often not available at the times when parents most needed it and they were not the people parents preferred as care providers for their children. Parents often relied on family and neighbors, people who could not be paid under the formal system. More recently, the Medicaid waiver program has been changed to allow parents to choose by whom, when, and where they want respite care provided. In some states they are allowed to use Medicaid funds to pay relatives and neighbors for providing respite.

By the turn of the 21st century, the waiting lists for community residences had become a problem on a large scale in the United States, as the numbers of adults living at home grew, though they want to live on their own in supported living arrangements. With the waiting lists came further recognition that families required support to maintain adults in their family homes until sufficient community services could be established, historically a slow process. In 2006, 429,000 families in the United States received family support services, an increase of over 300% since 1990. However, even with these increases only 8% of funds for people with DD and their families were allocated for family support in 2011. One important use of these funds is to help families obtain access to several of the programs reviewed here.

Gradually what has emerged in some states is a family support system made up of some core services offered by state-funded nonprofit centers and access to an array of many kinds of supports, some specialized for this group of families, others from generic agencies and services available to any family in their communities with sufficient means. The extent of choice and amount of control that families have varies greatly. Several states have formulated programs designed around a flexible system that provides access to goods and services for addressing many different family and individual needs while striving to empower families and family members with DDs to make their own choices.

One way to understand these newer values is to look at the standards that innovative states have agreed on for evaluating the quality of their family support service systems. Table 1.2 presents a set of indicators adopted by the National Association of State Directors of Developmental Disabilities (Bradley & Moseley, 2007). As of 2014, only 15 states had adopted these standards, but they are likely to be trendsetters if family support practices continue to grow based on new values. Several values are notable in these indicators: family empowerment, parent–professional partnerships, flexible access to an array of supports, capacity building to bolster family caregiving, individualization, an emphasis on access to generic community services and supports, and integration of the family into the community. Family-centered services for caregiving families exist in some parts of some states, are a work in progress in others, and are not yet on the horizon in still others.

In some states, governments have created regional agencies charged with developing and overseeing community-based services and to help provide access to generic community organizations. Studies under review in this book are discrete techniques and programs that are unlikely to be sufficient by themselves. They must take place in a broader

TABLE 1.2 NATIONAL CORE INDICATORS

The proportion of families reporting that they control their own budgets/supports (i.e., they choose what supports/goods to purchase).
The proportion of families who report that staff are respectful of their choices and decisions.
The proportion of families who report they choose, hire, and manage their service/support providers.
The proportion of families who feel that services and supports have helped them to better care for their family member living at home.
The proportion of families who report satisfaction with the information and supports received, and with the planning, decision-making, and grievance processes.
The proportion of families/guardians of individuals not living at home who report the extent to which the system supports continuing family involvement.
The proportion of families who report they are supported in using natural supports in their communities (e.g., family, friends, neighbors, churches, colleges, recreational services).
The proportion of families/family members who participate in integrated activities in their communities.
The proportion of eligible families who report having access to an adequate array of services and supports.
The proportion of families reporting that staff or translators are available to provide information, services, and supports in the family/family member's primary language/method of communication.
The proportion of families who indicate that services/supports provided outside of the home (e.g., day/employment, residential services) are done so in a safe and healthy environment.
The proportion of families who report that service and support staff/providers are available and capable of meeting family needs.
The proportion of families who report that services/supports are available when needed, even in a crisis.
The proportion of families who report that services/supports are flexible to meet their changing needs.
The proportion of families reporting that their support plan includes or reflects things that are important to them.
The proportion of families who report that staff who assist with planning are knowledgeable and respectful.
The proportion of families who report they are informed about the array of existing and potential resources (including information about their family member's disability, services and supports, and public benefits) in a way that is easy to understand.
The proportion of families who report they have the information needed to skillfully plan for their services and supports.

Source: National Core Indicators. Retrieved March 18, 2014, from www.nationalcoreindicators.org

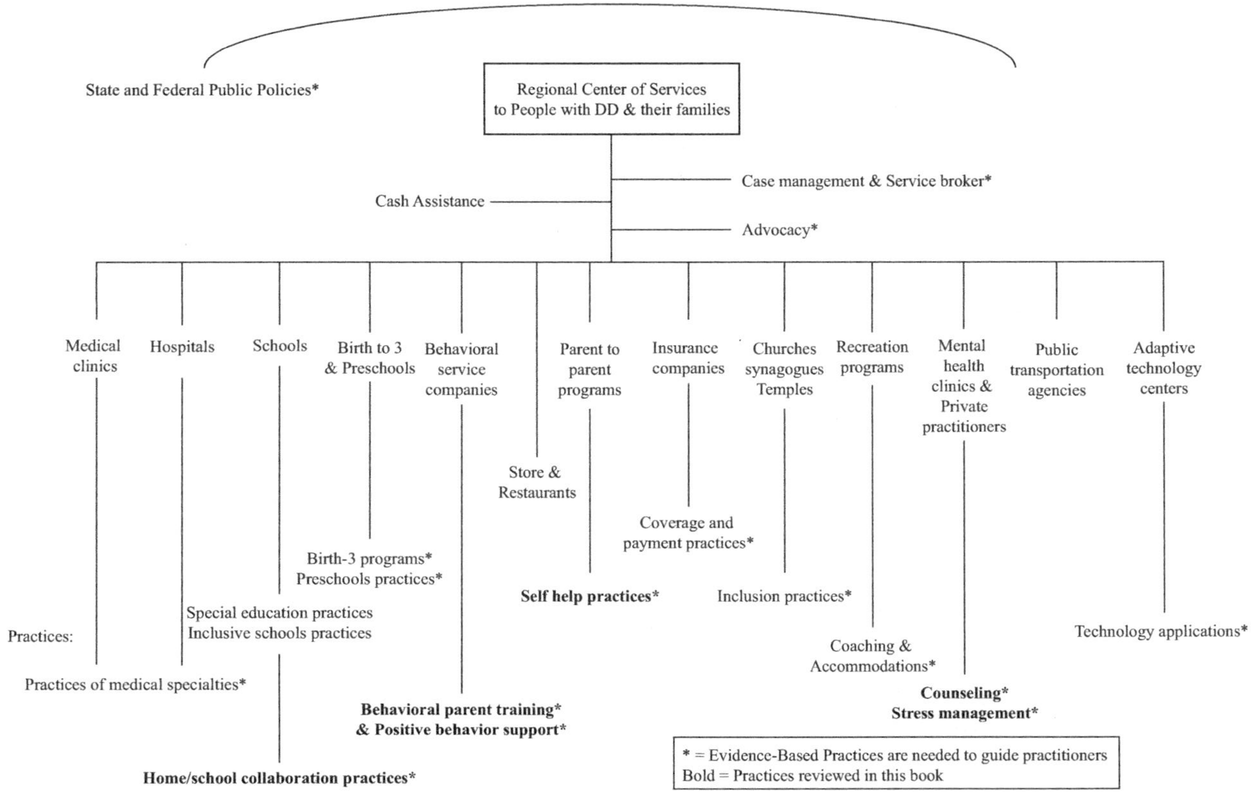

FIGURE 1.1 The place of evidence-based practices in a community-based system of family support.

community support system. By themselves, these interventions do not constitute a system sufficient to meet the many different needs that families identify, rather they inform practitioners in various parts of the system. Where then does the EBP movement intersect with the historic and service system evolutions we have described? Figure 1.1 shows where these practices fit into a larger system of community organizations functioning to offer many different forms of assistance, often to the whole community and sometimes exclusively for the families addressed in this book.

As seen in Figure 1.1, EBP is not limited to educational and social service programs. Any human service ought to be evidence based, and most have professional standards for determining when research gives a reasonable chance of success with intervention. Each of the components of a system of care should be studied in order to determine whether they are effective and whether some practices are more effective than others. Figure 1.1 illustrates a service system and where EBPs are needed within that system. Development and evaluation of interventions that meet standards for established and promising treatments are important steps in the evolution of family support services and have the potential to ultimately help improve the quality of life of caregiving families. The field of DDs has been marked by the promotion of invalidated and sometimes preposterous "treatments" ranging from fad diets to dolphin therapy. In this context, efforts to develop and validate science-based interventions represent an important effort to see that resources are channeled to practices that have a sufficient evidence base and reasonable probability for success. They can potentially inform stakeholders so that scarce resources can be allocated for beneficial and effective supports.

FAMILY SUPPORT FOCUSING ON POSITIVE OUTCOMES

With the contemporary view that some families adjust well with the right ecology of support, the goals of family support programs ought to reflect this knowledge. Dunst et al. (1993) and Singer and Irvin (1989) have argued that the goals of family support should be threefold: promotion, prevention, and amelioration. It should aim to promote a high quality of family life including finding benefits in caregiving, to prevent family stress and strengthen the capacity to cope with it, and to ameliorate suffering when it arises. Most of the practices reviewed in this book can contribute to this tripartite goal. Several have been used to promote positive outcomes, reduce existing stress, and directly ease suffering. Many of the interventions are forms of skills training aimed at improving quality of life. For example, a newly emerging program reviewed in chapter 2 is mindfulness-based stress management. The skills that are taught in these classes were originally developed as Buddhist aides to well-being, and they have also been used to prevent and reduce stress and help people with several different medical and psychological maladies.

In the chapters that follow we present a large and growing evidence base that offers considerable hope for families and policy makers. Forty years of research and policy development have led to an international effort to assist caregiving families with their crucial societal roles as sources of nurturance, support, and lifelong benevolence for individuals who are disadvantaged and too often shunted aside. These families constitute an invaluable national resource and as such are deserving of the most effective forms of support that the social sciences can develop and evaluate.

2

PSYCHOEDUCATIONAL GROUP PROGRAMS AS EVIDENCE-BASED PRACTICES

George H. S. Singer, Jiyeon Kim, Yeana W. Lam,

Mian Wang, and Kelsey Oliver

A body of research has grown incrementally over the past 40 years on ways to help parents of children with developmental disabilities with psychological and physical reactions to stressors related to caregiving. In this chapter we review those supportive practices that have been evaluated using group randomized experiments. Over this time span, our understanding of families of children with disabilities has expanded and shifted in its emphases in keeping with broader changes in the fields of social work, clinical psychology, and special education. One of the most consequential changes has been a belated recognition that families of children with intellectual disabilities (IDs) and/or autism vary greatly in how they adapt to life with a family member with these conditions. There are also many changes in adaptation as individual families change through the life course (J. M. Patterson, 1988). Understanding of these families has shifted away from a global assumption that a child's disability is inevitably a tragedy for families to recognition of a full range of responses including positive adaptation, perceived benefits, and strengthened families in addition to stress (Glidden & Schoolcraft, 2003). Formerly, under the unquestioned influence of the tragedy assumption, researchers solely measured dire impacts on parents and siblings, including mental health problems such as depressive and anxiety symptoms and stress-related physical illness. Measures of positive adaptation were virtually nonexistent in this literature until the early 21st century (Hastings & Taunt, 2002). A second related assumption was that these problems were the result of high levels of chronic stress that was generated by unusual caregiving demands based on the psychological and material costs of meeting the needs of the child with a disability. These two basic assumptions were reflected in research that compared groups of parents of children with ID and autism on measures of mental and physical health. This literature can be easily misinterpreted to support the tragedy assumption, risking a drastic oversimplification that can lead to the design of unnecessarily narrow sets of family supports with limited goals. On one hand, comparative studies with parents of typically developing (TD) children and parents of children with developmental disabilities (DDs) consistently show that mothers in the DD group have higher levels of emotional distress than mothers of TD children. A smaller body of studies suggests the same is true for fathers, although the difference between the fathers in the two groups is much smaller and the severity of the symptoms on average is lower than for mothers. On the other hand, there is considerable variability in the findings and the differences are relatively small between the TD and DD groups.

In this book we draw on meta-analyses whenever available. Singer (2006) conducted a meta-analysis of studies comparing groups of parents of children with DDs with parents of TD children on measures of depressive symptoms and found a significant but small effect size difference between the groups in the direction of more symptoms of depression in parents of children with DDs. These studies were conducted from 1984 to 2003 with little change in the outcomes over the years. While it is the case that in many (but not all) studies parents of children with DDs had statistically higher levels of depressive symptoms, the size of the difference when results were pooled was relatively small with an unweighted effect size of $d = 0.35$ and a 95% confidence interval between +.29 and +.39. The d score according to a commonly used metric is a modest one, not as large as might be suspected if impacts of parenting children with ID and autism were consistently severely detrimental. The confidence interval, a relatively narrow one, suggests that this finding of a fairly small effect size is robust. Furthermore, the outcomes of intervention research reviewed in this volume indicate that for many households the relevant helping professions have the necessary skills and knowledge to backstop families and support their resilience (Singer, Ethridge, & Aldana, 2007). The meta-analyses reported in this chapter show that interventions on average have sufficient efficacy to substantially close the gap between parents in the two different populations (Summers et al., 2007).

It is worth considering a few reasons why the research has been taken so negatively as evidence of extreme family hardship. First it is important to acknowledge that there are some families who are under utmost levels of stress usually because of a combination of ongoing life stress and severe problem behaviors or severe physical illness in their children with disabilities in a context of few services or ones that fall far short of their stated aims. These families often have the same kinds of extraordinary pressures to deal with as are common for very troubled families in general. But these families in extremity are a minority, many get better over time, and many benefit when high-quality supports are provided to them. There are additional stressors associated with parenting children in this population. Table 2.1 presents the stressors identified in a set of studies of parents.

Consistent with the findings regarding depressive symptoms, there is also evidence of negative medical impacts on parents of these children as measured by significant increases in parents' medical utilization compared with parents of TD children (Altman, Cooper, & Cunningham, 1999). But again, it is far too simplistic to assume that the medical impact is uniform or that it is necessarily large. Much of these outcomes have to do with how work is shared in the family and with the kind of resources parents have to get additional help with caring for their children. Research examining the relationship between time caring for children with several kinds of disabilities, found that as caregiving increased, mothers' daily negative mood and number of stressors followed suit. Further, diurnal samples of salivary cortisol revealed elevated levels of physiological stress (Seltzer et al., 2009) in mothers of children with ID compared to families of TD children. Again, it is important to see the extensive variability in these findings and to take care not to exaggerate their severity. If average findings are the only part of the data that practitioners heed, there is a problem. When writing about these families, researchers in the past focused on the averages but made little of the variability in the data. However, Singer estimated that approximately two in three parents of children with a DD had scores in the normal range

TABLE 2.1 CORRELATES OF DISTRESS IN MOTHERS OF CHILDREN WITH DEVELOPMENTAL DISABILITIES

Quine & Pahl (1985)	*Baxter (1989)*	*Bailey et al. (2007)**
1. Behavior problems in the child	1. Child's behavior problems in public	1. Behavior problems or autism
2. Nighttime disturbance	2. Behavior problems at home	2. Support from family or family cohesion
3. Social isolation	3. Explaining the disability to others	3. Maternal physical health
4. Adversity in the family	4. People's attitudes	4. Maternal coping style
5. Multiplicity of impairments	5. Physical health of the child	5. Diagnostic group
6. Difficulty in settling the child at night	6. Physical needs of the child	6. Mother's well-being or stress
7. Problems with the child's health	7. Obtaining help for the child	
8. Problems with the child's appearance	8. Intelligence of the child	
9. Money worries	9. Appearance of the child	
	10. Speech of the child	

*The most common predictors of depressive symptoms based on a review of 47 studies.

on measures of depressive symptoms (Singer, 2006), and Bailey, Golden, Roberts, and Ford (2007) estimated that three out of four parents were in this range. In either case, not only were the large majority of parents not highly distressed but also more recent research indicates that a substantial portion of these parents adapt well and rate their quality of life positively when researchers have gotten around to asking about the positive side of the picture (Hastings & Taunt, 2002).

Researchers in response to criticism from professionals who were parents of children with DD developed measures to tap into the characteristics of the families adapting well (Hastings & Taunt, 2002). Singer (2002) argued that much is to be learned from these families and that they can provide useful ways to understand how to help the minority of struggling parents. For example, Maul and Singer (2009) interviewed parents of children with autism to learn what kinds of accommodations they had created for their daily routines in order to meet the needs of their children with autism. A common adaptation involved how these parents modified their use of time by doing advanced planning, adjusting the amount of time they allocated to routines involving their children, and adjusting work schedules to accommodate to caregiving home-based routines. These ways of adjusting the temporal dimension of family life could be modeled and taught to other parents. There is much to learn from successful family adaptation.

Several researchers have conducted interviews with parents of children with disabilities and identified positive statements about the long-term impact of the child on the family (Bayat, 2007; Hastings, Allen, McDermott, & Still, 2002). Hastings et al. (2002) also investigated correlates of positive perceptions in 48 parents of children with ID. They found that mothers viewed their children with ID as sources of happiness and fulfillment, as bringing the family closer together, and as sources of personal growth. The parents were more likely to make these types of affirmations if they used cognitive reframing as a coping strategy and received support from family and friends. This combination of social support and cognitive reframing are common elements in the stress management practices reviewed in this chapter.

Parents of children with autism and ID also show variability in their appraisal of how their children impact their personal and family well-being. Many parents report that despite difficult episodes and crises, their children with autism spectrum disorder (ASD) are positive contributors to their quality of life and that over time sadness and distress are replaced by feelings of love and a sense of accomplishment in raising these children (Bayat, 2007). Bayat (2007) interviewed and surveyed parents of children with ASD and found evidence of resilience. In a sample of 167 parents of children with ASD 28% described the impact of the child with ASD on their family in exclusively positive terms, and an additional 34% described both positive and negative impacts, whereas 30% reported only negative impacts. One family's report of family benefits in Bayat's (2007) study emphasized the way the experience made the family closer and stronger:

> While the initial diagnosis was devastating, ultimately it did bring our family closer together. We work together to support our children (with ASD) and close ranks when necessary to protect them. Our priorities have shifted and we no longer sweat the small stuff. (Bayat, 2007, p. 709)

Another mother reported on both positive and negative impacts describing the effect on her family this way:

> My son's autism has made our family life tougher, emotionally and financially. Each member has to devote additional time and effort to help him, and learn how to live peacefully in such an environment. Through working together, we all learned how to help my son together. In some sense, this also makes our family closer, because an individual cannot handle the toughness alone. (Bayat, 2007, p. 709)

The important contribution of research on benefit finding adds two important dimensions to how professionals and eventually the public view these families. It ought to alter perceptions among parents and practitioners about what outcomes of family support services should be (Singer, Biegel, & Ethridge, 2009). It has been an assumption until recently that because children with disabilities were thought to inevitably impose chronic stress on their families, the best outcomes that could be reasonably expected would be to reduce family and individual distress; however, the research on benefit finding suggests that family support programs ought to aim higher. One goal of family support should be to help families attain positive outcomes through the right kinds of support provisions. Specifically, it is no longer sufficient to simply reduce depressive symptoms, stress, or ill health without positively promoting a better quality of life. The second implication of the finding is for the design of interventions. Since benefit finding is an obtainable outcome, the question arises as to what forms of support will help parents and other family members move from distress to bonadaptation, a term used by Antonovsky (1987) to describe positive outcomes from life stress.

What makes the difference between resilient and more distressed parents and families? Theories of the stress response in individuals and such processes at the more complex family level provide a framework for making sense of studies about the important variables that mediate and moderate stress responses at both the individual and the family levels of analysis (Folkman & Lazarus, 1984; McCubbin & Patterson, 1983). It is important to identify these predictors of stress responses in order to determine whether interventions are designed to address them.

The double ABCX theory of stress is a multivariate model of the stress process applied to families. It describes responses to stressful conditions as an interaction of an event or pressure from the environment. The (A) term represents these stressful events or conditions (B), represents resources including, for example, social support, education levels, support from formal service agencies, socioeconomic status (SES), and prior experience in dealing with the stressor. The C term represents cognitive appraisal of the stressful event and resources available to cope with it. The X term in the theory stands for the outcome of the family's encounter with a stressor which may be a crisis or a new form of positive adaptation. Since its original development, the basic theory has evolved with recognition that stress processes can lead to growth, strengthening, and other positive outcomes (J. M. Patterson, 2002). Some parents and siblings, for example, report that their family works as a team and is closer because of the child with a disability.

McCubbin and Patterson modified the basic ABCX framework by doubling each term to account for background and immediate levels of the variables. A represents current stressors (A) and difficult background conditions or ongoing levels of stress to the family (a). The preexisting coping repertoire and supply of resources (b) was added to the B term. Preexisting cognitive styles or systems such as religious faith (c) were combined with the currently available cognitive repertoire.

Researchers have devoted considerable attention to identifying sources of stress (Aa) in the model. Table 2.1 presents findings from three such studies. This line of work is important because it is often necessary to know if the stressor is something that may be preventable or if it can be ameliorated with supports. Researchers have attempted to identify and rank specific aspects of parenting a child with ID. The list in the leftmost column of Tabe 2.1 is derived from interviews of parents of children with multiple disabilities (Quine & Pahl, 1985). The list in the middle column comprises items used in an assessment by Baxter (1989) based on a review of the literature at the time. The list in the rightmost column is drawn from a review of research on predictors of parental depression and lists variables that significantly accounted for levels of parental depression (Bailey et al., 2007). This last study is an important review because it was published more recently than most and it covered 45 studies in which parents of TD and ID or autistic children were compared. These stressors from the review by Bailey et al. are ranked by the severity of their impact on parents' mental health based on multiple regression studies.

An examination of this table shows some important commonalities. The importance of behavior problems as sources of stress is a consistent finding in the research literature and is one of the most common reasons that parents seek help from the service system (Floyd & Gallagher, 1997). Behavioral parent training, for example, is an intervention designed to reduce problem behavior and increase a child's adaptive skills, one that has an impressive evidence base as reviewed in this book.

The availability of effective in-home behavior intervention services may be an important contributor to family quality of life in families of individuals with ID or ASD (Seltzer, Greenberg, Floyd, Pettee, & Hong, 2001). However, there are shortages of trained personnel for these services, and there is no uniform pattern of funding for them across the states in the United States (Braddock et al., 2013). Some states like California and Massachusetts make them widely available through regional center systems dedicated to serving individuals with DD and their families. Others provide little or no support to families.

The ABCX theory emphasizes the importance of cognitive appraisal in the stress process. The C term includes the ways that people appraise events as threatening or not and their perceptions of the resources they have available for dealing with challenging events. Changes in the meanings that people assign to the environment can reduce the likelihood of feeling threatened by events. These cognitive changes can also modulate the impact of stressors and they can guide instrumental actions that effectively deal with challenging events. When people under stress deliberately revise or restructure the way they think about a stressor they may choose to think about circumstances in a way that reduces or eliminates the perception that an event is a threat. Cognitive coping may also be used after a stressor and subsequent stress response have occurred in order to adaptively deal with its psychological and physiological impact. One of the well-studied versions of this kind of self-controlled cognitive modification is known in the literature as *cognitive reframing* (Tunali & Powers, 2002). Hastings et al. (2002) found that a predictor of maternal positive attributions about their children was the extent to which they used cognitive reframing as a way to guide and alter their perceptions on their children.

The term for resources (B) in the ABCX theory includes parents' coping skills and social support. This element in the double ABCX theory has been specifically addressed in studies that focused on training parents in groups to implement several different skills including, among others, problem-solving, communication, behavior management, and social skills. One way that researchers have attempted to increase family resources is by adding to their social support system. The psychoeducational methods reported in this chapter were all conducted as group treatments; groups of several parents learned skills together and interacted in a safe environment in which parents could learn from each other and sometimes develop new friendships. Finally, the outcome, the X term, if it is a state of crisis or high stress, is addressed in the interventions that teach stress-reduction techniques such as relaxation and mindfulness training. They are meant to both help to prevent stressors from happening but also to moderate the fight and flight responses typical in stress reactions. Many of the intervention practices reviewed in what follows include multiple elements that address stress as framed by the double ABCX theory.

PSYCHOEDUCATIONAL GROUP PROGRAMS

The psychoeducational approach starts with the assumption that programs that are generally effective for people with other sources of stress are likely to also be helpful to parents. These methods represent a transfer of intervention methods from a larger population of people experiencing stress from many common sources to family care givers of individuals with ID and autism. As a consequence, many of the programs described in this chapter are generic interventions that have been evaluated with several different groups in addition to the population of concern in this book. These programs share many commonalities but are distinct enough to fall into discriminable groupings. We have categorized the interventions into three groups: (1) stress management training (SMT), (2) cognitive change interventions derived from cognitive-behavioral therapy (CBT), and (3) coping skills instruction (CSI). Stress management training includes older relaxation-based programs and more recent mindfulness-based approaches.

COMMON FEATURES

Before describing the unique characteristics of each kind of program, we first discuss features that they share in common. The commonalities are to be expected, because these interventions bear a strong family resemblance derived from many common elements and a shared theoretical framework.

Psychoeducation

The interventions reviewed in this chapter all involve teaching small groups of parents skills for coping. Psychoeducation is an approach to supporting parents that emphasizes provision of information and instruction on skills for changing internal as well as social functioning (Lincoln, Wilhelm, & Nestoriuc, 2007). Psychoeducational programs provide support to parents through an educational process. Rather than equating support with therapy or treatment, the programs under review here emphasized teaching parents skills, some that involve self-regulation, others that have to do with social interactions with others including parenting. The emphasis on education is important, because there is no reason to believe that this group of parents on average suffers from mental illness. Belonging to a family with a child or sibling with a DD does not automatically confer patient status. Families are best viewed as learners who have requested support rather than patients. Many experience high levels of stress, but stress is common in the general US population. Many of the procedures are commonly used for parents of TD children who experience chronic pressures like underemployment, a highly demanding job, a troubled marriage, or challenges in parenting TD teenagers (Crnic & Greenberg, 1990). The educational approach is also relevant because much stress is amenable to skilled self-management that does not require the kinds of intensive self-examination common in forms of psychotherapy; instead these skills can be learned through ordinary educational processes of explanation, demonstration, guided practice, and independent practice in generalization settings.

Cognitive-Behavioral Framework

The psychoeducational programs discussed here have a strong a family resemblance because they are rooted in a common framework on the stress process (Folkman & Lazarus, 1980) and in cognitive-behavioral theory (Dobson, 2010). They share a set of common core principles: (1) cognitive activity affects behavior, (2) cognitive activity can be monitored and changed, and (3) changes in cognitive activity can lead to positive changes in behavior (Dobson, 2010). The cognitive-behavioral approach differs from psychodynamic theories, which give central importance to an individual's history, particularly their childhood experiences, and sometimes to cathartic expression of emotions. Cognitive-behavioral therapies (CBTs) have been developed and tested for depression, generalized anxiety disorder, panic disorder and agoraphobia, social anxiety, obsessive-compulsive disorder, preparation for medical procedures, spinal cord injury, and post-traumatic stress disorder, and they have also been used to support parents of children with DDs to manage stress and to adapt positively. Several different approaches to CBT have been developed and evaluated. Again they share several features. Based on a review of one CBT in treatment of HIV, Crepaz et al. (2008) identified the following common features of CBT: (1) altering irrational cognitions, (2) correctly appraising internal and external stressors, and (3) developing adaptive behavioral coping strategies. Cognitive-behavioral therapy has also been used for stress management, and it is usually in this context that it has been applied to supporting parents of children with disabilities. In this research literature, it has been the basis for several different interventions consisting of combinations of multiple components.

Coping Skills Instruction

Coping is the focus of a large body of research in psychology and related social sciences (Zeidner & Endler, 1996). Many of the treatments for parents of children with DDs provide instruction in coping skills as part of the psychoeducational approach to supporting families. Coping consists of efforts to address a stressor or to prevent stress. Early research on coping skills suggested that there are three major ways that people take action when stressed. These are problem-based coping, avoidance, and emotion-focused coping. Subsequently, this simple triadic term has been more fully developed and expanded to include additional ways that people prevent stressors from taking place and garner social support to help them when needed (Taylor et al., 2000). Coping skills are a broad class of behaviors, which are usually sequences of activities aimed at preventing stress or at reducing stress reactions. A long-standing taxonomy of coping skills divides them into three major categories: (1) emotion-focused coping, (2) action-focused coping, and (3) avoidance (Folkman & Lazarus, 1980). In the first two kinds of coping, people under stress respond to stressors in order to reduce, control, or prevent them in the future (Zeidner & Endler, 1996). In avoidant coping, people seek to escape from a situation or to suppress or cover up painful emotions and thoughts. The researchers who created and evaluated the programs described in this chapter chose different sets of coping skills. Nonetheless, the programs all share some commonalities. The skills were broken into steps and taught through modeling and practice with feedback. The skills pertain to personal internal or external actions that are thought to be useful in managing stress. Further, they can be taught in a brief period of time and are readily assigned as homework for practice in family homes.

Self-Monitoring

Observation of one's thoughts, feelings, and actions are core components of many stress management programs. For example, in the stress management program described by Singer, Irvin, and Hawkins (1988) the participants identified what caused them to experience stress reactions. Moreover, the basic premise of CBT is that people can monitor their own thoughts and feelings, identify the thoughts that contribute to dysfunction, and challenge them (Dobson, 2010). This process requires self-monitoring, which can be taught and practiced as a skill. The stressor and cognitive responses to it have to be defined clearly so that parents know what it is they are working to monitor and change. A diary form given to parents provides a place for them to identify the circumstances in which they felt stressed, the signs of stress in their bodies and minds, and the intensity of the stress reaction. The form also provides a place for them to note problematic thinking associated with stress.

Group Programs

The programs in this chapter were all delivered to small groups of parents rather than as individual therapy. Most were led by professionals with training in running groups. An exception was a study by Dykens, Fisher, Taylor, Lambert, and Miodrag (2014), who had professionals train and supervise parents to lead their mindfulness-based stress management programs. Groups have several advantages. Support groups are more economical for financially strained service programs. At their best they facilitate development of new peer-to-peer relationships, which sometimes become long-term sources of mutual aide. The group setting allows parents to hear from people who have experienced similar difficulties and successes leading to a reduction in perceived social isolation or stigma. When parents report on their application of skills taught in the group they can serve as models for one another. In a group setting they can also share information that may be particularly salient given their common experiences and needs. In order to maximize the possibility of mutual support developing in the groups, some researchers report deploying several strategies. Gammon and Rose (1991) reported that in their coping skills psychoeducational program they scheduled unstructured breaks in meetings with a snack food available to create an opportunity for parents to get to know one another without the formal structure of the group. During the training sessions they encouraged parents to share similar experiences and to provide encouragement to one another. Singer, Irvin, and Hawkins (1988) asked parents to agree to a set of rules of etiquette aimed at reducing criticism and increasing mutual encouragement between group members. They also asked parents each week to describe to one another their commitments for the week to practicing skills taught in the meetings as homework before the next meeting. These commitments to a group have been associated with better treatment compliance in some related areas such as behavioral medicine (Levy & Feld, 1999). Gammon and Rose (1991) quoted parents who had been through their program who subsequently emphasized the particular value that group interaction had for them; hearing from and supporting each other was a major benefit of the program. The consensus in the studies reviewed in this chapter is that parents can help one another through well-managed group programs. There is no evidence that we could find suggesting that group programs are definitely superior to individual support but rather that the benefits of group programs seem evident to providers and parents when they evaluate the service.

Homework

Homework assignments are widely used by group leaders as a way to practice cognitive-behavioral skills, promote self-management, and mediate generalization in psychoeducational programs. A 1999 survey study found that most therapists reported using homework assignments as part of their therapies (Kazantzis & Deane, 1999). A meta-analysis of 22 studies reported positive effects of using homework for treatments addressing a wide range of psychological and social problems (Kazantzis, Deane, & Ronan, 2000). They estimated that the overall effect size for homework assignments was $d = 0.36$, indicating that it has a small but robust impact on therapy outcomes. Most of the studies reviewed were cognitive-behavioral treatments for anxiety and depression. Table 2.2 presents examples of homework assignments from three different cognitive-behavioral

TABLE 2.2 EXAMPLES OF HOMEWORK FROM THREE COGNITIVE-BEHAVIORAL PROGRAMS FOR PARENTS OF CHILDREN WITH DEVELOPMENTAL DISABILITIES

Singer, Irvin, & Hawkins (1988)	*Nixon & Singer (1993)*	*Gammon & Rose (1991)*
Class 1: Participants are given a log form and asked to rate their stress level and to record stressful situations.	Class 1: Participants keep a daily record of dysfunctional thoughts, record stressful situations, negative feelings, automatic thoughts, and cognitive distortions.	Class 1: Class participants record daily hassles in a notebook.
Class 2: Keep daily record of stressors, practice PMR with an audio recording, and try to practice PMR once without the audio recording.	Class 2: Keep a daily record of dysfunctional thoughts and attempts at rational response to automatic thoughts and cognitive distortions.	Class 6: Keep the hassles diary with notes on distorted thoughts, coping statement to counter these thoughts, and a record of expressing feelings as presented in class. Work on individual achievement goals
Class 6: Record PMR practice, rate level of relaxation, note stress responses during the week, not successes in coping with stress.	Class 6: Keep daily record of dysfunctional thoughts focusing on guilt feelings and self-blaming cognitive distortions and automatic thoughts.	Class 9: Continue work on individual achievement goals, keep hassles diary with negative self-thoughts and coping statements, read a handout on basic human rights, read handout on maintenance of change.

interventions for parents of children with disabilities. These common elements were used as components of the interventions we review in this chapter.

THE PROGRAMS

The intervention programs have been grouped into three categories: (1) SMT, (2) CBT, and (3) CSI. Developing a useful taxonomy of these practices is difficult because they share many similar basic approaches. For example, the Singer et al. (1989) SMT program included weekly practice of progressive muscle relaxation (PMR), practice of self-monitoring and challenging negative automatic thoughts, and teaching coping skills to use in daily life, such as Benson's relaxation response (Benson, 1974). We classified psychoeducational program as SMT if a form of relaxation was taught and practiced as a regularly scheduled activity in 80% or more of the class meetings. Three programs fell into this category: mindfulness-based stress management training (MBSMT), cognitive-behavioral stress management training (Singer et al., 1988; Singer et al., 1989; Singer et al., 1994), and Schultz and Schultz's Care for Caregivers (N.C. Schultz & Schultz, 1997). The category that is most clearly distinguished from the others is CBT. In these programs the sessions were almost exclusively devoted to self-monitoring, challenging distorted or unduly negative thoughts, and developing more realistic or more positive thoughts to replace them (Greaves, 1997; Nixon & Singer, 1993). Though most of the other programs included some cognitive change elements, these were usually presented as one among several coping skills that were taught and practiced by parents during group meetings. Similarly, coping skills education was a component of several programs. When the preponderance of time and topics were devoted to skills training, we assigned programs to the CSI category. When the whole group of studies was analyzed using meta-analysis methods, each of the three groups was distinctively different from the others. Tests of homogeneity of variance supported the integrity of these three categories of programs.

STRESS MANAGEMENT TRAINING PROGRAMS

Stress management training programs share in common an emphasis on teaching participants skills for relaxation. In the general literature on stress management the forms of relaxation have included physical exercise, stretching, yoga, PMR, meditation, deep breathing, and guided imagery. All of these methods have been effective for reducing the average stress levels in people experiencing stress from many different sources. In the programs reviewed in this chapter two forms of relaxation were at the center of the treatment programs: (1) mindfulness meditation, and (2) PMR. New meditation-based treatment methods for stress and the positive psychology movement have influenced researchers in developing and evaluating ways to support people undergoing a variety of difficulties.

MINDFULNESS-BASED STRESS REDUCTION PROGRAMS

A major line of research on stress focused on mindfulness-based stress reduction (MBSR) (Kabat-Zinn & Hahn, 1994). Mindfulness as a way of preventing and coping with stress has been tested on individuals with a wide range of concerns. Mindfulness is an open, aware state of mind in which thoughts and feelings as well as sensory stimuli are observed in the present moment in a nonjudgmental, accepting way regardless of whether or not these thoughts and perceptions are pleasant, neutral, or painful. Some researchers believe mindfulness is made up of two components: The first involves bringing attention to bear on what is in the mind in the present, and the second is viewing experiences with acceptance regardless of their valence (Bishop et al., 2004; Kabat-Zinn & Hahn, 1994). Mindfulness derives from Buddhist meditation practices. It has been extracted from its religious origins and adopted in clinical psychology as a secular practice. Given its effectiveness with several different populations, it makes sense that researchers have begun to evaluate mindfulness as a treatment for parental stress and distress in families of children with ASD.

Dykens and her colleagues (2014) conducted the largest randomized trial to date of an intervention directly aimed at helping parents of children with developmental disabilities with stress-related distress. Because it is an exemplary study in the literature on interventions for families of individuals with DDs, we describe it in some detail here. Readers who would prefer an abbreviated description of the study are advised to turn to the tables at the end of this chapter. The study was primarily designed to evaluate MBSR as a way to support parents of children with autism or with other DDs. The rationale for the study was the evidence of elevated stress and related mental and physical health problems in this group of parents compared with parents of TD children. Further, the authors noted that previous randomized controlled trials (RCTs) aimed at reducing caregiver stress had relatively small sample sizes and did not primarily serve families of individuals with autism, who were the central focus of this study, although a substantial percentage of the participants were parents of individuals with ID. The strengths of this study include both the treatment model and the research methodology.

Program

The central treatment was MBSR, developed by J. Kabat-Zinn. Mindfulness-based stress reduction is a positive, psychoeducational approach that does not focus on pathology and emotional distress. It taught specific breathing, meditation, and movement techniques, including paying attention to the breath, deep belly breathing, the relaxation response, self-observation without self-evaluation, Qigong (gentle movements), and the sitting, body scan, and loving-kindness meditations. The researchers designed ways of making the group classes accessible to parents by scheduling them in the afternoon and evening, locating them in community centers near the parents' residences, and providing childcare during the meetings. The instructors who led the mindfulness classes were parents of children with DDs who were supervised by a clinical social worker. Consequently, there was a strong parent-to-parent component in the intervention, in keeping with previous research demonstrating the benefits of peer support for parents of children with special needs (Ireys, Sills, Kolodner, & Walsh, 1996; Singer et al., 1999). We review parent-to-parent programs in chapter 5, suggesting that peer-to-peer programs hold promise as part of a system of family support. The comparison group received an online positive psychology program, positive psychology practice (PAD) (Seligman, Steen, Park, & Peterson, 2006). Table 2.3 lists the major components of both treatments.

Methodology

Many of the studies reported in this chapter were conducted in the 1990s and earlier. Since then, standards for conducting RCTs have been widely promulgated in medicine, psychology, and education. Dykens and her colleagues met a set of standards for conducting RCTs, the Consolidated Standards of Reporting Trial (CONSORT), developed to improve the quality RCTs in medicine (Schulz, Altman, & Moher, 2010). There are several advances in methodological quality in this study. Dykens et al. made a unique contribution to the literature in recruiting a large and diverse sample of families with demographic characteristics that represent the range of ethnic, racial, and economic diversity in the 21st-century United States. Seventy percent of the parents were Caucasian, 15% were African American, 9% Hispanic, and 6.5% Asian. Furthermore, close to one in five participant families were from low-income households. Participants were followed for up to 8 months after the initial baseline assessment, a relatively long follow-up period in this literature. However, by week 18, almost half of the participants failed to return the assessments. Nonetheless, the study provides some valuable data on maintenance of effect.

TABLE 2.3 THE COMPONENTS OF MINDFULNESS-BASED STRESS REDUCTION AND POSITIVE PSYCHOLOGY PRACTICE

Mindfulness-Based Stress Reduction	*Positive Psychology Practice*
Paying attention to breath	Tempering negative emotions
Deep belly breathing	Recruiting character strengths and virtues
Relaxation response	Using strengths in new ways
Self-observation without evaluation	Practice gratitude
Qigong (gentle movements)	Practice forgiveness
Sitting meditation	Practice grace
Body scan	Practice optimism
Loving kindness meditation	

Source: From Dykens et al. (2014)

The measures used in this study were all standardized and have known psychometric properties. Three of the measures have established clinical cutoff scores, allowing the authors to report on the percentage of parents who were thought at baseline to have clinically significant depressive symptoms, anxiety symptoms, or parenting stress, although these data was not reported for the follow-ups. The primary measure in the study was the Parent Stress Index (short form) (Abidin, 1990). It has become one of the most widely used measures in studies aiming to reduce stress. Both treatments were associated with improvements in the major outcome measures. These gains were maintained up to 8 months after the treatment. The Beck Depression Inventory (BDI) (Beck, Steer, & Brown, 1996) was used to measure depressive symptoms. It has a long history of use and has substantial evidence regarding key psychometric properties (Beck, Steer, & Garbin, 1988). The Beck Anxiety Inventory (BAI; Steer & Beck, 1997) and the Insomnia Severity Index (Bastien, Vallières, & Morin, 2001) were used to assess two common reactions to stress. Dykens et al. also used measures of positive adaptation, an important improvement in the treatment literature: the Ryff Scales of Psychological Well-Being (Ryff, 2014) and the Life Satisfaction Scale (Diener, Emmons, Larsen, & Griffin, 1985) were used to tap parents' positive adjustments. The researchers administered these measures several times, allowing them to develop growth curve analyses that compared improvements in outcomes at baseline, during the intervention, and post-test, as well as follow-ups at roughly 3, 5, and 8 months post treatment. The use of growth curve modeling from repeated measures is another unique methodological contribution of this study.

The authors of the report did not emphasize the outcomes in the comparison group, but we believe they also may have an important potential in a service system for this population of families. The PAD comparison group also showed consistent gains on most of the outcome measures. In some instances the PAD participants appear to have benefited more than the parents who received MBSR. Further, additional research on PAD is warranted, given its potential as a cost-effective treatment. It was delivered entirely online, and likely is considerably less expensive than MBSR to deliver. It holds promise as a cost-effective way to provide some support to parents who cannot otherwise access psychoeducational support programs. The content of the two programs that were compared in this study are shown in Table 2.3.

The study by Dykens and colleagues provides an important standard for future research on social and psychological support programs for families of children with ASD and other DDs. As with any study, there are features of the study that should be improved in what must be continuous efforts to produce high-quality research. The study did not report a treatment manual for either intervention. As with any journal article, the space for explaining the treatments was very limited, so that without recourse to manuals it is difficult to gain a more thorough understanding of the treatments. Arguably, future research should include a no-treatment or treatment-as-usual comparison group so that between-group effect sizes can be determined. Dykens reported a different effect size than we calculated for the other group comparison studies in this book. Throughout the book we reported the comparison of mean scores between treatment and control groups, these are between groups comparisons. This kind of comparison was not available in Dykens et al.'s study. She did report within-group pretest-posttest comparisons for the two forms of treatment. These effect sizes for the MBSM treatment and the PAD treatment respectively were d = 1.03 and .58 for depression, .88 and .44 for anxiety, and 1.10 and .26 for insomnia. We did not enter this data into our meta-analysis for the studies in this chapter because the effect sizes are not measuring the same kinds of comparisons. Nonetheless, these within group comparisons suggest strong impacts of the MBSM treatment. Finally, the measures could be improved by using data that goes beyond self-report, including direct observations of affect and parent–child interactions by independent observers, physiological measures such as cortisol levels for parents and children, and clinical interviews evaluating depression and anxiety. There is always room for improvement in any research, and we do not wish to downplay the value of MBSR for parents of children with autism that has been so effectively demonstrated in this high-quality study.

In order to meet the criteria for acknowledging a practice as established, additional evidence is required. To meet these criteria the intervention must be replicated in at least one other study that is a well-designed randomized controlled experiment using the same treatment with a similar sample of participants.

A Second Randomized Controlled Trial of Mindfulness-Based Stress Reduction

An earlier study provides the additional support required to evaluate MBSR as an evidence-based practice with at least short-term benefits. It was a small randomized trial of mindfulness training plus additional meditation-based positive psychological practices. Benn, Akiva, Arel, and Roeser (2012) evaluated a manualized mindfulness training program with parents of children with special needs and with special educators. Prior to randomization, parents and educators were divided into two different groups. Parents and teachers were then randomly assigned to treatment or waiting list control groups. As a result, at baseline researchers were able to compare 12 treated parents with 13 parents on a waiting list and 19 treated special educators with 16 teachers in a waiting list group. At post-test, because of attrition, the numbers were reduced to 19 and 9, respectively, for the treatment and waiting list educators and 11 and 13 for the two groups of parents. The intervention consisted of 2 weekly, 2.5-hour meetings over a 5-week period and 2 full days of a group retreat. As with the stress management programs described earlier, the program included homework assignments, which were the basis for parental discussion at meetings. The sessions involved didactic presentations by professionally trained group leaders, mindfulness practices including deep breathing, awareness exercises, and mindful stretching followed by group discussions. Table 2.4 presents the content of each meeting.

The table shows that, in addition to mindfulness, participants learned about and practiced directing acceptance and loving kindness toward themselves, practicing compassion

TABLE 2.4 SUMMARY OF SESSIONS, TOPICS, AND ACTIVITIES IN MINDFULNESS TRAINING CURRICULUM

Session	*Topic*	*Content*
1	Introduction	Mindfulness introduction; guided visualization; written reflection; raisin exercise.
2	Perceptions	Setting intentions, moods and thoughts exercise; stress didactic and discussion; body scan; silent eating; emotions didactic; mindful stretching; breath awareness.
3	Responding vs. Reacting	Mindful stretching; body scan; stress reaction cycle and coping didactic and discussion.
4	Pleasant, Unpleasant, and Neutral Affect	Breath awareness and awareness of sound; events calendar charting and discussion.
5	Exploring Forgiveness	Mindful stretching; awareness of breath, sounds, and physical sensations; forgiveness didactic and dyad exercise; guided visualization.
6	Working with Conflict	Mindful stretching; awareness of breath and thoughts; aikido of communication role play.
7	Compassion and Kindness	Mindful stretching; awareness of breath, sounds, sensations, thoughts, emotions and mental states; kindness and compassion discussion; eyes on exercise; kindness meditation.
8	Working with Anger	Choiceless awareness meditation; anger didactic; relived anger exercise; anger triggers/dyads and discussion, anger profiles.
9	Silent Retreat	Awareness of the breath and choiceless awareness; mindful stretching; body scan; walking meditation; guided visualization; mindful eating; mindful movement to music; sitting meditation; walking meditation; kindness meditation; walking meditation with kindness on the go.
10	Working with Fear	Mindful stretching; breath awareness and choiceless awareness; working with fear didactic and discussion; relived fear exercise; fear dyads.
11	Beginnings and Endings	Body scan; guided visualization; mindful stretching; community resources and discussion of continuation of practice; personal reflections.

Note. All sessions were 2.5 hours long except for Sessions 2 and 9, which were 6 hours long.

Source: Benn et al. (2012, p. 3)

and forgiveness of others, mindful walking and eating, and mindfulness for coping with fear. Part of one session was also devoted to teaching communication skills for avoiding enmeshment in conflict with others. There were several dependent variables as measured by reliable self-report scales. These included mindfulness, stress, anxiety, depression, negative affect, positive well-being, personal growth, and self-compassion. Measures were administered as a pretest, a posttest and a follow-up 2 months later. Participants in the intervention groups showed statistically significant improvements on all variables except for positive affect. Most effect size differences, the *d* statistics, were in the moderate-to - large range from .40 to .79. An important finding is that at follow-up the effect sizes were even larger on several of the outcomes indicating further improvement after the end of the treatment. Although the numbers of participants in this study was relatively small, the research meets high standards for a randomized trial.

Overall Evaluation of Mindfulness-Based Stress Reduction

Rigorous published studies with randomized control designs allow us to evaluate this intervention as an evidence-based practice for supporting families of children with ID or ASD at least in the short term. There is a large and growing evidence base for the benefits of mindfulness training in the general population as a treatment for stress (Chiesa & Serretti, 2009). Given these outcomes, a practitioner can be reasonably confident that mindfulness will be useful for some, perhaps many, families of concern in this book. We regard it as an established treatment given the existing evidence.

COGNITIVE-BEHAVIORAL STRESS MANAGEMENT TRAINING

A second approach to stress management has also been tested with parents of children with DDs. Cognitive-behavioral stress management training (CBSMT) consists of multiple component packages of relaxation, cognitive coping skills, and active behavioral coping skills. Cognitive-behavioral stress management training has been investigated in RCTs with parents of children with moderate/severe ID, autism, and traumatic brain injury (TBI) (Singer et al., 1988; Singer et al., 1989; Singer et al., 1993; Singer et al., 1994; and the Care for Caring Parents Program (C. L. Schultz et al., 1993) in which each session included practicing deep breathing as a way to decrease or suppress a full stress response.

Singer, Hawkins, and Irvin's Cognitive-Behavioral Stress Management Training Program

In the following discussion we present the major themes in the cognitive-behavioral stress management intervention studied by Singer and colleagues at the Oregon Research Institute. Stress management was conceptualized and presented as a set of psychoeducational skills taught to groups of 8 to 12 parents through short lectures, group discussions, homework, and in-class practice of relaxation techniques. The program's eight weekly meetings were conceptualized as educational sessions rather than as therapy or as support group meetings and were advertised as such.

Two hallmarks of the cognitive-behavioral approach to stress management training (SMT) are its focus on skills acquisition and homework practice for generalization. The classes were presented by a clinical psychologist and a doctoral level special educator, who mainly acted as leaders and instructors. In subsequent replications the intervention was presented by a PhD-level special educator and by social workers. The classes followed an agenda that was posted each week for all to see. The content of each class was predetermined based on the treatment manual (Hawkins, 1985). The leaders were responsible for keeping the group on track according to weekly lesson plans and for managing the direction of the meeting. Leaders guided discussions based on parents' reports of stressors and coping efforts during the week based on a diary they kept. The emphasis during discussions was on successful coping efforts. In addition to these homework-based discussions, classes consisted of brief lectures focused on a new coping skill, guided relaxation training, and guided imagery. Classes closed with parents making a specific commitment as to the amount of time they promised to practice STM skills during the coming week. Homework assignments were designed to encourage generalization of the stress management skills to their daily environments. These assignments were very important in influencing the focal point of group discussions. Unlike a more loosely structured form of group therapy or a support group, parent's discussions in the meetings were centered on the homework assignments, which often brought to light specific stressors as well as successful and unsuccessful ways of trying to cope with them.

The emotional tone of the meetings and the leaders was one of friendliness and hopefulness. The leaders were knowledgeable and accepting of the contributions children with disabilities often make to family life as well as the challenges that caregiving families may encounter. After gaining some experience with these families, the leaders of the program did not assume that having a child with a severe disability was necessarily damaging to the family or even the main source of stress in some families. It was not unusual for parents to attend the classes because they were concerned about stress related to raising a TD teen who was the sibling of a child with a disability or to attend in order to address long-standing insomnia and work stress. One way of shaping the positive tone of the meetings was to ask parents to enter into a set of agreements about how the classes would be conducted. These included being supportive of one another, providing a comfortable way for parents to demur when called on if so inclined, keeping the discussions at the meeting confidential, and allowing one another equal time to talk. The group leaders also asked the group for permission to manage the time allotted to activities on the class schedule.

The program was designed to teach coping skills in addition to muscle relaxation and to encourage parents to use these in their daily lives. Table 2.5 presents the content of the eight class sessions for the program.

Evaluation of Cognitive-Behavioral Stress Management Training

In two of the Singer et al. studies, parents were randomly assigned either to a no-treatment waiting list (Singer et al., 1988; Singer et al., 1989) or to an information/attention-only comparison group (Singer et al., 1993). This program has some important strengths including treatment manuals, fidelity of implementation data, standardized dependent measures, publication in peer-reviewed journals, and replication studies. The developers published two studies that used randomized group assignment. In the 1988 study, Singer

TABLE 2.5 CONTENT OF CLASS SESSIONS IN HAWKINS'S STRESS MANAGEMENT TREATMENT PROGRAM

Session Number	*Content*
Session 1	Greetings and introductions. Ground rules are presented and agreed on: respectful communication, confidentiality, allowing others to speak. Minilecture on stress. Parents give examples of how they feel under stress. Importance of identifying specific stressors. Explanation of a self-monitoring log.
Session 2	Review of the group agreements; Play a game to help participants with each other's names; Review homework assignments; Introduce relaxation; Demonstrate relaxation and debrief the experience; and Discuss homework and have group members make a public commitment to complete some assignments.
Session 3	Overview of session; Review of homework; Practice PMR and debrief; Discuss other forms of relaxation; Introduce Comfort Checks as a beginning coping skill; Assign homework and obtain a public commitment to practice.
Session 4	Review of homework; Brief relaxation practice; Introduction of how thoughts can affect emotion; Describe self-talk; decrease negative thinking and increase positive thinking; Assign homework and obtain a public commitment to practice.
Session 5	Review of homework; Review examples of 3-Step Thought Analysis; Brief relaxation practice; Discuss Comfort Checks and how to use them to decrease negative talk; Introduction of Thought Stopping; Assign homework and obtain a public commitment to practice.
Session 6	Review of homework; Description of Covert rehearsal; Combination of relaxation practice with covert rehearsal practice; Discussion of social support; Participants share their current social support; Assign homework and obtain a public commitment to practice.
Session 7	Review of homework; Review of Covert rehearsal and introduce using this technique for reducing fears; Combination of relaxation practice with Covert rehearsal practice; Discussion of increasing social support contacts; Participants share their current social support; Assign homework and obtain a public commitment to practice (p. 53).
Session 8	Review of homework; Practice PMR; Discussion of ideas for managing time; Provide tips for maintaining the skills they have learned; and Debrief the participants to find what were the most helpful concepts learned during these sessions (p. 59).

Source: Singer et al. (1988)

and colleagues compared a waiting list control group with their SMT program, finding significant differences on measures of depressive symptoms and anxiety symptoms. The effect size difference for depressive symptoms was .27. In a second study, CBT-SMT was one component of a multicomponent intervention that also included behavioral parent training, case management services, and respite care; it is reviewed in chapter 5 on multiple component interventions (Singer et al., 1989). We evaluate this program as promising.

PROGRESSIVE MUSCLE RELAXATION

Singer et al. (1988) chose PMR as the relaxation technique taught to parents. In addition to the broad evidence base for its efficacy, brief forms of PMR have been tested for use in everyday stressful circumstances, providing a way to generalize the relaxation response to the natural environment (Carlson & Hoyle, 1993). Progressive muscle relaxation includes the practice of tensing and releasing skeletal muscles to learn the sensations associated with tension and its release and the feeling of muscles that are relaxed or have normal tone. A review and meta-analysis of the research on relaxation training as a treatment for anxiety found that it had a consistent positive effect with a moderate effect size, $d = 0.57$ (Manzoni, Pagnini, Castelnuovo, & Molinari, 2008). A review of the behavioral medicine literature specifically on the brief form of PMR used in the Singer et al. study reported an average positive effect size of $d = 0.76$ for treatment of several illnesses including migraine, essential hypertension, and chronic low back pain. These maladies are commonly associated with stress (Carlson & Hoyle, 1993).

PROGRESSIVE MUSCLE RELAXATION AND GUIDED IMAGERY

As part of each class parents were led through a short form of PMR and were guided to imagine a restful scene. Guided imagery is a procedure that has also been widely used in cognitive-behavioral stress management programs and in behavioral medicine (Van Kuiken, 2004). In reviewing the medical literature, Van Kuiken (2004) identified four different approaches to guided imagery that can be provided in a group or individual session, by audiotape, or by self-prompting. The form used in the Singer et al. studies was *pleasant imagery*, a format in which participants provided their own content with broad instructions to imagine or remember a pleasing and relaxing environment. As with PMR, guided imagery was taught as a skill that can be learned and transferred to other settings and circumstances. Parents are assigned PMR and guided imagery practice as homework.

THE CARE FOR CARING PARENTS PROGRAM

C. L. Schultz et al. (1993) developed and tested a stress management and coping skills intervention for parents of children with DDs. The program has a published manual for group leaders (N. C. Schultz & Schultz, 1997) and an accompanying book for parents with material presented in the meetings. Similar to Gammon and Rose in its psychoeducational approach, the treatment consisted of 2-hour group sessions for fathers and mothers led by the authors. No more than 12 parents were permitted per group. The groups met weekly for 6 weeks. The goals of the program are presented in Table 2.6; it shows the wide-ranging scope of topics and skills presented. The authors stressed the importance of facilitating groups in which parents found a warm and supportive milieu and had an opportunity to establish new social ties with each other. The sessions were a combination of didactic presentations, discussions, and practice exercises.

TABLE 2.6 CONTENT OF CARE FOR CARING PARENTS PROGRAM

Session Number	*Contents*
Class 1	Welcome and a statement of group guidelines. A structured discussion of the impact of parenting children with disabilities. Positive and negative demands and rewards are elicited. Leader presents a theory of parent caregiving and its impact on the whole person. Interaction of cognition and external events is emphasized in the stress process. Parents are encouraged to identify and monitor internal sources of pressure and external pressures. Schultz & Schultz's theory of caregiving is presented in common language, and parents are asked to comment on each element. Parents invited to state topics they would like discussed in classes. Small groups discuss effective coping skills and experiences including social support. Parents identify helpful attitudes, beliefs, or values and share experiences of them. Parents are encouraged to build their coping repertoire over the 9 weeks of classes. Leader guides parents through a deep breathing exercise for relaxation. Parents are given homework exercises based on the class topics.
Class 2	Leader presents a review of previous week. A model of how family's function is presented and discussed. Problem-solving is presented and discussed. Idea of a varied repertoire of coping skills is emphasize and discussed. Relaxation practice: guided visualization and peaceful breathing. Whole group and small groups discuss impacts of caregiving on the whole family. Parents invited to talk about loss and grief. Explain positive adaptation and elicit examples of the process. Parents are guided through creating a family genogram while the leader describes family interaction. A 7-step cognitive-behavioral self-change process is presented. Parents are encouraged to set a personal goal for themselves and their families. Assign reading and exercises from parent handbook.
Class 3	Discussion of efforts to accomplish goal from previous week and family change efforts. Guided imagery and deep breathing are practiced. A social-ecological model is presented. Parents draw an eco-map around their genograms. Parents are guided to discuss troubled and helpful relationships from outside the family. Parents prioritize an external relationship to change. The leader presents importance of self-affirmations and self-care. The leader explains assertiveness and has parents respond to vignettes. Homework from a parent's manual is encouraged.
Class 4	Discussion of progress on internal and external goals. Parents encouraged to share their effective strategies. Leader lectures on communication and challenges to it. Parents are guided through a model of listening in different levels of responsiveness. During a break parents share family photos. A cognitive behavioral model of emotion is presented in common language. The importance of emotions in stress and coping. The topic of grief is revisited and parents are encouraged to express their feelings of grief in dyads. A brief form of deep breathing to use in crisis situations is presented and practiced.
Class 5	A model of communication is presented including problem-ownership, assertiveness, empathic listening, and problem-solving. Assertiveness is revisited. A six-step cognitive-behavioral assertiveness sequence is presented. Leader guides a discussion of conflict resolution. A 6-step problem-solving process is presented. In dyads, parents give examples of personal conflicts and generate possible solutions. Parents are guided through identifying a network of support with an emphasis on professional and organization-based resources. Deep breathing and muscle relaxation are practiced.

(*continued*)

TABLE 2.6 (CONTINUED)

Session Number	*Contents*
Class 6	The group compiles a list of community resources. The importance of rest and relaxation is emphasized. A form of relaxation chosen by the group is presented and practiced.
Class 7*	The leader gives a presentation on stress and leads a discussion with an emphasis on the role of subjective reaction in the stress process. A cognitive-behavioral model of stress is presented and discussed. Stress management is presented and discussed. In small groups parents discuss ways to deal with stress. The leader emphasizes skills from previous classes for managing stress. A model for preventing stress with an emphasis on taking time to build relationships that buffer stress.
Classes 8 & 9*	These sessions follow a different structure. The whole group convenes and parents select one of six topical groups to join while at the class. The gather into common interest groups. The choice of topics is: (1) extended deep muscle relaxation, (2) longer term continuation of the Care for Caring Parents group, (3) involvement in existing organizations, (4) advocacy, (5) legal and guardianship issues, and (6) living with loss and grief. The leader's manual includes an additional section for the group on a cognitive-behavioral adaptation to grief and loss. The manual also presents outlines for a special group meeting on couples' relationships.

*Classes 7, 8, & 9 are offered at monthly rather than weekly intervals.

The Care for Caring Parents Program (Schultz & Schultz, 1997) is one of the most fully developed interventions for parents. It is unique in that it is based on a comprehensive theory of effective caregiving, which the authors first developed based on their clinical experience with family caregivers of elderly family members. Although they derived their own theory, the intervention package they created has many similarities to the other coping skills programs reviewed here. One unique feature of this program, which did not appear elsewhere, was psychoeducation about grief and adjustment to loss. The Care for Caring Parents Program has been used widely in New Zealand and has a commercially available manual (Schultz & Schultz, 1990). The leader's manual provides several figures to help guide discussion and introduce new concepts and practices. Table 2.6 summarizes the content of each session of the program.

The researchers chose the General Health Questionnaire (GHQ-28) (Goldberg & Hillier, 1979) as their primary measure. Two factors have been identified for this 28-item measure: (1) inability to perform one's current social roles, and (2) appearance of a new major stressor. There is a substantial evidence base used to calculate basic psychometric properties. A 2(parent gender) × 2(groups) analysis of covariance (ANCOVA) with pretest scores as the covariate found a statistically significant difference in the two groups at post-test of $F(1, 50) = 4.95$, $p = .03$. The effect size, d, was 0.385. This effect size is modest but consistent with many of the studies in this literature.

OVERALL EVALUATION OF STRESS MANAGEMENT TRAINING

We have evaluated this group of research studies in two different ways. In the first, the studies using MBSMT are grouped together and evaluated using meta-analytic techniques. This treatment is supported by sufficient evidence to designate it as an established program. Practitioners can be reasonably confident that it can be helpful to many parents of children with disabilities at least in the short term. The second way of looking at these studies is to consider all of the stress management programs as making up one category. The approach emphasizes the similarities in the various programs including their repeated practice sessions of relaxation training, their focus on acquiring related coping skills, and their attention to identifying sources of stress. When examined in this way SMT can be considered to be an established practice.

COGNITIVE-BEHAVIORAL THERAPY APPROACHES

The two studies in this grouping share in common an emphasis on the core components of CBT: self-monitoring, identification of dysfunctional thoughts, and challenging and replacing these cognitions with more functional thoughts. Cognitive-behavioral therapy is an approach to treating and preventing mental health conditions including stress reactions to discrete life events as well as for treating problems linked to chronic stressors. It is based on the belief that private events, thoughts, and feelings, mediate the relationship between the environment and behavior. Extensive reviews have been published, including as of 2005, 16 meta-analyses synthesizing 332 published outcome studies. When compared with a waiting list control or no-treatment control group, the effect size for CBT for adult unipolar depression was $d = 0.82$, indicating a large effect. Studies using similar comparisons also yielded an effect size of $d = 0.82$ for generalized anxiety (Butler, Chapman, Forman, & Beck, 2006).

Cognitive therapies have been developed and tested for depression, generalized anxiety disorder, panic disorder and agoraphobia, social anxiety, obsessive-compulsive disorder, preparation for medical procedures, spinal cord injury, and post-traumatic stress disorder, and as detailed in this section, they have also been used with some effectiveness to support parents of children with DDs to manage stress and to adapt positively (Dobson, 2010). Several different approaches to CBT have been developed and evaluated. They share a set of common core principles: (1) cognitive activity affects behavior, (2) cognitive activity can be monitored and changed, and (3) changes in cognitive activity can lead to positive changes in behavior (Dobson, 2010). Two published studies have reported on CBT programs for parents of children with DDs.

NIXON AND SINGER'S PROGRAM: A TREATMENT FOR EXCESSIVE SELF-BLAME AND GUILT

Nixon and Singer (1993) conducted research on a group cognitive-behavioral intervention aimed at reducing parental self-blame and guilt and associated depressive symptoms. Nixon conducted the study as his dissertation and was responsible for its content. When compared with the other published evaluations of interventions, this one is somewhat different in that it was entirely devoted to helping parents identify and alter cognitive distortions that were assumed to lead to excessive self-blame about the children's disabilities. Beck's (1976) theory of cognitive distortions provided the foundation for the treatment method. In his research on psychopathology Beck identified a set of eight cognitive distortions including, for example, polarized thinking and catastrophizing. He demonstrated that CBT could effectively help people to identify distorted thinking and to alter it by challenging and replacing with more realistic cognitions.

Nixon and Singer (1993) were specifically concerned about inappropriate ways that parents might blame themselves for children's disabilities and for children's problem behaviors. They reviewed literature on characterological self-blame and behavioral self-blame. Behavioral self-blame is a thinking process in which an individual identifies behavior that he/she judges to be inappropriate or mistaken and makes attributions about these acts rather than about the actor. A parent who left a bottle of medications where his/her child could reach it would attribute the problem to the action and conclude that he/she must be more careful in the future. A parent caught up in character-based blame would assume that he/she left the bottle in reach because he/she is an incompetent person. Behavioral-self-blame implies that behavior can be improved in the future, whereas character-based blame is viewed as immutable. Table 2.7 shows the content of each of the sessions in the program by Nixon and Singer.

Nixon recruited 50 mothers of children with moderate/severe disabilities through public schools in a large metropolitan area. Thirty-four mothers participated in the treatment group, and 16 in a no-treatment waiting list group. They were parents of children with ID of an average age of 9.3 years. Some of the children also had a diagnosis of ASD in addition to ID. The children all attended public school programs for students with severe disabilities. The comparison group received the intervention after posttest data was collected from the initial cohort. Six couples participated, but the data from men were excluded because they were not independent spouses' data. The treatment consisted of five meetings of 2 hours each. The group sessions consisted of guided discussions in which the therapist, a counseling psychologist, encouraged participants to express their thoughts and feelings about their roles as parents. When parents made unduly self-blaming attributions or expressed cognitive distortions, the therapist challenged these and asked the group to discuss these challenges and to suggest alternative ways of thinking about the topic. Nixon's account of the group process emphasized the importance of the group dynamics in helping parents to change their views. Parents were able to help one another with facilitation by the therapist.

The dependent measures were published scales with established psychometric properties. These included the Situational Guilt Scale (Klass, 1987), a measure of self-blame, and the Attributional Style Questionnaire (Peterson et al., 1982), which measures the tendency to choose specific causal explanations for negative and positive events. Finally, the Beck Depression Inventory (Beck et al., 1988) was used to measure depressive symptoms. The researchers randomly assigned parents to treatment and control groups. Pretest

TABLE 2.7 TOPICS DISCUSSED IN NIXON AND SINGER'S COGNITIVE-BEHAVIORAL THERAPY PROGRAM

Session Number	*Content*
Session 1	Overview. Brief lectures on cognitive distortions and automatic thoughts. Parents respond to vignettes illustrating distorted thinking and are asked to identify it. In small groups parents generate examples of problematic events in parenting and ways they think in a distorted way about them. Self-monitoring is explained and parents are given homework to use a handout diary form to note stressful circumstances and the ways they thought about them.
Session 2	Review and discuss homework. Minilecture on reality testing and techniques for disputing distorted thinking. Minilecture on ways to dispute "should statements". All or nothing thinking and alternatives to it. In-group parents provide examples of these ways of thinking and generate alternatives. Homework is assigned: record stressful events and automatic thoughts about them; also, record examples of alternative self-talk.
Session 3	Review homework. Minilecture on exaggerated personal control. Parents are given the Belief in Personal Control Scale to fill out about themselves. These are the topic of small-group discussions. Minilecture and small-group discussion on techniques for dealing with exaggerated personal control. Minimization of personal control is presented and discussed in small groups and ways develop a more realistic sense of personal control are presented and discussed in groups. Homework assignments are to record stressful situations, affect, automatic thoughts, alternative cognitions, and an evaluation of their efficacy.
Session 4	Review and discuss homework. The minilecture centers on how people explain negative events. Discussions of self-blame as a way to provide an explanation for an event that may be out of a parent's control or may have ambiguous causes. Self-blame as a way to preserve a belief in a just world. Blaming the victim is discussed as a cognitive distortion. The therapist presents ways that parents have reported the cause of children's disability in previous research. Examples of helpful and unhelpful explanations are discussed. The focus of the homework for the week is on guilt feelings, ways to challenge the thinking behind them, and evaluating their efficacy.
Session 5	Review and discuss homework. The meeting centers on parents' expectations for the parental role and the guilt that is linked to unrealistic expectations. The ten cognitive distortions are reviewed and examples are presented regarding the parental role. A minilecture focuses on types of guilt: causal guilt, parental-role guilt, and moral guilt. Techniques for dealing with overly generalized guilt attributions are presented and discussed.

Source: Nixon & Singer (1993)

and posttest data from the two groups were analyzed using ANCOVA with pretest data as covariates of the posttest data. After participating in the treatment program, parents reported statistically significant improvements on all measures. In discussing the treatment, Nixon and Singer emphasized the ways in which groups contributed to helping individual parents change. Within the structured format of the five classes, parents were able to support one another. Nixon and Singer (1993) suggested that social comparison processes accounted for part of the efficacy of the treatment in combination with the cognitive-behavioral approach. There are some important shortcomings in this study.

GREAVE'S RATIONAL EMOTIVE PARENT EDUCATION PROGRAM

Greaves (1997) provided a similar second study of a cognitive change program by evaluating the Rational-Emotive Parent Education Program (REPE). Greaves used a published manual, *Reason and Emotion in Psychotherapy-Revised* (Ellis, 1994). The similarity of the Nixon and Singer intervention and Greaves's is readily apparent. The major contribution of this study is in its research design. It provides crucial evidence for efficacy because it compared REPE with an existing treatment with evidence for effectiveness. He randomly assigned mothers of children with Down syndrome to one of three groups, an REPE group of 21 parents, an applied behavior analysis (ABA) parent training group of 17 mothers, and a no-treatment control group of 16. The REPE group received eight sessions. The ABA comparison group had a similar format for group meetings composed of short lectures followed by discussions, with the crucial difference being content focused on parenting skills rather than on helping parents with their thoughts and emotions. Both interventions were advertised as stress management programs and met the same number of sessions with the same duration. The ABA group received lectures and participated in discussions about the principles of operant conditioning, the use of baselines, extinction, punishment, and positive reinforcement.

The dependent variables in Greaves's study were parent's stress, parental dissatisfaction, and their negative emotions. Dissatisfaction was measured using the Cleminshaw-Guidubaldi Parent Satisfaction Scale (Cleminshaw & Guidubaldi, 1985). Parental stress was measured using a compilation of scales by Bernard (1990). Negative emotions were measured with the Profile of Mood States (POMS) (McNair, Lorr, & Droppelman, 1971). Compared with the no-treatment control group and the ABA group, parents participating in REPE showed significantly less stress and negative affect after the treatment. They also reported less depression and significantly higher ratings on their sense of competence. Taken together, the Nixon and Singer study and Greave's research meet the standards as established practices. That is, they have been evaluated with two randomized trials, one comparing the practice with another established intervention. Further, the quality of the research and the availability of a treatment manual provide reasonable confidence that there is evidence supporting the use of these methods to help parents with aspects of cognitive adaptation.

COPING SKILLS TRAINING PROGRAMS

Coping skills are ways of actively responding to prevent or address stressors or modulate their impact. Several kinds of psychological and social skills have been studied and evaluated as treatments for people experiencing stress and stress-related mental and physical health problems (Holahan, Moos, & Schaefer, 1996). Coping skills instruction

TABLE 2.8 COPING SKILLS ADDRESSED IN FOUR CLINICAL TRIALS

Kirkham & Schilling (1990)	*Gammon & Rose (1991)*	*Davis & Rushton (1991)*	*Erguner-Tekinalp & Akkok (2004)*
Cognitive coping	Cognitive restructuring	Social problem-solving	Self-monitoring of stress and stress reactions
Interpersonal communication	Individual goal attainment	Information/referral to other resources	Progressive muscle relaxation
Social support enhancement	Interpersonal skills training	Empathetic listening	Identification of common stressors and stress responses
Environmental change project	Group-based treatment		Cognitive restructuring/coping
Problem-solving			

is a pervasive approach to a variety of treatments for many different conditions. Coping skills have included cognitive responses such as reframing and active strategies including problem-solving, assertiveness training, goal-setting, recruiting social support, and planning. The coping skills of parents of children with disabilities have been studied extensively (Glidden, Billings, & Jobe, 2006). Table 2.8 illustrates the different coping skills addressed in the four randomized trials reviewed in this section.

KIRKHAM AND SCHILLING'S LIFE SKILLS TRAINING PROGRAM

Kirkham and Schilling (1990) conducted one of the most important of the studies in this series. It is notable because of the large number of participants, the use of a treatment-as-usual comparison group, and follow-up at 2 years after the end of the intervention. Over a 2-year period, 215 parents of children with developmental disabilities between ages 2 and 14 were followed after receiving either a coping skills training program or a treatment as usual counseling program. The components of the Life Skills Training Program were: (1) cognitive coping skills, (2) interpersonal communication (3) problem solving, (4) an environmental change project, and (5) social support enhancement. As in other programs, the meetings consisted of some didactic instruction, modeling, rehearsing skills by practicing in the group, and homework aimed at transfer of training to parents' daily lives. Two social workers co-led groups for nine 2-hour meetings held twice a week. The participants were mothers of children between the ages of 2 to 14 years. The children experienced several different DDs including 19% with ID.

Cognitive Coping

The cognitive coping component appears to be a variant on standard CBT, identifying and replacing distorted or overly negative thoughts and feelings. Kirkham and Schilling

(1990) state that they first encouraged parents to talk about difficulties they faced raising children with special needs. Group leaders helped parents identify their thoughts and feelings that could add to the stress in a particular set of circumstances. Parents were asked to create lists of personal coping strategies. These included self-praise and reminders of their children's positive characteristics. Parents were given a homework assignment to practice using their positive internal talk at home.

Interpersonal Communication

The aim of this component was to teach parents skills for building personal social support networks and for advocating for services for their children. The group leaders used structured lessons; parents actively practiced each skill in the group meetings and were given homework to practice them outside of the meetings. The interpersonal skills included active listening, reading nonverbal cues, and ways to deal with criticism. Parents were guided to identify ways to make initial contacts via telephone, express appreciation to others, accept it, and request or offer help. In addition, the group talked about ways to introduce sensitive topics about their children's disabilities and how to gauge listeners' reactions. These communication skills appear to be especially well suited to address the needs of individuals who are exposed to social stigma because of their children's disabilities. The focus on teaching skills to interact with professionals is a particularly important contribution of this study.

Social Support Enhancement

Minilectures were designed to teach how to identify people in parents' social networks and to recognize different levels of support, ranging from close and personal relationships to acquaintances. They also discussed negative relationships and were given homework assignments to take action to change the ratio of positive to negative connections to a more favorable one. Parents were coached to develop individual plans for working on increasing positive relationships. They wrote contracts with a buddy in the group who offered alternative solutions to relationship difficulties and encouraged one another to carry out the plans.

Environmental Change Project

Uniquely among all of the programs we have reviewed, the Life Skills Training Program incorporated group action to work toward social change in parents' local communities. We believe this component is an important one that ought to be replicated as part of future studies. Its importance derives from research on empowerment, which shows that group solidarity and successful change efforts can benefit parents psychologically (Swift & Levin, 1987). The group leaders facilitated discussions of possible mutual goals and then assisted parents to break a project into one manageable step. Tasks were assigned as part of the homework and parents reported on their progress at each meeting. Examples of projects they planned and enacted were developing a speaker's bureau centered on presentations by local service professionals to parents in the community about the services their agency provided. Another project involved creating brochures with information about children with special needs intended for friends and relatives of other families with children with special needs.

Problem-Solving

As in the other coping skill programs we review here, one major component of Kirkham and Schillings's (1990) program was instruction of problem-solving skills. Group leaders taught a problem-solving model. The group then talked about several problems and used the method to generate solutions for these difficulties. Participants solved several real-life problems during the program. The researchers did not describe the particulars of the problem-solving routine. Parents wrote contracts with each other to encourage addressing frequent problems at home. They reported on their efforts at subsequent meetings.

Comparison Group

Parents who were randomly assigned to the comparison group participated in meetings that were designed as treatment-as-usual support groups. The groups met and discussed family relationships and benefits and costs of working with professionals. Meetings were made up of discussions, sharing of resources, and giving and receiving mutual support for other parents. The group invited a guest speaker to talk about living with a disability, and they shared favorite books on parenting. These are activities that one would expect to see in a parent support group. One of the main differences between this usual treatment and the experimental program centered on skills training. The treatment for the experimental group was a skills-building program, whereas the comparison group had the opportunity for gaining social support and useful information without any direct instruction of coping skills. This design allows some inferences to be drawn about the differences between the two approaches to supporting parents, skills based versus informational and social support without instruction on coping skills.

Evaluation at Post-Test and 2-Year Follow-Up

The program was evaluated using measures of parental stress, depression, self-reinforcement attitudes, and satisfaction with several aspects of life, and knowledge about communication. A short form of Holroyd's (1974) Questionnaire on Resources and Stress was used to test stress levels related to the children with disabilities. The Beck Depression Inventory, one of the most widely used measures of depressive symptoms was meant to gauge parent's stress related mental health. The Inventory of Parents Experiences (Crnic, Greenberg, Ragozin, Robinson, & Basham, 1983) has six factors measuring different aspects of the respondents' social support network. A knowledge test made up of vignettes requiring various communication skills was used to assess knowledge of skillful interpersonal interactions.

Kirkham (1993) published follow-up data collected between 20 and 26 months after the original posttest. This is the only published psychoeducational treatment study with relatively long follow-up data. For this reason, we present the outcome data in detail. The data presents a useful example of the limitations of statistical significance testing and the alternative ways of understanding the data offered by effect size analysis. Multiple regression analyses were used to analyze the data. At the 2-year follow-up, 49% of the original participants returned the questionnaires, 76 of the original 153. Kirkham (1993) attempted to control for the differences between the people who returned follow-up assessments and those who did not. We believe that the measure of depressive symptoms is the central outcome of this study, because elevated depressive symptoms have been repeatedly identified as among the most common mental health problems associated with caregiving stress. On the Beck Depression Inventory (BDI), the mothers in the treatment group at posttest had lower depression levels than the control group but the difference was not statistically significant level ($R^2 = .451, p < .08$) but at follow-up the people who returned from the skills group had significantly lower levels of depressive symptoms than the treatment as usual group ($R^2 = .429, p < .03$).

These results represent the best data available on the relatively long-term impact of coping skills training for parents. Attrition in the long-term follow-up is problematic, but nonetheless, for the parents who did return the questionnaires 2 years after the end of treatment, the results are modest but represent improvement over baseline levels. The evidence suggests that a CSI may be an effective form of support for reducing depressive symptoms over time, up to 2 years post treatment. However, given the attrition, these results are suggestive but not yet fully convincing. The evidence suggests to us that research ought to investigate the additive benefits of periodic contact with families including booster sessions in order to better maintain outcomes. Most individuals with autism or ID live with their parents well into middle age, so long-term support for caregivers is an essential goal of a social support program for these families.

GAMMON AND ROSE'S COPING SKILLS TRAINING PROGRAM.

Gammon and Rose (1991) studied the impact of a coping skills education program on parents of children with DDs including ID and other conditions such as spina bifida, learning disability, and attention deficit hyperactivity disorder. They randomly assigned parents to a treatment group ($n = 24$) and a no-treatment control group ($n = 18$). Parents met in groups of four to eight for 2 hours, once a week for 10 weeks. The treatment components were (1) cognitive restructuring, (2) problem-solving, (3) individual goal attainment, and (4) interpersonal skills training.

Cognitive Restructuring

Cognitive restructuring has appeared in the previously reviewed studies. This part of the intervention followed the methods recommended by Ellis (1970) and Beck (1963,

1984) for identifying, refuting, and replacing self-defeating thoughts with self-enhancing ones. This part of the program appears to be virtually identical to the CBT skills taught in the programs described by Nixon and Singer (1993) and Singer, Irvin, and Hawkins (1985). Cognitive-behavioral therapy has been successful in treating several common psychological problems, so it is fitting that these researchers all employed the same practices. The second set of coping skills in the Gammon and Rose intervention was problem-solving based on the work of D'Zurilla and Goldfried (1971). It has become a widely accepted step-by-step approach to addressing problems through definition, generation of alternatives, implementation, and evaluation. It has a long history of efficacy for treating several problems and populations (D'Zurilla & Nezu, 2009).

Individual Goal Attainment

The intervention package also contained instruction in individual goal attainment. These authors believed that learning to set realistic and measurable goals would help parents with efforts to change their own behavior and to evaluate the outcomes of these efforts. The instruction aimed to teach parents how first to assess a baseline level of the behavior they want to change, second to decide what changes are desirable, and third to decide on criteria so an observer could evaluate how successful their efforts would be. This procedure has a substantial evidence base supporting its value to people who want to modify their own actions and as a way to evaluate individual changes in a variety of rehabilitation settings (Sugavanam, Mead, Bulley, Donaghy, & VanWijck, 2012).

Interpersonal Skills Training

The third intervention component was interpersonal skills training (Bellack, Hersen, & Turner, 1976). The researchers believed that because parents had to deal with difficult social interactions with service providers, they needed to gain or improve skills at communicating effectively with professionals. They also recognized that improved interpersonal skills would help with personal relationships. The instructional sequence had eight steps, beginning with teaching how to identify interpersonal behaviors. These were taught using role-playing and didactic instruction. A second step involved identifying difficult situations that were unique to individual parents. Parents subsequently set goals for addressing these troubling circumstances. They thought through critical moments for acting in new ways in situations and deciding on what the new alternative behavior would be. The next part of the instructional sequence involved role-playing the problematic situation and then rehearsing new responses to it. They rehearsed through role-playing and received feedback from the group leader. After this rehearsal, they discussed the targeted situations for change, and as a last step they set homework assignments around practicing the skill in increasingly difficult situations using an easy-to-hard sequence. This procedure has been used widely in research on depression and other mental health problems, medical education, and business management (e.g., Corrigan, 1991).

Evaluation

The program was evaluated using a combination of self-report paper and pencil measures and analogue role-play based assessment. The former included the POMS (McNair et al., 1971) as a measure of depressive and anxious symptoms and the Questionnaire on Resources and Stress (Holroyd, 1974) to assess stress associated with parenting children with disabilities. The extent to which parents learned and used new problem-solving skills was measured with the Problem-Solving Inventory (PSI; Heppner & Petersen, 1982). It has three scales focused on personal control, problem-solving, and approach-avoidance. The role-play situations were used to measure performance on making assertive requests, making statements of positive self-regard, expressing feelings, giving negative feedback, use of defensive techniques, and assertive refusal. Goal attainment scaling (GAS) was used to evaluate parents' progress on individual goals formulated by parents during one of the early group meetings. Compared with the control group, the parents in the intervention group showed significant improvement on the measures of problem-solving skills and interpersonal skills as measured by role-play scenarios. Further, they showed greater goal attainment than parents in the no-treatment comparison group. Contrary to the authors' expectations, the intervention did not lead to improved outcomes on the POMS total score or the QRS. The study contributes to the cumulative evidence supporting the benefits of group psychoeducational coping skills instruction for parents of children with DD.

THE SOCIAL PROBLEM-SOLVING SKILLS PROGRAM

Davis and Rushton (1991) published an elegant study evaluating social problem-solving skills training for parents of children with moderate to severe delayed development. The authors presented a theoretical framework for the design of their intervention. They defined the aim of their intervention broadly. "For interventions to be successful, it was assumed . . . that parents had to be helped to adapt to their circumstances generally including their child's disability" (p. 91). They believed that positive adaptation to life circumstances required a clear understanding of their children and disabilities, self-acceptance, and acceptance of their role in the family. To this end, they provided an in-home intervention. Fourteen parents, including one Bangladeshi-speaking parent, received 60 hours of in-home parent education over a 10-week period. This training is manualized (Buchan, Clemerson, & Davis, 1988). Visitors made weekly visits at first and then at longer intervals over time. Data on the number of visits and their duration was not available. Home visitors were trained to listen with empathy, to prompt discussions, and to establish a trusting relationship so that they could explore problems raised by the parents.

The visitors followed the parents' lead regarding the stressor or problem they discussed. When parents identified a problem, the intervention centered on social problem-solving with its traditional components: clarifying problems or events, setting goals, making plans, and carrying out action. The home visitors also provided information and referral to other resources when needed. There was no explicit instruction about how to care for the children with disabilities; rather, the focus was on difficulties faced by the parents. They worked with two groups of parents, Bangladeshi immigrants to England and English-speaking families. Twenty-eight Bangladeshi parents were randomly assigned to a treatment ($n = 16$) or no-treatment control group ($n = 12$), and 52 English-speaking families were divided into groups of 31 and 21, respectively. Children ranged in age from 1 to 15 years, with an average age of 5 years. Half of the children experienced cerebral palsy, 12% had Down syndrome, and the remaining children had developmental delays from several different conditions. This study is notable for the breadth of its outcomes, which included parental evaluations of their own well-being, perceived social support, quality of their relationship with their spouses, understanding of their children and how to help them, and positive as well as negative views of their children. Unusually, the outcomes also included children's developmental progress and problem behaviors. The intervention was not specifically focused on the children, but in both treatment groups they showed significantly higher gains in development and reductions in problems behaviors compared with children in the control groups.

The measures used to evaluate outcomes were a mix of rating scales developed by the Davis, based on a procedure called the repertory grid technique, a well-established method for assessing beliefs about specific constructs (Fransella, Bell, & Bannister, 2004). Davis had used these measures in a previous study in which she provided some evidence for concurrent validity. Nonetheless, these measures are not widely used in current psychological intervention research and the psychometric properties of the particular scales used in this study are unknown. Fortunately, the authors also used well-established measures including the Malaise Inventory (Rutter, Tizard & Whitmore, 1970), the Griffiths Mental Development Scales (Griffiths, 1954), and the Behavior Screening Questionnaire (Richmond et al., 1982).

At the end of the intervention, the Bangladeshi-speaking parents had statistically higher ratings on perceived social support ($d = 4.3$), parenting self-efficacy ($d = 0.97$), reduction in depression ($d = -.86$), positive ratings of the spousal relationship ($d = 1.17$), and increased joy in caring for their children ($d = 1.17$). Change scores on developmental measures showed significantly more intellectual development and reductions in behavior problems for children in the treatment group. For example, on the rating scale for children's problem behavior, the treatment group's change scores improved by 12 points as compared with a change of -3.3 in the control group, indicating that children in this group showed little change in their problem behaviors. Children's gain scores were higher on several developmental outcomes as determined from the Griffiths Scales of Mental Development (Griffiths, 1970) and reductions in behavior problems. By contrast, the working-class English-speaking parents did not show gains on as many outcomes as the Bangladeshi parents but also had significant increases in perceived social support and increased positive attributions about their children. Children in this group had positive change scores significantly greater than children in the control group on their mental age, and personal-social development. This study provides partial evidence for the efficacy of coping skills training. The focus on a non-English-speaking immigrant population and on low-income English-speaking parents helps to extend the generalizability of coping skills training. The use of measures of positive views of their children is also unusual in the treatment literature, indicating that support for parents can positively impact their view of their children. This study adds further evidence that parent-focused interventions that do not involve parent training can lead to improvements in children development and behavior. Although there are some methodological weaknesses in the description of the intervention and perhaps in some of the measures used, this study contributes to the weight of the evidence for coping skills training as an established intervention.

ERGUNER-TEKINALP AND AKKOK'S COPING SKILLS TRAINING PROGRAM

A study from Turkey evaluated the impact of a coping skills training program on parents of children with autism (Erguner-Tekinalp & Akkok, 2004). The authors implemented a psychoeducational program that aimed to teach coping skills including identification of stressors and stress reactions, problem-solving training, training in self-monitoring and management of self-defeating cognitions, and skills for obtaining social support. The program also included PMR, but there was insufficient information in the study to determine whether it met our criteria for a stress management treatment—weekly in-class practice of a relaxation procedure. There are three notable features of the evaluation research on this coping skills training program. The participants were all parents of children with autism. The study was developed and conducted in Turkey. Furthermore, it is the only study that used hopelessness as an outcome variable. The authors' choice of the original form of the Questionnaire on Resources and Stress (Holroyd, 1974) and use of three short author-written assessments were problematic. The former has been criticized for conceptual confusion (Glidden et al., 2006). The latter consisted of only three Likert scales written by the authors, who did not provide any psychometric data. Nonetheless the measure of hopelessness, the Beck Hopelessness Scale (Beck, Weissman, Lester, & Trexler, 1974) is a standardized measure with known psychometric properties.

EVALUATION OF COPING SKILLS PROGRAMS

Evaluation of these studies as a group poses a dilemma. If they were all considered as one form of intervention they would readily meet the criteria for established practices. All were effective in moderating psychological distress in parents, and all were evaluated with sufficient rigor to permit confidence in the findings. As a general approach practitioners should feel encouraged that teaching coping skills can be an effective way of supporting some parents. However, we are unable to rate a family of interventions, and current standards require close replication of programs in two or more studies to categorize any program as established. Because no two studies are sufficiently alike to count as replications, we must limit the rating of the programs reviewed here to assigning the individual studies to the category of promising. In the short term, these approaches have been reasonably effective for mothers of children with ID or autism. There is insufficient evidence

TABLE 2.9 SUMMARIES OF STUDIES ON PSYCHOEDUCATIONAL GROUP PROGRAMS

Author(s)	*Design/Intervention components/ Manual/ Fidelity*	*Participants (Sample, Age, Ethnicity)/Setting*	*DV Measures*	*Treatment Effect(s)*
Benn et al. (2012)	• A randomized controlled trial • To assess the efficacy of a 5-week Mindfulness Training (MT) • MT intervention: the SMART-in-Education (Stress Management and Relaxation Techniques) program was provided. 36 hours of didactic and group discussion activities, mindfulness practices, and homework assignments delivered over nine 2.5-hour sessions and 2 full days. • Control: a waiting list control • Manualized: SMART-in-Education (Stress Management and Relaxation Techniques) program, Cullen & Wallace, 2010) • Fidelity reported (program completion rates, MT session attendance, reported estimates of frequency of homes practice, participants' satisfaction on sessions, and qualitative reports on instructor adherence to the format, content, and process of curriculum delivery by research assistants	PARENT • 25 parents of children with special needs, mean age of 47 years (27–55 years), 23 females and 2 males, 18 (72%) college degree or higher education, 5 (20%) minority status CHILD • Ages 5–23 years • 12 ASD, 8 Attention-deficit/ learning disability, and 6 cognitive or health impairment	PARENT • Mindfulness: Five Facet Mindfulness Questionnaire • Anxiety: State–Trait Anxiety Inventory (STAI) for Adults • Stress: Perceived Stress Scale • Depression: Center for Epidemiological Studies Depression (CES-D) Scale • Positive and Negative Affect: Positive and Negative Affect Schedule • Forgiveness: a state forgiveness questionnaire • Personal growth: subjective well-being derived from Ryff and Keyes's Psychological Well-Being Scale • Self-compassion: a 26-item scale validated by Neff • Empathic concern: a seven-item subscale of the Interpersonal Reactivity Index • Parenting self-efficacy: Everyday Parenting Scale • Quality of parent–child interaction: Parenting Stress Index	PARENT • MT intervention groups showed statistically significant improvements on all variables of self-reported mindfulness except for positive affect. • Most effect size differences, the d statistic, were in the moderate range from .79- .40. • The effect sizes were even larger on several of the outcomes at the follow-up assessment. (see Table 2.10)

Davis & Rushton (1991)	• A randomized controlled trial • To evaluate the effect of a social problem solving skills training for parents with disabilities • Social problem solving skills training: 60 hours of weekly in-home parent education over a 10 week period by professionals as a parent advisers • Control: a no-treatment control • Manualized (Davis, Buchan, & Clemerson, 1987) • No fidelity reported	• 80 families of children with disabilities, most fell into the lower socio-economic range • Bangladeshi families: 16 Intervention and 12 Control • English-Speaking families: 31 Intervention, 21 Control • UK	PARENT • Malaise Inventory • Malaise Inventory • Support questionnaire—General support CHILD • Behavior problems • Child Grid – Positiveness • Griffiths Mental Development—General quotient	PARENT • Parents in the intervention group improved significantly on all of the items with the exception of the sensory-motor support item CHILD • Children showed improvements in behavior and development
Dykens et al. (2014)	• A randomized controlled trial • To examine the effects of Mindfulness-Based Stress Reduction (MBSR) intervention on mothers of children with autism or other developmental disabilities • Intervention: Six 1.5-hour weekly sessions of MBSR treatment where parents were taught breathing, meditation, movement techniques, relaxation response, and meditation • Comparison: Six 1.5-hour weekly sessions of positive psychology practice where parents were taught to reduce negative emotions and increase optimism MBSR implemented by parents supervised by professionals. • Manual available (Kabat-Zinn et al.) • Fidelity examined but measures not reported	• 243 mothers of children with autism (65%) or other developmental disabilities (35%) • 69.6% White, 14.7% African American, 9.2% Hispanic, 6.5% Asian or other • Children's mean age 10.85 years, range 2-54 years • US	PARENT • Parenting Stress Index-Short Form • Beck Depression Inventory • Beck Anxiety Inventory • Insomnia Severity Index • Ryff Scales of Psychological Well-Being • Life Satisfaction Scale	PARENT • Mothers in both treatment and comparison groups exhibited reduced stress, anxiety, and depression and improved in parent-child interactions, sleep, and life satisfaction. Depression, anxiety, and life satisfaction improvements sustained at 6-month follow-up. Intervention mothers showed greater gains in depression, anxiety, sleep, and satisfaction compared with comparison group mothers. Only effect sizes for within groups pre-post comparisons were available because there was not a no treatment control group. Within group d for depression was .88 for mindfulness group and

(continued)

TABLE 2.9 (CONTINUED)

Author(s)	*Design/Intervention components/ Manual/ Fidelity*	*Participants (Sample, Age, Ethnicity)/Setting*	*DV Measures*	*Treatment Effect(s)*
Ergüner-Tekinalp & Akkök (2004)	• A randomized controlled trial • To investigate the efficacy of parent-mediated communication-focused treatment (PACT) vs. routine care • Intervention: participating parents were provided the coping skills training (eight group sessions, 1.5 hour twice a week). The program consisted of understanding stress and its effects, discussion of general coping strategies, problems solving skills, relaxation training, positive thinking, and developing social support. • Control: the informative written materials about skills and techniques applied in the Intervention were provided. • No manual reported • No fidelity reported	PARENT • 20 mothers of children with autism • Intervention: age 30–52 years (M = 42.45; SD = 7.02) • Control: age 29–46 (M = 39.10; SD = 1.82) CHILD • Intervention: age 12–19 (M = 15.2; SD = 1.93) • Control: age 11–17 (M = 14.0; SD = 1.82) • Turkey	PARENT • Questionnaire on Resources and Stress (QRS) • Beck Hopelessness Scale (BHS) • Coping Strategy Indicator—Avoidance • Coping Strategy Indicator (three subscales; Problem Solving, Exploring Social Support, and Avoidance)	PARENT Intervention's effect on use of social support and hopelessness levels was positive and statistically significant. • No difference was reported between two groups on use of problem solving, avoidance, and stress levels.
Gammon & Rose (1991)	• A randomized controlled trial • To evaluate the effectiveness of a coping skills training programs (CSTP) of parents of children with DD vs. no-treatment control • Intervention: parents were provided a group-format of the CSTP training (ten 2-hour weekly sessions) involving problem-solving, achieving personal goals, interpersonal skills training, and cognitive restructuring. • Control: no-treatment control • Manualized • No fidelity reported	• 42 parents of children with developmental disabilities including ID and other conditions (spina bifida, learning disability, cerebral palsy, and attention deficit hyperactivity disorder) • Intervention: n = 24, mean age = 38.9 years • Control: n = 18, mean age = 37.8 years • US	PARENT • Problem-solving skills: Problem-Solving Inventory • Interpersonal communication skills: Role-play test • Self-regards: Role-play test • Stress: Profile of Mood States, Questionnaire on Resources and Stress • Individual goal attainment: Individualized goal attainment scaling	PARENT • Problem-solving skills, interpersonal communication skills, and perceptions on goal achievement are higher in the CSTP training group than the control group. • No difference reported in parents' use of expressions of positive self-regard, and both of two measures of stress.

Greaves (1997)	• A randomized controlled trial • To investigate an effect of a Rational-Emotive Parent Education Program (REPE) vs. a comparative-treatment control (Applied Behavior Analysis; ABA) vs. a no-treatment control • REPE training: eight sessions emphasized core irrational beliefs and their hypothesized links with the stress response • ABA training: eight seminars included the principles of ABA (operant conditioning, the use of baselines, the role of extinction, punishment, and reinforcement) • Control: no-treatment control • Manualized • No fidelity reported	• 54 mothers of young children attending an early intervention center for Down syndrome (21 in the REPE, 16 in the ABA, and 17 in the control group) • Australia	PARENT • Two single questions asking about stress with child care • Parent Dissatisfaction scale • Stress Reaction • Feeling Scale • Profile of Mood States • Parenting Stress Index	PARENT • The REPE showed significant reductions in Profile of Mood States and Parenting Stress Index compared with both control groups.

(*continued*)

TABLE 2.9 (CONTINUED)

Author(s)	*Design/Intervention components/ Manual/ Fidelity*	*Participants (Sample, Age, Ethnicity)/Setting*	*DV Measures*	*Treatment Effect(s)*
Kirkham & Schilling (1990)	• A randomized controlled trial • To compare the effects of a life skills intervention and a traditional parent support group for parents of children with disabilities. • Life skills training: participants were provided nine 2-hour sessions involving coping skills training, interpersonal communication, problem-solving, environmental change project, social support enhancement, in groups of 10–12. • Control: a traditional parent support group (family relationships and the advantages and disadvantages of working with professionals) • Manualized • No fidelity reported	PARENT • 230 mothers of children with a variety of developmental disabilities • Ages 22–69 years (mean age = 34 years), 92% White, 70% married, and 94% high school graduate CHILD • Ages 2 to 14 years, 62% males • 19% mental retardation, 19% learning disabled, 13% neurological impairment, 13% language delay, 10% cerebral palsy, 6% epilepsy, 4% emotional disturbance, 4% hearing impairment, 4% autism, 2% visual impairment, and 6% other diagnoses. • US	PARENT • Questionnaire on Resources and Stress (QRS-F) • Beck Depression Inventory (BDI) • Self-Reinforcement Attitudes Questionnaire (SRA) • Inventory of Parent Experiences (IPE) • Communication	PARENT • Participants in the intervention group showed statistically significant gains on their self-reinforcement ability and satisfaction with their social networks and reduction of their stress levels compared with the traditional parent support groups
Nixon & Singer (1993)	• A randomized controlled trial • To investigate the effect of a group cognitive-behavioral treatment focusing on self-blame and guilt in parents with disabilities vs. a waitlist control • Intervention: five 2-hour sessions on cognitive distortions using group instruction, discussions, and homework • Control: a waitlist control • No manual reported • No fidelity reported	PARENT • 40 parents of children with disabilities (34 females and 6 males) CHILD • Mean age 9.3 years • Children had intellectual deficits • US	PARENT • Self-blame and guilt: Situational Guilt Scale • Internal negative attributions: Attributional style Questionnaire • Automatic thoughts: Automatic Thought Questionnaire • Depression: Beck Depression Inventory	PARENT • Significant differences between two groups were found in self-blame and guilt, internal negative attributions, automatic thoughts, and depression (effect sizes .39, 1.11, .34, and .34, respectively)

C. L. Schultz et al. (1993)	• A randomized controlled trial • To examine the effectiveness of a stress management and coping skills intervention using a psychoeducational approach • Intervention: six 2-hour sessions on coping skills strategies and topics, didactic presentation, discussions, practice exercises, and homework (see Table 2.6) • Control • Manualized • Fidelity not reported	PARENT • 54 parents of children with developmental disabilities CHILD • Ages 2.8 to 20.5 years • Mean age = 8.6 years (SD = 5.1)	PARENT • General Health Questionnaire (GHQ-28) • Inventory of Socially Supportive Behaviors	PARENT • A significant difference in parents' mental health was found between the intervention and comparison groups (GHQ-28 effect size 0.385). More modest effect sizes found for the other measures of social support and parent stress.
Singer et al. (1988)	• A randomized controlled trial • To assess the effects of parent stress management program • Intervention: eight sessions on cognitive reframing, relaxation, and self-monitoring • Control: a waitlist control • Manualized • Fidelity inferred	PARENT • 36 parents of children with developmental disabilities CHILD • Ages 4 to 16 years	PARENT • Beck Depression Inventory	PARENT- Intervention group parents were found to have a greater reduction in depressive and anxiety symptoms posttreatment compared to control group parents (effect size 0.27).

TABLE 2.10 RESULTS OF META-ANALYSIS OF PSYCHOEDUCATIONAL GROUP PROGRAMS

					Intervention		*Comparison*			
Study	*Measure*	*Group*	*Outcome*	*Study Type*	*N*	*M (SD)*	*N*	*M (SD)*	*P*	*D*
Benn et al. (2012)—Post	Center for Epidemiological Studies Depression (CES-D) Scale—Post	Parent	Mental Health	Stress Management	12	30.03 (8.03)	16	36.69 (10.46)		0.510
	Five Facet Mindfulness Questionnaire—Post	Parent	Stress	Stress Management	12	3.61 (0.08)	16	3.33 (0.07)		0.520
	Perceived Stress Scale—Post	Parent	Stress	Stress Management	12	1.97 (0.58)	16	2.25 (0.55)		0.400
	OVERALL									0.476
Benn et al. (2012)—Follow-Up	Center for Epidemiological Studies Depression (CES-D) Scale—Follow-Up	Parent	Mental Health	Stress Management	12	30.82 (9.10)	16	35.51 (9.83)		0.270
	Five Facet Mindfulness Questionnaire—Follow-Up	Parent	Stress	Stress Management	12	3.70 (0.06)	16	3.43 (0.07)		0.570
	Perceived Stress Scale—Follow-Up	Parent	Stress	Stress Management	12	2.04 (0.45)	16	2.42 (0.56)		0.790
	OVERALL									0.538

Davis & Rushton (1991)	Behavior problems	Child	Child Behavior	CBT	16	18.70 (9.20)	12	24.90 (13.30)		0.558
	Child Grid—Positiveness	Child	Child Behavior	CBT	16	47.80 (14.50)	12	45.30 (16.80)		0.161
	Griffiths Mental Development—General quotient	Child	Child Behavior	CBT	16	36.80 (21.30)	12	33.00 (23.00)		0.172
	Malaise Inventory	Parent	Mental Health	CBT	16	7.30 (5.20)	12	13.30 (4.20)		1.249
	Support questionnaire—General support	Parent	Social Support	CBT	16	5.90 (0.70)	12	2.10 (0.80)		5.108
	OVERALL									0.777
Ergüner-Tekinalp & Akkök (2004)	Beck Hopelessness Scale (BHS)	Parent	Mental Health	Coping Skills	10		10		0.000	1.754
	Coping Strategy Indicator—Avoidance	Parent	Stress	Coping Skills	10		10		0.188	0.612
	Coping Strategy Indicator—Exploring Social Support	Parent	Social Support	Coping Skills	10		10		0.009	1.309
	Coping Strategy Indicator—Problem-Solving	Parent	Stress	Coping Skills	10		10		0.689	0.182
	Questionnaire on Resources and Stress (QRS)	Parent	Stress	Coping Skills	10		10		0.254	0.527
	OVERALL									0.811

(*continued*)

TABLE 2.10 (CONTINUED)

					Intervention		Comparison			
Study	*Measure*	*Group*	*Outcome*	*Study Type*	*N*	*M (SD)*	*N*	*M (SD)*	*P*	*D*
Gammon & Rose (1991)	Problem-Solving Inventory	Parent	Stress	Coping Skills	24		18		0.002	1.031
	Profile of Mood States	Parent	Mental Health	Coping Skills	24		18		0.160	0.446
	Questionnaire on Resources and Stress (QRS)	Parent	Stress	Coping Skills	24		18		0.110	0.510
	OVERALL									0.651
Greaves (1997)	Berger Anger and Guilt scale	Parent	Mental Health	CBT	21	15.78 (0.00)	16	-1.56 (0.00)	0.049	0.677
	Measurement of Parental Stress Response	Parent	Stress	CBT	21	1.13 (0.00)	16	0.06 (0.00)	0.049	0.677
	Parent Dissatisfaction scale	Parent	Mental Health	CBT	21	4.23 (0.00)	16	0.56 (0.00)	0.049	0.677
	Parenting Stress Index (PSI) Parent Domain Total	Parent	Stress	CBT	21	19.91 (0.00)	16	-3.31 (0.00)	0.049	0.677
	Profile of Mood States	Parent	Mental Health	CBT	21	27.27 (0.00)	16		0.049	0.677
	OVERALL									0.677

Kirkham (1993)	Beck Depression Inventory (BDI)	Parent	Mental Health	Coping Skills	143	7.08 (5.90)	72	9.85 (8.45)	0.404
	Inventory of Parent Experiences	Parent	Social Support	Coping Skills	143	11.92 (2.64)	72	11.40 (2.82)	0.191
	Questionnaire on Resources and Stress (QRS)	Parent	Stress	Coping Skills	143	27.48 (17.30)	72	31.67 (20.71)	0.227
	Self-Reinforcement Attitude	Parent	Self-Esteem	Coping Skills	143	2.08 (0.29)	72	2.21 (0.32)	0.433
	OVERALL								0.313
Kirkham & Schilling (1990)	Beck Depression Inventory (BDI)	Parent	Mental Health	Coping Skills	143	6.59 (5.80)	72	7.83 (6.97)	0.200
	Inventory of Parent Experiences	Parent	Social Support	Coping Skills	143	11.99 (2.68)	72	11.61 (2.57)	0.143
	Questionnaire on Resources and Stress (QRS)	Parent	Stress	Coping Skills	143	26.11 (18.30)	72	28.55 (18.42)	0.133
	Self-Reinforcement Attitude	Parent	Self-Esteem	Coping Skills	143	1.98 (0.35)	72	2.12 (0.33)	0.408
	OVERALL								0.220
Nixon & Singer (1993)	Situational Guilt Scale (SGS)	Parent	Mental Health	CBT	18	257.10 (41.30)	16	286.00 (64.40)	0.541
	Automatic Thoughts Questionniare (ATQ)	Parent	Mental Health	CBT	18	51.40 (13.30)	16	60.40 (16.40)	0.607
	Attributional Style Questionnaire—Internal (ASQ-IN)	Parent	Mental Health	CBT	18	23.10 (6.10)	16	29.00 (5.60)	1.005
	Beck Depression Inventory (BDI)	Parent	Mental Health	CBT	18	10.60 (7.10)	16	13.60 (8.70)	0.370
	OVERALL								0.370

(continued)

TABLE 2.10 (CONTINUED)

Study	Measure	Group	Outcome	Study Type	Intervention		Comparison		P	D
					N	*M (SD)*	*N*	*M (SD)*		
C. L. Schultz et al. (1993)	General Health Questionnaire (GHE)	Parent	Mental Health	Stress Management	15*	16.00 (8.75)	39	20.74 (13.28)		0.387
	Inventory of Socially Supportive Behaviors	Parent	Social Support	Stress Management	15	70.18 (22.43)	39	71.24 (17.34)		0.056
	Schedule of Recent Events	Parent	Stress	Stress Management	15	177.87 (110.40)	39	153.48 (131.45)		0.193
	OVERALL									0.212
Singer et al. (1988)	Beck Depression Inventory (BDI)	Parent	Mental Health	Stress Management	18	7.40 (5.90)	18	9.00 (6.10)		0.270
	OVERALL									0.270
All Studies										
		Child								0.294
		Parent								0.495
			Child Behavior							0.294
			Mental Health							0.498
			Self-Esteem							0.420
			Social Supports							0.946
			Stress							0.363
				CBT						0.770
				Coping Skills						0.356
				Stress Management						0.363
	CBT OVERALL									0.480

Note. *Data for mothers only. Fathers not included because data not independent from mothers.

TABLE 2.11 AVERAGE EFFECT SIZES OF INDIVIDUAL PSYCHOEDUCATIONAL GROUP PROGRAMS AND THE OVERALL EFFECT SIZES

Study	*Measures*	*d*	*95% CI*
Benn et al. (2012)—Post	B + E	0.476	[0.038, 0.915]
Benn et al. (2012)—Follow-up	B + E	0.538	[0.097, 0.979]
Davis & Rushton (1991)	A + B + D	0.777	[0.405, 1.15]
Ergüner-Tekinalp & Akkök (2004)	B + D + E	0.811	[0.396, 1.226]
Gammon & Rose (1991)	B + E	0.651	[0.288, 1.014]
Greaves (1997)	B + E	0.677	[0.378, 0.976]
Kirkham (1993)	B + C + D + E	0.313	[0.17, 0.455]
Kirkham & Schilling (1990)	B + C + D + E	0.22	[0.078, 0.362]
Nixon & Singer (1993)	B	0.622	[0.276, 0.968]
Schultz et al. (1993)	B + D + E	0.212	[-0.133, 0.556]
Singer et al. (1988)	B	0.27	[-0.386, 0.926]
Overall		0.48	[0.341, 0.618]

d and 95% CI

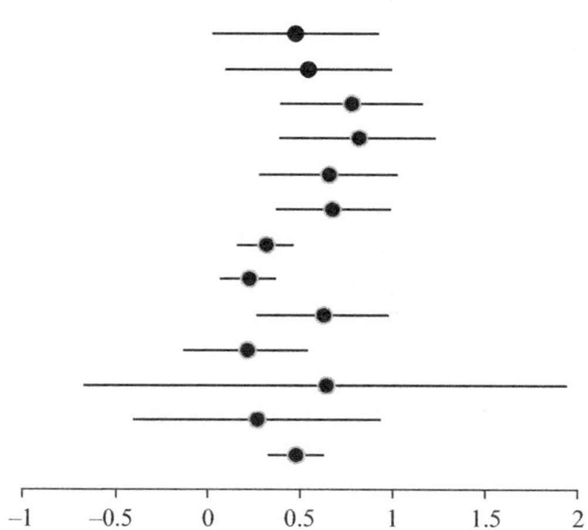

Note: A = Child Behavior; B = Mental Health; C = Self-Esteem; D = Social Support; E = Stress

Note: Study by Dykens et al. not included because we could not calculate the same effect size comparison of a treatment with no treatment control group as used with other studies.

to indicate longer-term impacts. Further research is needed to develop ways to individually tailor the selection of coping skills. Also needed are replications, follow-up studies, and evaluations with fathers and other family members as subjects. Two studies provide evidence for the external validity of coping skills training (Davis & Rushton, 1991; Erguner-Tekinalp & Akkok, 2004). The former demonstrated efficacy with Bangladeshi immigrants to London, and the latter provided some evidence for efficacy from Turkey.

SUMMARY, META-ANALYSIS, AND OVERALL EVALUATION OF PSYCHOEDUCATIONAL PROGRAMS

The basic components of the studies evaluated in this chapter are summarized in Table 2.9. It shows that there are now several published randomized experimental evaluations of psychoeducational group programs and gives a picture of the limitations in these studies in diversity of participants, lack of follow-up studies, and a predominant focus on mothers. It also shows that treatments that have been effective for many life challenges can be effective for this specific population. Transfer of treatment approaches appears to be a viable strategy for future research.

When analyzed using meta-analytic methods, the average effect sizes, *d*, for CBT-based interventions was .77, for coping skills programs, .36, and stress management, .36. Overall the average effect size for these psychoeducational interventions was $d = 0.48$. This level of effect can be interpreted as impressive, given what was previously considered to be the intractable nature of the problems parents faced. These effect size results are described in Table 2.10, with further information about the confidence interval of each study's effect size listed in Table 2.11 along with a total average *d* and its 95% confidence intervals. As will be seen in Chapter 5, subsequent research indicates that the interventions reviewed in this chapter are likely to have more substantial effects when they are combined as part of multicomponent intervention packages, which in some cases have evidence of effect sizes much larger than those attained through single treatments. Initial follow-up evidence suggests that the benefits may endure up to 2 years post treatment, though these longer-term outcomes must be viewed as preliminary. Given the quality and extent of the evidence, overall we rate psychoeducational support programs as highly promising and one of the specific programs as an established practice, namely MBSM. Practitioners can have reasonable assurance that these approaches to supporting parents can benefit many, particularly mothers and particularly in the short term.

The one program reviewed in this chapter that meets the criteria for established practices, is MBSM (Benn et al., 2012; Dykens et al. 2014). The quality of the evaluations and the degree of sameness in the independent variables allows us to assign this approach to the category of an established practice. There is also more evidence for external validity, in that Dykens and colleagues evaluated MBSM on a large and diverse sample of parents. In the short term, this approach can be efficacious in helping parents with psychological distress and improving well-being.

3

BEHAVIORAL PARENT TRAINING AS EVIDENCE-BASED PRACTICES FOR FAMILIES OF CHILDREN WITH DEVELOPMENTAL DISABILITIES

Mian Wang, Yeana W. Lam, Jiyeon Kim,

George H. S. Singer, and Robin Dodds

Behavioral parent training (BPT) has long been considered as an evidence-based treatment to children with a wide array of social, emotional, and behavioral disorders (Kazdin, 2005; Pfiffner & Kaiser, 2010). Although the effectiveness of BPT has been demonstrated in a number of target populations and yielded successful clinical results on both child and parent outcomes, little is known about the results of BPT and level of evidence to treat children with developmental disabilities (DDs) and their families in the literature. In this chapter, we provide an overview of BPT, summarize the key findings from relevant research literature of treatment effect of BPT on children with social, behavioral, and emotional disorders, and then synthesize and analyze the empirical evidence of BPT on children with DDs and their families.

AN OVERVIEW OF BEHAVIORAL PARENT TRAINING

Behavioral parent training refers to a variety of training programs or models that focus on providing training on a common set of behavioral strategies for parents to help them become change agents for their own children. Despite diverse terminology, the ramifications of the BPT approach have common theoretical underpinnings and shared intellectual roots. Many BPT programs and models target training parents in a number of core topics such as antecedent-based strategies of attending, giving proper commands, planning ahead, and environmental modification, and consequence-based strategies of praise and positive reinforcement, extinction, differentiated reinforcement, and mild punishment (Pfiffner & Kaiser, 2010). But professional trainers might choose to cover different topics in training in correspondence with specific problems of a given child and family. The training procedures are well developed, typically involving a process where a professional trainer teaches a set of behavioral strategies to parents either individually or by group in different formats and different settings, and the parents then apply the learned skills with their children at home. Since its formal beginning in the late 1960s (Kazdin, 2007), BPT has grown to be one of the most widely used behavioral interventions for children with disabilities and their families (Singer, Goldberg-Hamblin, Peckham-Hardin, Barry, & Santarelli, 2002).

EVOLUTION OF BEHAVIORAL PARENT TRAINING AND ITS THEORETICAL UNDERPINNINGS

Behavioral parent training grew out of a behavioral modification tradition from the 1920s (Graziano & Diament, 1992). It then evolved to become a parent-directed rather than clinician-directed model to change children's behaviors and promote other skills. According to Kazdin (2007), the development of BPT is rooted in three important theoretical underpinnings: operant conditioning (Skinner, 1953), applied behavior analysis (ABA; Baer, Wolf, & Risley, 1968), and coercive process or contingency theory (G. R. Patterson, 1965; G. R. Patterson, Chamberlain, & Reid, 1982). As first introduced by Skinner (1938), operant conditioning refers to a concept of organism learning (for both animals and humans) that reveals the influence of environmental events on a behavior. In other words, it depicts and interprets how behavior is influenced by various antecedents (things existing before the behavior) and is also contingent on certain consequences (things following the behavior). In operant conditioning, behavior is an operant because it "operates on the environment" as a response to the stimulus (Kazdin, 2007, p. 22). Most operant behaviors, including humans' everyday-life behaviors, are influenced by things occurring before or following after the behavior. Behaviors are believed to increase or decrease as a function of antecedent and consequent events.

Early laboratory research of operant conditioning and applications of operant conditioning principles were extended to treat children with disabilities exhibiting clinical, social, and educational problems in the early 1960s. Its rapid growth in applications gave rise to a new area of study and practice, ABA. Applied behavior analysis emphasizes the application of operant conditioning principles in the process of identifying, assessing, and modifying a target behavior of concern. The core of ABA is that trained professionals conduct a functional analysis to assess the relationship between a target behavior and the environment to generate a hypothesis about the function(s) of the target behavior. Based on this analysis, behavioral techniques surrounding the antecedent-behavior-consequence contingency (A-B-C contingency) are applied to change the target behavior of concern (Cooper, Heron, & Heward, 2007). Since the 1970s, ABA has been applied widely in clinical setting to treat children with challenging behaviors and children with DD (particularly autism). As the emphasis was made to extend the applications of ABA in home settings, it spawned the early efforts of behavioral parent training (Baker & Brightman, 1984; Lovaas, Koegel, Simmons, & Long, 1973).

Moreover, in the same era when ABA began to evolve, the research and clinical work on the development of aggressive and antisocial behavior also gained increasing attention (G. R. Patterson, 1965). In a research effort to understand the mechanism of aggressive child behavior in home environments, G. R. Patterson et al. (1982) studied child–parent interaction in the home through observations, focusing particularly on how parents give commands, attend to child deviant behavior but not to appropriate behavior, and overly and inconsistently use punishment. He found that mutual actions and reactions of the child and parent often form a sequence of interactions associated with escalation of aggressive behaviors in frequency and intensity, which is characterized as a coercive process.

The framework of the coercive process has not only shed light on understanding the role of parent in disciplinary practices of child aggressive behavior (G. R. Patterson, 1982; G. R. Patterson et al., 1982), but also lent support to the importance of training parents about how to interact with their child effectively. Therefore, the seminal work of Gerald Patterson on the coercive process has made special contributions to the emergence and growth of BPT, particularly setting the foundation for the development of the Parent–Child Interaction Therapy (PCIT) model (Bagner & Eyberg, 2007).

Over the course of BPT evolution, there have been numerous variations of BPT, and different terms have been used by researchers to emphasize distinctive features of their tailored programs or models. For parents of children with DD, chief among these different BPT models are parent training, which consists of parents as teachers and parents as advocates programs to train parents in behavioral principles and management skills (Baker, Brightman, & Blacher, 1997); parent management training (PMT), which comprises specific and systematic treatment procedures to teach parents the behavioral principles of operant conditioning and behavioral strategies in order for them to change children's behaviors at home (Kazdin, 1997; 2007), and parent behavioral training (PBT), which is akin to BPT, focusing on training parents to become a cotherapist or mediator of their child's behavior changes by learning a set of common behavioral strategies (Forehand et al., 1979; Graziano & Diament, 1992). Due to the similarity of these different programs, we count all of them under the umbrella term BPT, which refers to procedures designed to help parents become agents of change for their child's behaviors at home through learning behavioral principles and applying behavioral strategies. According to Kazdin (1997), BPT programs bear some common characteristics: Through training, parents are taught to observe and monitor child behavior, to give clear commands, to reinforce appropriate behavior positively, and to ignore or punish inappropriate behavior.

CORE TOPICS AND PROCEDURES OF PARENT TRAINING

Despite the diversity in training format and duration of BPT programs, there are some underlying elements and core topics across different training packages or programs. The key purpose of training is to train parents to become a therapist for their children in order to provide treatment in natural settings, over extended periods of time, and get it integrated into everyday routines. Many BPT training programs embrace a common psychoeducational approach to teaching parents parenting skills for establishing conditions that elicit and shape children's prosocial (positive) behaviors.

Behavioral parent training programs are often well structured, where professional trainers (e.g., therapists or clinicians) follow manuals or use programmed instructions (when no specific manuals were developed) to teach parents special topics, involve parents in role-playing activities or other exercises, and assign homework to parents after each session. The length of BPT programs varies depending on the severity of child and family needs. But a BPT program typically comprises 8 to 14 weekly sessions with each session lasting about 1 to 2 hours (Kazdin, 2007). Based on the general ABA principles such as reinforcement, extinction, and punishment, a series of behavior techniques and skills are taught to parents over the course of BPT training. Skills typically include behavioral shaping principles of positive reinforcement (e.g., giving rewards to a child for appropriate behaviors), attending to wanted behaviors (e.g., paying attention to the good things a child does), ignoring unwanted behaviors (e.g., not giving attention to a child's inappropriate behaviors), and using mild punishments (e.g., time-outs, natural consequences, and loss of privileges) (Kazdin, 1997, 2007). Pfiffner and Kaiser (2010) provided an excellent summary of all core training session topics of BPT: psychoeducation background information, attending and ignoring, praise/positive reinforcement, token economy/point system, giving effective instructions, time-out, response-cost procedures, developing a homework plan, home-school report cards, managing behavior in public places, "Grandma's rule" (Premack contingencies), and anticipating future behavior problems. Despite an incomplete list of all training topics, this summary covers most of commonly shared topics and elements of BPT across different programs and models.

In addition to group BPT, behaviorists often work directly in environments where problem behavior occurs. Using Moes and Frea's study (2002) as an example where BPT is contextualized in a positive behavior support (PBS) intervention for children with autism, we illustrate what constitutes the key procedures and core training topics of BPT and how they are embedded in natural home environment. Home-based PBS is an offshoot of BPT that uses multiple behavioral approaches in treating problem behaviors. This form of intervention often seeks to fit within the existing family environment and characteristics; it also has the goal of enhancing family's general quality of life. According to Moes and Frea (2002), BPT consists of an assessment and intervention phase. The assessment phase, which occurs during the 5-week baseline period, begins with a functional assessment to learn more about the nature of the challenging behavior and skills deficits of most concern to the family. The functional assessment begins with an initial interview with families conducted in their home to identify family routines in which their child's challenging behaviors and skill deficits are most problematic. During the initial interview, parents are also asked to answer questions about their child's problem behaviors using a functional assessment interview (FAI). The objectives of the FAI concern (1) development of a clear description of the problem behaviors, (2) identification of general and more immediate physical and environmental factors that predict the occurrence and nonoccurrence of the problem behaviors, (3) identification of the potential functions of the behaviors in relation to the outcomes or consequences that are maintaining them, and (4) development of summary statements describing relationships among situations, behaviors, and their functions. The routines identified as most problematic by parents are then chosen as the specific contexts for making ongoing observations during baseline, assessment, intervention, and follow-up phases of the study.

The next step in the functional assessment process is to carry out direct observations (e.g., at least two observations) within the identified family routines to further evaluate the antecedents and consequences associated with problem behaviors, collect baseline data on the frequency and severity of problem behaviors, and better understand these family routines (e.g., participants, resources and constraints, competing demands on parents, strengths and needs of family members).

After the BPT team (e.g., behavioral therapist, supervisor, clinical manager) have reviewed the assessment data, a subsequent interview with the family is conducted in order to review the reliability of information gathered from the informant and direct observation methods, gain answers to any remaining questions, and have parents describe what they would like the target routines to look like if their child's challenging behaviors and skill deficits were resolved. For example, parents of a child who refuses to sit at the dinner table might say that they want to have a dinner routine in which all family members sit together, pass food family-style, and talk pleasantly. The routine will vary according to parents' culture or family history. Once this information is gathered, the intervention planning process begins, aimed at developing clear behavioral goals associated with reducing or eliminating the child's problem behavior and teaching them meaningful replacement behaviors or alternative skills. Corresponding intervention strategies are selected to develop a behavioral support plan focusing on the use of (1) proactive strategies that decrease the likelihood that challenging behavior will occur, (2) teaching strategies that give children with autism a more adaptive ways of getting their needs met (e.g., replacement behaviors) so that they become successful in their interactions with family members (e.g., by using desirable alternative skills), and (3) reactive strategies that help maintain the health and safety of the child and family as well as teach the child that challenging behavior no longer leads to desirable outcomes. For instance, the first step for a child who runs away when called to the dinner table might be coaching the parent to quietly take the child by the hand and lead him to the table, prompting him to sit down and praising him. The second step involves teaching the child better ways to get attention from the parents at dinnertime instead of running away. The parents might be taught to ask him questions, to respond to him with more enthusiasm or affection, and to more frequently comment about what he is doing at the table or what he did during the day. If the child does bolt without eating his food, he might be led back to the table and be told to eat one bite of the food before he can leave the table. The amount of the food required to leave would be gradually increased. These intervention strategies are proceduralized and written up into a PBS plan to be reviewed with the family. In week 6 of BPT, the PBS plan is reviewed with the family and adjustments of goals and strategies are made as needed. In week 7, the intervention phase begins, with BPT sessions at least twice a week on a mutually agreeable schedule with at least one of the home visits occurred in the targeted routines.

Behavioral parent training is implemented by a behavioral therapist and his or her supervisor. The behavioral therapist's duties include conducting weekly parent training sessions (e.g., two sessions per week for a total of 5 hours). These duties consist of reviewing child behavioral goals and discussing corresponding intervention strategies designed to resolve problem behavior. They also entail teaching meaningful replacement behaviors and alternative skills, implementing and modeling the use of these strategies during contrived and natural family routines, as well as coaching families and providing feedback on their use of these strategies. Supervisor duties associated with the project include weekly field visits (e.g., 2 hours per week) to the participating families' homes to ensure fidelity of implementation of the behavioral therapist's parent training intervention. "Fidelity of implementation" means the extent to which a program is carried out according to a treatment manual or an individualized plan. Supervisor *responsibilities* also consist of participating with behavioral therapist and counseling staff (for those families who need the positive family therapy intervention) on implementation of the parent training intervention and carrying out probe data collection practices (e.g., videotaping parent training intervention sessions).

BEHAVIORAL PARENT TRAINING AS EVIDENCE-BASED PRACTICE FOR CHILDREN WITH DEVELOPMENTAL DISABILITY AND FAMILIES

Over the decades, special education and disability research has made great strides in identifying and developing evidence-based practices to help children with DD develop their functional academic skills, appropriate social skills, and functional life skills that can lead to their full participation in the community, independent living, and quality of life (Snell & Brown, 2006). Many of the treatment models are based on ABA. More and more studies particularly look into the issues of involving parents in the treatment process as change agents. Therefore, a substantial literature on BPT for children with DD has emerged.

By following the search procedures described in chapter 1, we conducted a thorough literature search on BPT programs for children with DD in a number of common databases (see the list in chapter 1). In addition to the use of search terms about parents and DD as described in chapter 1, search terms used as either a single term or a combination of terms also included training components (e.g., "setting events," "antecedents," "prompts," "planned activity training," "scheduling," "compliance training," "skill teaching," "positive reinforcement," "praise," "token economy," "negative reinforcement," "extinction," "differentiated reinforcement," "response cost," "time-out," and "punishment") and parent training models ("parent training," "behavioral parent training," "parent behavioral training," and "parent management training"). Following the articles selection procedures and inclusion criteria of evidence-based practice studies defined in chapter 1, we eventually chose a total of 56 qualified articles fallen into two categories: randomized control trials (RCTs) or quasi-experimental designs (QEDs) in which an alternative to randomization was used to assign subjects studies (15 studies) and single-subject design (SSD) studies (41 studies) that present solid empirical evidence for BPT as evidence-based practice.

EVIDENCE OF BEHAVIORAL PARENT TRAINING: RANDOMIZED CONTROLLED TRIALS AND QUASI-EXPERIMENTAL DESIGN STUDIES

As a result of the search process, a dozen RCTs and QED studies were identified regarding the effectiveness of BPT programs. A total of 15 RCT or QED studies were included in a research synthesis, and only 13 were eligible for the meta-analysis. In the research synthesis below, 15 RCT or QED studies were categorized into: Typical BPT, Step to Independence, Parent–Child Interaction Therapy, Parents Plus, and BPT for sleeping problems. These studies are summarized in Table 3.1.

Typical Behavioral Parent Training

Tavormina's (1975) intervention study makes an early case for the importance of BPT. In this study, the effects of a PBT condition were compared with the effects of parent reflective counseling condition. While true random assignment did not occur, mothers were assigned to the intervention groups or the control condition based on their availability to attend certain days of the week (behavioral vs. reflective intervention) or a later month (waitlist control group). The BPT group used the text *Parents Are Teachers: A Child Management Program* (Becker, 1971), and the clinicians taught parents to use operant techniques, mainly praise and positive contingent reinforcement, as well as observing target child behaviors. The BPT group employed a variety of training methods: discussion,

TABLE 3.1 SUMMARIES OF RANDOMIZED CONTROLLED TRIALS/QUASI-EXPERIMENTAL DESIGN STUDIES ON BEHAVIORAL PARENT TRAINING

Author(s)	*Design/Intervention Components/Manual/ Fidelity*	*Participants (Sample, Age, Ethnicity)/Setting*	*Dependent Measures*	*Treatment Effect(s)*
Bagner & Eyberg (2007)	• RCT • To increase prosocial behaviors while decreasing inappropriate behaviors • Weekly individual training to mastery and daily practice on differential reinforcement during child-directed play and positive attention and consequences (praise or time-out) during parent-directed play • Manualized (*Parent–Child Interaction Therapy* [PCIT]) • Fidelity procedures reported	• 30 families of children with ID and comorbid ODD (ages 3–6) • 67% White, 17% African American, 13% biracial, 3% Hispanic • Setting: clinic	PARENT • Parenting Stress Index • Therapy Attitude Inventory CHILD • Child Behavior Checklist • Eyberg Child Behavior Inventory PARENT & CHILD • Dyadic Parent–Child Interaction Coding System	More child compliance in treatment group and fewer externalizing and disruptive behaviors post intervention.
Baker & Brightman (1984)	• Quasi-experimental group design • To increase parents' knowledge and application of skills • Presentations, modeling, discussion, role-playing, consultation on behavioral teaching and behavioral management • Manualized (*Steps to Independence*) • No fidelity reported	• 15 families of children with DD (mean age 5) • No race/ethnicity information reported • Setting: PT at regional center	PARENT • Behavioral Vignettes Test • Teaching Proficiency Test • Advocacy Information Questionnaire • Parent Talk	Behavioral teaching group showed significant improvement in application of skills and small increase in knowledge of advocacy information.

Brightman, Baker, Clark, & Ambrose (1982)	• RCT • To train parents to manage child problem behaviors and to teach child self-help skills • Group or individual training on self-help skill teaching, behavior management, play and language skill teaching • Manualized (*Steps to Independence*) • No fidelity reported	• 66 families of children with mild to severe DD (ages 2–15) • No race/ethnicity information reported • Setting: community center	PARENT • Behavioral Vignettes Test • Modified training proficiency scale • Follow-up interview CHILD • Observations of self-help and play skill teaching • Child performance inventory: self-help • Child behavior problem checklist	Treatment families experienced significant gains in behavioral principles knowledge, proficiency in self-help teaching, observed play skill teaching. Treatment children had fewer behavior problems. No significant differences found between treatment groups (group vs. individual training).
Chadwick, Momcilovic, Rossiter, Stumbles, & Taylor (2001)	• RCT • To reduce problem behavior • Group or individual training on behavioral analysis and behavioral techniques • No manual reported • No fidelity reported	• 62 families of children with severe learning disabilities (cerebral palsy, Down syndrome, autism, and epilepsy; mean age 8) • 15% African, 16% Afro-Caribbean, 53% White, and 16% Other. • Setting: community center or home	PARENT • Parenting Stress Index • Intervention Evaluation Questionnaire CHILD • Disability Assessment Schedule	Short-term decreases in child problem behavior for individual training. No differences among groups at 6-month follow-up. No differences in parental stress among groups.

(*continued*)

TABLE 3.1 CONTINUED

Author(s)	*Design/Intervention Components/Manual/ Fidelity*	*Participants (Sample, Age, Ethnicity)/Setting*	*Dependent Measures*	*Treatment Effect(s)*
Feldman & Werner (2002)	• Quasi-experimental group design • To decrease problem behavior and parental stress • Individual parent training on data collection, differential reinforcement, errorless procedures, extinction, response cost • No manual reported • No fidelity reported	• 36 families of children with DD (mean age 11) • No race/ethnicity information reported • Setting: PT at home	PARENT • Questionnaire on Resource and Stress Short Form • Beck Depressive Inventory • Social Support • Parental Self-Efficacy • Therapist Rating of Parental Behavior Management Skills • Consumer Satisfaction CHILD • Child Behavior Management Survey FAMILY • Family Quality of Life	Reduced child problem behaviors and parental stress, higher parental self-efficacy on behavioral teaching.
Griffin, Geurin, Sharry, & Drumm (2010)	• Quasi-experimental group design with sequential block sampling • To promote child development and positive parent–child interactions • Video-based group trainings with discussion and role-play; individual trainings with video-feedback during play sessions • Manualized (*Parents Plus Early Year Programme*) • No fidelity reported	• 117 parents of children (ages 3–8 years) with behavioral/ emotional difficulties and DD • No race/ethnicity information reported • Setting: clinic and home	PARENT • Parental Stress Scale CHILD • Strengths and Difficulties Questionnaire FAMILY • Observations of interactions • Parent-Defined Problems and Goals	Significant improvement in total child difficulties, hyperactivity, and problem behaviors that maintained at 5-month follow-up for treatment group. Greater parental goal attainment for treatment group. No differences between DD and behavioral groups.

Jang et al. (2012)	• RCT • To increase family members' knowledge of ABA • Web-based electronic training, with visual and auditory notes and videos, on autism, ABA, antecedents- and consequences-based interventions • No manual reported • Parents must meet passing score to proceed with next training module	• 24 family members of children (ages 3–11) with autism • No race/ethnicity information reported • Setting: Web-based	PARENT • Researcher-developed exam on ABA principles	Intervention family members' knowledge of ABA principles significantly increased from pre- to post-intervention.
Kashima, Baker, & Landen (1988)	• RCT • To increase children's self-help skills and parents' behavioral knowledge • Live training or video training on behavioral teaching, creating behavior plans, reinforcement, and problem-solving • Manualized (*Steps to Independence*) • No fidelity reported	• 61 families of children with ID (mean age 6) • 55.7% Caucasian, 26.2% Hispanic, 13.1% Asian, 4.9% Black • Setting: PT at regional center	PARENT • Behavioral Vignettes Test • Teaching Proficiency Test • Teaching Interview • Program Evaluation CHILD • Mini-Performance Inventory (child behavior measure)	Significant increases in children's self-help skills. Live and video training associated with gains in parents' behavioral knowledge, with live training outperforming video training. Gains reported on behavioral teaching but not behavioral proficiency.

(*continued*)

TABLE 3.1 CONTINUED

Author(s)	*Design/Intervention Components/Manual/ Fidelity*	*Participants (Sample, Age, Ethnicity)/Setting*	*Dependent Measures*	*Treatment Effect(s)*
Hand, Raghallaigh, Cuppage, Coyle, & Sharry (2012)	• RCT • To reduce behavioral problems and promote child development • Group-based training with video, discussion, role-play • Manualized (*Parents Plus Children's Programme*) • No fidelity reported	• 29 parents of children (ages 6–12 years) with developmental delay • 5 parent English learners • Setting: clinic	PARENT • Parental Stress Scale • Kansas Parental Satisfaction Scale CHILD • Strengths and Difficulties Questionnaire FAMILY • Parent-Defined Problems and Goals	Significant improvements in total child difficulties, conduct problems, parent stress, and parent- and child-directed goal attainment for treatment group, compared with control group.
Prieto-Bayard & Baker (1986)	• RCT • To increase child self-help skills, parents' behavioral teaching, modification, and management skills. • Group training in Spanish with lectures, demonstrations, role-play, videos, discussions, and individual consultations on behavioral techniques and management, self-help, and play skills • Manualized (*Steps to Independence*) • No fidelity reported	• 20 parents of children (ages 3–16) with DD (e.g., Down syndrome, autism, cerebral palsy) • All parents monolingual Spanish-speaking; 75% immigrants from Mexico within last 10 years • Setting: regional center	PARENT • Verbal Behavioral Vignettes Test • Teaching Proficiency Test • Teaching Interview CHILD • Child Behavior Checklist	Improved child self-help skills. Increased sophistication of behavior management and teaching and knowledge of principles but no improvement in behavioral teaching proficiency.

Quinn, Carr, Carroll, & O'Sullivan (2006)	• Quasi-experimental group design (DD group vs. conduct problem group • To improve child behaviors and to promote child development • 6 weekly group sessions with video and role-play about parental attention, praise, rule-setting, planned ignoring, time-out, and teaching play skills • Manualized (*Parents Plus Programme*) • No fidelity reported	• 39 parents of children (ages 4–7 years) with significant conduct problems or DD • No race/ethnicity information reported • Setting: clinic	PARENT • General Health Questionnaire-12 • Kansas Parental Satisfaction Scale • Perceived Social Support Scale • Parenting Stress Index CHILD • Strengths and Difficulties Questionnaire • Child Behavior Checklist FAMILY • Family Assessment Device • Family Inventory of Life Events and Changes • Questionnaire on Resources and Stress	Psychological distress increased for DD group from post-treatment to follow-up. DD group reported meeting child-directed goals more successfully and were more likely to use learned parenting skills than behavioral group. No significant differences in difficult child behaviors or total parenting stress over time between groups.

(*continued*)

TABLE 3.1 CONTINUED

Author(s)	*Design/Intervention Components/Manual/Fidelity*	*Participants (Sample, Age, Ethnicity)/Setting*	*Dependent Measures*	*Treatment Effect(s)*
Quinn, Carr, Carroll, & O'Sullivan (2007)	• Quasi-experimental group design (DD and conduct problem vs. control) • See Quinn et al. (2006)	• 41 parents of children (ages 4–7 years) with significant conduct problems or DD • No race/ethnicity information reported • Setting: clinic	PARENT • General Health Questionnaire-12 • Kansas Parental Satisfaction Scale • Perceived Social Support Scale • Parenting Stress Index CHILD • Strengths and Difficulties Questionnaire • Child Behavior Checklist FAMILY • Family Assessment Device • Family Inventory of Life Events and Changes • Questionnaire on Resources and Stress	Improvements in total child behavioral difficulties that maintained at 10-month follow-up for treatment group.

Solomon, Ono, Timmer, Goodlin-Jones (2008)	• Quasi-experimental group design • To train parents to reduce child problem behaviors • Parents trained individually in child-directed interaction (e.g., positive attention, ignoring) and parent-directed interaction (e.g., clear, direct commands, reinforcement, time-out) with modifications for ASD (e.g., addressing circumscribed interests) • Manualized (*Parent-Child Interaction Therapy* [PCIT]) • Fidelity procedures reported	• 19 boys (ages 5–12) with ASD and their parents • No race/ethnicity information reported • Setting: home	PARENT • Parenting Stress Index CHILD • Eyberg Child Behavior Inventory • Behavior Assessment System for Children FAMILY • Dyadic parent–child interaction coding	Child behaviors reported to be less problematic for intervention group, compared with control. Child adaptability increased significantly for intervention group, but not for control. Parents reported children to be less atypical following treatment. No changes in parent stress reported.
Wiggs & Stores (2004)	• RCT • To improve settling, night waking, early waking, and cosleeping behaviors • Brief parent advice session on bedtime routines, standard extinction and reinforcement • No manual • No fidelity procedures reported	• 46 children with Down syndrome (age 7 months to 4 years 9 months) • 18 children without disabilities (comparison-ages 12 months to 5 years 5 months) • No race/ethnicity information reported • Setting: PT in a group	PARENT • Knowledge of Behavioural Principles as Applied to Children Questionnaire CHILD • Composite Sleep Problem Score (settling problems, night waking, early waking, sleeping with parents) • Actometry readings of sleep-wake patterns • Sleep of Young Children Questionnaire	Treatment group mothers scored significantly higher on their knowledge of behavioral principles and on knowledge of sleep problems. Children increased their time asleep and decreased the number of wake episodes.

(*continued*)

TABLE 3.1 CONTINUED

Author(s)	*Design/Intervention Components/Manual/ Fidelity*	*Participants (Sample, Age, Ethnicity)/Setting*	*Dependent Measures*	*Treatment Effect(s)*
Tavormina (1975)	• Quasi-experimental group design • To train mothers behavioral techniques • Mothers trained using group discussion, role-play, modeling, and feedback to provide positive contingencies, to observe child behavior, and to apply principles to child's own target behaviors in eight weekly sessions • Manualized (*Parents Are Teachers: A Child Management Program)* • No fidelity procedures reported	• 51 mothers of children with DD • 2% (n = 1) Black, 98% White • Setting: PT at clinic; CI at home	PARENT • Hereford Parent Attitude Survey CHILD • Missouri Behavior Problem Checklist • Mothers' rating of target behavior • Mothers' report of frequency of occurrence of target behaviors at second baseline phase FAMILY • Behavior observations of mother–child interactions • Social validation survey	Treatment groups improved on multiple measures compared with control group, but behavioral group tended to outperform reflective counseling group, particularly in maternal causation, decreasing child aggression, and total appropriate interactions.

Note. ABA = applied behavioral analysis; ASD = Autism Spectrum Disorder; CI = child intervention; DD = developmental disabilities; ID = intellectual disabilities; ODD = oppositional defiant disorder; PT = parent training; RCT = randomized controlled trial role-play, and modeling continually throughout the 8-week-long sessions averaging 1.5 hours weekly to help the participating mothers learn how to apply the behavioral principles and strategies to the target behaviors they each faced. For the reflective counseling training, clinicians led parents in discussions about concerns of raising a child with a disability. Sessions also focused on awareness and understanding of their child's feelings. It was found that both treatment groups improved on multiple measures as compared with the control group and that the behavioral and counseling groups did not differ in the outcome measures of confidence, acceptance, understanding, or trust of the parent, total score for child behavior problems, and sleep disturbance and inhibition. However, compared with the mothers in the counseling group and the waitlist control group, the 19 mothers in the BPT group exhibited greater positive change in parent attitude (i.e., extent to which she saw herself as a change agent in child's behavior), parent-reported child aggression, researcher-observed parents' response to child behavior (appropriate antecedent-response during play), researcher-rated target behavior ratings, and parent-reported emotional reactions to child. Parents in the BPT group also reported greater perceived family functioning and overall treatment effectiveness on their child at the termination of the study. The behavior training was related to parental cognitive changes as well as significantly greater child behavioral changes. The results of Tavormina's study seem to suggest that BPT alone outperforms counseling alone, even in measures of parents' emotional coping.

In a more recent study by Feldman and Werner (2002), completers of a BPT program were compared with those on a waitlist. Eighteen families of children with DDs were randomly selected from "graduates" of the program and were then compared—on child and parent outcome measures—with 18 similar families on the program's waitlist. Program graduates had been instructed in the home setting by behavioral consultants for 3 to 6 months on a weekly basis. Consultants conducted functional assessments and individualized the treatment plans for each family. Parents were then trained to record behavioral data and implement strategies related to a number of behavioral principles, including antecedents, errorless procedures, replacement skill training, noncontingent and differential reinforcement, extinction, response interruption and redirection, and response cost. As behavioral objectives were met, trainings were faded; that is, the number of trainings was reduced as parents mastered these strategies and no longer needed instruction. Parent and child measures were collected once: post-invention for program graduates and pre-intervention for those on the waitlist. Compared with the waitlist control group, the treatment group scored lower on child problem behaviors and parental stress. The treatment group parents also scored higher on self-efficacy on changing child behavior than did control group parents. The groups, however, were not significantly different on parental depressive affect and social support. While observational data showed that the treatment group's objectives were met at the time of discharge, not all parents were competent in implementing behavioral strategies at home. An obvious limitation is that random assignment did not occur before the start of intervention, and thus, Feldman and Werner's study cannot be considered a true RCT study.

One persistent research question in the BPT literature is about the effect of training delivery format on parent and child outcomes. In other words, the question *Does the training approach matter?* calls for an answer. While there is evidence for the benefit of individualized, supervised practice to parents of infants and toddlers with DD (Hudson, 1982), this does not necessarily suggest that individual-based training is superior to group-based training, particularly for families of older children. Chadwick et al.'s (2001) intervention study sought to examine the difference between individual-based and group-based training with parents of children ages 4 to 11. In this less rigorous RCT design study, Chadwick et al. (2001) randomly assigned parents in two adjacent boroughs to group training or individual training. Parents from a third borough were all assigned to a third group, which received no intervention and served as the control group. Group interventions were held at community centers for five 1.5- to 2-hour sessions, while individual-based interventions occurred at the families' homes with five to seven sessions lasting 1 to 2 hours each. The treatment group parents were exposed to behavioral analysis, strategies to teach appropriate behaviors, and ways to identify factors related to child behavior. The authors report that based on the postintervention measures, the individual-setting group outperformed the group-setting intervention parents and the control group in reducing children's problem behaviors and that the treatment group parents found the intervention useful. However, these differences did not maintain at the 6-month follow-up. Furthermore, at post-test, no significant differences were found in parental stress among the three groups. The failure of BPT to reduce parental stress is a finding that we encountered in other studies that follow.

Researchers continue to address the issue of effective training approaches by incorporating new, ever-more cost-efficient technology in 21st century BPT programs. Jang et al. (2012) tested the use of a Web-based electronic training (i.e., eLearning) program for parents of children with ASD. The purpose of the program was to equip parents with an understanding about their children's disability and with foundational knowledge of ABA treatment. In this RCT study, 28 participating family members (24 mothers, two fathers, and two grandmothers) of children with ASD, ages 3 to 11 years, were randomly assigned to the intervention group and to a waitlist control group. Those in the intervention group gained access to the eLearning training immediately after taking the online pretest, whereas the control group only began training after the conclusion of the treatment group's intervention. The program consisted of a self-paced, 1-week 30- to 40-hour online training that participants accessed from their own computer. It covered 15 topics, including an introduction to ASD, ABA, discrete trial training, prompting and fading, shaping and chaining, functions of behavior, and antecedent-based and consequence-based interventions. These topics were organized in nine modules taught through didactic visual and auditory notes, as well as through videos, which participants could review multiple times. Only after meeting criteria in all quizzes (85%), given at the end of each module, could participants proceed to the final test. A comparison of the pre- and postintervention test between groups showed that the intervention group made a significant (27 percentage point) improvement in their test scores, demonstrating an increased understanding of ABA procedures. Following the completion of training for the waitlisted group, both groups' test performance was analyzed together; results indicated that all participating family members made significant gains after training. These are promising outcomes for technology-mediated BPT that may substantially mitigate the cost of training. However, unlike previous studies, which also considered more distal child behavior results, Jang et al.'s intervention study only examined proximal parent outcomes. It behooves future research to measure associated changes in the child behavior, and in parent–child interactions, in addition to parent knowledge. As seen in the studies reviewed already, changes in parents' knowledge do not necessarily translate into changes in children's behavior. More direct, in vivo practice with coaching for parents may be necessary (e.g., Hand et al., 2013).

Given the evidence from two RCT studies and two QED studies conducted by four independent research groups, it seems that typical BPT programs, regardless of the format of parent training and the way of delivering parent training, have demonstrated a strong treatment effect on both child and parent outcomes. So we are confident to suggest that typical or traditional BPT programs are established practices for children with DD and their families.

Steps to Independence

In the 1970s and 1980s, Baker, Brightman and colleagues ran a series of group studies—experimental and quasi-experimental in nature—to test the effectiveness of their *Steps to Independence* program (Baker, Brightman, Heifetz, & Murphy, 1976) for children with developmental disabilities. The *Steps to Independence* program employs BPT to teach parents behavioral management skills to correct children's problem behaviors and also to increase children's self-help skills (e.g., dressing, toileting, grooming). It teaches parents how to make and follow task analyses of everyday activities such as hand washing and dressing. Parents learn a system of prompts and how to fade them so children can ultimately perform the skills without assistance. Prompts include moving a child through a task with hand on hand guidance, showing how to perform the skill by demonstration, and giving clear verbal instructions. Research on parents' stress in this population indicates that some of the problems with high levels of stress and depressive symptoms are associated with children's problem behaviors and extra caregiving demands that often involve self-help (Roach, Orsmond, & Barratt, 1999). Self-help skills are a necessary part of normal home routines. When children require extra assistance with them, they can set the stage for problem behaviors, particularly noncompliance. These parent–child encounters around self-help can also trigger coercion (Lucyshyn et al., 2004).

Brightman and colleagues (1982) tested their program in multiple training formats. The 66 participating families were randomly assigned (with the exception of three families) to a group training ($n = 37$), individual training ($n = 16$), or waitlist control group ($n = 13$). The treatment group families received a large group orientation meeting, which was followed by nine training sessions held at community centers. Individual parent training sessions took place in community-based centers for 1 hour each session, and parents were able to bring their children to rehearse the skills taught and to obtain feedback from trainers. The group sessions lasted 2 hours each session, and featured mostly didactic instruction; still, group sessions contained various training methods like media, role-playing, small group discussion, and problem-solving. The trainers covered self-help skill teaching strategies in the first hour sessions and developing and implementing problem behavior management programs in the next three sessions. Teaching language and play skills was the emphasis in the final two sessions. All families were also provided the *Steps to Independence* manuals, as well as weekly homework assignments between sessions to practice addressing child problem behaviors and teaching self-help skills.

The outcomes measures used in Brightman et al.'s (1982) study included a researcher-developed assessment of behavior principles knowledge, a researcher-modified training proficiency scale, observations of parents' facilitation of self-help and play skills, a performance inventory of the children's self-help skills as reported by the parents, and a checklist of child behavior problems. Immediately following the training, the treatment group parents demonstrated significant improvements in behavioral management principles knowledge, training proficiency, and teaching play skills, as compared with the control group parents. The children with DD in the treatment group families were also found to have significantly fewer behavior problems. However, there were no significant differences in performance between parents receiving individual training and those in the group training format. Such findings seem to be consistent with what Chadwick and colleagues (2001) found at follow-up to their intervention. As group training used fewer training resources, Brightman and colleagues (1982) concluded that the group training format was the more cost-effective technique.

In subsequent studies of the *Steps to Independence* program, trainers used the group format but included individual consultations to retain some of the benefits of individualized attention to families. Other studies by these scholars explored additional interests, such as the effectiveness of parent advocacy training compared with the original behavioral management training program. In Baker and Brightman's (1984) study, 15 families were randomly grouped into a behavioral training program and an advocacy training program. Both programs provided training to the participating parents for 2 hours weekly in a total of 7 weeks. Although the advocacy training group is not a traditional control group, this quasi-experimental study still sheds light on the usefulness of this BPT program. Using some of the same measures as Brightman et al.'s (1982) investigation, the researchers here found that behavioral training parents showed significant improvement on the application of behavioral management skills on a skills test and also displayed a slight increase in parent advocacy knowledge.

Subsequently, the Baker and colleagues' curriculum was converted to a video-based training program. Kashima, Baker, and Landen (1988) evaluated the potential benefits of such an approach in an RCT design study. The 61 parents in their intervention study were first randomly assigned to a standard live training, a video-based training, or a waitlist control group and then participated in a preintervention assessment. Those in the intervention groups received four weekly group trainings that covered assessing self-help skills, using behavioral strategies, using reinforcers, and problem-solving. Specific to the live training group, trainers were clinicians experienced with teaching the program and used lectures, group exercises, demonstrations, discussion, and video clips. The video training comprised videos showing content and explaining activities similar to that presented in the live training. Inexperienced trainers then facilitated group exercises based on the video content. When comparing the performance of the three groups, Kashima et al. (1988) reported that both the video and live training produced gains in parents' application of behavioral teaching assessed through the parents' anecdotal accounts about teaching these behaviors to their children but not through a behavioral proficiency test. Yet in an assessment of behavioral knowledge, while both treatment groups outperformed the control group, the live training was associated with greater gains compared with the video training group. Most importantly, Kashima and colleagues' study found that both the live and video training groups reported improvements in children's behaviors, especially in the targeted skill. While parent knowledge outcomes appeared to favor the live training condition, there was evidence that child outcomes were comparable between the live training approach and the more cost-effective video-based training.

When the live training and the manual for this program was adapted for Spanish-speaking families, Prieto-Bayard and Baker (1986) also observed gains made in the sophistication of the behavioral management and teaching and parents' knowledge of behavioral modification principles and in children's acquisition of self-help skills. In this study, participants were monolingual, Spanish-speaking parents of 20 children with DD, who were randomly assigned (except for one participant) into the intervention or waitlist control group. This is one of the few studies in the literature we review in this book with a group of parents from an ethnic minority, non-English-speaking population. Following the curriculum used by Brightman et al. (1982), the trainers implemented 10 weekly 2-hour sessions that incorporated lectures, videos, and discussion. Trainers also offered incentives to participate (e.g., children's toys, small transportation stipend), modeled appropriate parent teaching, and supervised parents' use of strategies with their children. As mentioned, following intervention, children from the treatment group significantly increased their use of self-help skills, and parents improved in their knowledge of behavioral principles. While parents' proficiency in teaching seemingly did not improve, there was evidence of gains in the sophistication of teaching methods used. Across all four studies, the *Steps to Independence* program of BPT has demonstrated improvements in both parent knowledge and child behavior. Although there is a manual developed for all parent training components across these studies, no fidelity of treatment information was reported in any of aforementioned four studies. Table 3.1 presents more details about the studies described above. According to the criteria of categorization of EBPs introduced in chapter, it seems clear that three RCT studies and one QED study conducted by two independent research teams provide strong support to the claim of *Steps to Independence* program as an established practice for children with DD and their families. One important contribution of Baker and colleagues' studies on *Steps to Independence* program is that BPT program can teach parents to work on children's adaptive skills as well as problem behaviors. This use of BPT is particularly important for children with moderate/severe disabilities, who often have substantial deficits in adaptive behaviors.

Parent-Child Interaction Therapy

In the same vein, the PCIT program focuses on both enhancing behavioral management skills and stimulating more positive relationships between the mother and child. Bagner and Eyberg (2007) revealed the evidence of PCIT effectiveness on child behavior in their RCT study. Thirty families of children with intellectual disabilities and comorbid oppositional defiant disorder were randomly assigned into a treatment group or waitlist control group. The treatment group parents were then trained in the PCIT program for 1 hour per week for approximately 12 weeks until they mastered the techniques for both child-directed and parent-directed interactions. Through the training, the parents were instructed to use differential reinforcement of child behavior during child-directed play. For parent-directed interactions, the training focused on decreasing inappropriate behaviors by giving positive attention to appropriate behavior and time-out for noncompliance. The postintervention data suggest that the child outcomes were more positive than parent outcomes. No significant differences were found between two groups on the measure of maternal distress about behaviors. Yet the observational data showed that the treatment group children were significantly more compliant, compared with the control group. The mothers in the treatment group also reported significantly fewer child externalizing and disruptive behavior problems at follow-up, 4 months after intervention.

In a pilot study, Solomon et al. (2008) recruited 19 children with ASD, ages 5 to 12, and their parents to be involved in a PCIT training intervention. The study employed a design with semirandomization: Eligible child participants were first matched with similar others (based on age, cognitive level, and types of behaviors) and then a treatment participant was randomly selected from each matched pair. The nonselected children served as the waitlist control group. While the treatment largely followed the same procedures as Bagner and Eyberg's (2007) intervention, Solomon and colleagues also made adjustments to address social behaviors particular to children with ASD, including restricting perseverative talk, as well as allowing parents to redirect children to more interactive activities during the child-centered phase of the program. Parents were also instructed to deliver a generous amount of praise when their children initiated interactions. The analysis of the data indicated some positive results for the intervention. Treatment parents rated a significant decrease of problematic behavior following the intervention, in comparison with the waitlist control group, which did not experience a similar decline. In comparison with the waitlist group, the treatment group parents reported significantly more adaptability in their children and reported that they perceived their children to be less atypical. However, the data suggested that both groups of children experienced similar changes in the intensity of problem behaviors, as well as changes in hyperactivity, conduct problems, aggression, leadership, and social skills. As was found in Bagner and Eyberg's PCIT study, no changes in parent stress were reported following this intervention.

Based on the categorization criteria of EBPs introduced in chapter 1, it seems that one RCT study and one QED study conducted by two independent research groups have given evidence to categorize *Parent-Child Interaction Therapy* program as a promising practice for children with DD and their families. However, parent stress has often shown to be unresponsive to parent training interventions, even though children's problem behaviors typically improve. Evidence of this pattern was found in evaluations of another BPT program, Parents Plus.

Parents Plus

The Parents Plus intervention consists of a group-based course, with therapists introducing instructional content on video. Its two videos were developed specifically to be used in Ireland, with the actors' scripts written in Irish idiom (Quinn et al., 2006). Along with the videos, program materials also include a facilitator's manual and handouts for parents.

The original course was divided into eight weekly sessions of 2 hours each, with the last session serving as a review of learned skills and a discussion of special interest topics. However, researchers often conducted the course in six to nine sessions, adjusting the length of training to accommodate parents' and children's needs. During group sessions, trainers typically (1) welcomed parents, (2) reviewed parents' progress with skills learned from previous sessions, (3) introduced new topics using video, (4) facilitated group discussions and activities, and (5) assigned homework and helped parents plan in practicing learned skills. The topics from the videos presented in group sessions revolve around the primary goals of the Parents Plus program: (1) promoting child development targeting child play, communication, and language skills; and (2) encouraging positive parent–child interactions and parenting strategies when managing problem behaviors through using praise and ignoring, following through on rules, and using routines (Sharry, Guerin, Griffin, & Drumm, 2005). To address behavior problems, parents are urged to consider a plan of action to discipline their children and a plan of prevention to keep the behavior from occurring.

One team of researchers evaluated Parents Plus and sought to compare treatment effects on children having developmental needs with children having only behavioral needs. Quinn and colleagues (2006) studied the program with parents of preschool-age children. In this quasi-experimental study, a group of parents of children with DDs (n = 23) were compared with a group of parents with children having conduct disorders (n = 24). The intervention group received six group sessions of Parents Plus training. Researchers discarded the training component focusing on rewards, which they believed to be more appropriate for older children. The program was also abridged for the convenience of parents and parents' time commitments.

All measures were taken at three time points: pre-intervention, post-intervention, and follow-up 10 months post-treatment (Quinn et al., 2006). There appeared to be no significant differences in parent adjustment to difficult child behavior or in total parenting stress over time between the disability group and the conduct problems group. However, parents' psychological distress increased from post-intervention to follow-up for the disability group, whereas it decreased over the same period of time for the conduct problems group. Parents of children with disabilities, on average, were able to meet child-centered goals overtime more so than parents of children with conduct problems. Furthermore, parents of children with DDs rated themselves as significantly more likely to use the learned parenting skills following the intervention compared with the conduct disorder group. Researchers hypothesized that, for the DD group, learning new parenting strategies helped enhance parents' goal attainment and confidence in using these new skills; however, having to manage behavior without the help of ongoing training negatively affected these parents' psychological health.

One major shortcoming of Quinn et al.'s (2006) intervention study was a lack of a true control group. This was partly addressed in Quinn et al.'s (2007) next study. Participants of the study were parents of children ages 4 to 7 with DD and parents of children with behavior problems. The researchers compared the results of 22 parents assigned to the Parents Plus training with those of 19 waitlisted parents on a number of measures. Group assignment was based on which participating early intervention clinic the parents were referred to by their children's multidisciplinary team. As in the previous study, Quinn and colleagues shortened the Parents Plus course to six sessions, foregoing the instructional component about implementing rewards. After intervention, the treatment showed greater reductions in parental adjustment to children's behavioral difficulties, compared with the control group, and this difference was significant. This improvement maintained at the 10-month follow-up. Although researchers also noted improvements over time in conduct problems, parent satisfaction, parent resources and stress, and parent- and child-centered goal attainment, these changes were not significantly different from those reported by the control group. Furthermore, no significant changes were found in child behavior problems nor in parental social support. No changes were noted in parent stress processes, either. Unlike their earlier study, the researchers did not conduct an analysis of the difference in treatment effect by disability group (DD group vs. behavioral problems group).

The original developers of the Parents Plus program ran a series of intervention studies with children with DDs, as well. Their Parents Plus Early Years program specifically trains parents of young children up to 6 years old with behavioral and developmental issues (Sharry et al., 2005). The program consists of group sessions that follow the Parents Plus curriculum, as well as accompanying individual sessions. In the first evaluation of the program, Sharry and colleagues (2005) conducted eight 2-hour group sessions and included five individual sessions. Child-centered play and establishment of home routines were two major areas of emphasis during the individual sessions, but these were personalized to the family. Video feedback was also a critical feature of the individual sessions. With the support of a trainer, parents rehearsed skills discussed in the group sessions; these practice sessions are adapted to fit individual goals of the parent. The therapist video-recorded interactions between the parent and child and then reviewed the video with the parent during the home-based individual session. The feedback provided to parents typically focused on positive parenting behaviors. For example, the therapist will point out effective strategies the parent employed in the video to reinforce those desired skills. Parents' own videos were often incorporated in the group trainings as examples of the topics relevant to the lesson. Similar to the group training, the therapist helped the parent to plan and apply learned strategies at the close of each individual session.

Griffin et al. (2010) conducted a controlled study of the Parents Plus Early Years program. This study had a sequential block design, assigning parents to the treatment group or to the waitlist comparison group based on the date of referral to intervention. Four clinics were recruited to be involved in the study, resulting in 65 parents allocated to the treatment group and 52 to the comparison group. Rather than eight group sessions, Griffin and colleagues only held seven of these sessions, with the same number of individual trainings. Once again, video feedback was a major component of the individual sessions, allowing an opportunity for parents to think about their interactions with their children and for therapists to reinforce positive parenting skills. Following intervention, parents in the treatment group exhibited a significant reduction in total child difficulties, child hyperactivity, and parent-reported problems, when compared with the waitlisted group. Improvements in child behavior maintained at the 5-month follow-up. Not only that, treatment parents also reported greater goal attainment than control group parents. No between-group differences in parent improvement were found for child conduct problems and child emotional symptoms. Once again, no significant differences were found in parent stress. Furthermore, an analysis of measures between treated parents of children with developmental disabilities and parents of children with conduct problems was conducted, and no differences were found across measures. The researchers' findings suggest that treatment parents, on average, made progress, regardless of their children's presenting difficulty.

It was not until Hand et al.'s (2013) study that a true RCT was conducted to test to the efficacy of Parents Plus. Sharry's research team examined the program's effectiveness on a slightly older group of children (ages 6 to 11) with developmental and behavioral difficulties. This RCT involved parents of children with solely DDs (e.g., intellectual disability, autism). For this study, 16 parents assigned at random to the Parents Plus Children's Program (PPCP) intervention group completed the treatment, while 13 parents randomly assigned to the control group completed the study. There were eight weekly group sessions to introduce positive disciplining and positive parenting skills. Taking into account feedback from parents and because two participating parents reported having mild intellectual disabilities themselves, modifications were made to the Parents Plus intervention. The trainers incorporated video clips from the Parents Plus Early Years program featuring children with special needs to enhance the relevance of the instructional content. Reading materials for parents included more visual representations, materials were read aloud more often, and therapists-in-training provided one-on-one support to parents with literacy needs. The authors argue that, while individual sessions were not provided, the one-on-one support during group sessions may have been a more effective approach. The results of this study indicated that treatment parents observed significant improvements in their children's total difficulties and conduct problems, which was not reported by wait-listed parents. Parent- and child-centered goal attainment showed significantly larger gains for treatment group parents than for control group parents. Unlike in the results for previous Parents Plus studies, the parents in this intervention rated themselves lower on the Parent Stress Index compared with the control group.

In general, parent stress has proven to be unresponsive to parent training interventions, even though children's problem behaviors often improve. That reduced parental stress was an outcome in Hand et al.'s (2013) study perhaps speaks to their intervention's effectiveness in diligently tailoring the program to meet the parents' specific needs (e.g., through the inclusion of visual aids, literacy assistance, and relevant video clips). Stress might also need to be directly targeted, as it is in the stress management interventions presented in chapter 2 or as in the multicomponent interventions that are discussed in chapter 5. In summary, four studies including one RCT study and three QED studies done by three independent research groups have given adequate evidence to suggest *Parents Plus* to be an established practice for children with DD and their families.

Behavioral Parent Training Interventions for Sleeping Problems

Behavioral parent training interventions have also targeted poor sleeping behaviors of children with DD, although a majority of such interventions are SSD studies. One parent education package was evaluated by an RCT-design study in the treatment of young children with Down syndrome in England (Stores & Stores, 2004). As part of a brief parent training on behavioral techniques to encourage good sleep habits, Stores and Stores (2004) conducted a random assignment study of 46 children with Down syndrome between the ages of 6 months and 5 years. Parents in the treatment group attended a 90-minute advice session run by one of the authors in small groups of around five parents with similarly aged children. Topics included rewarding desired behavior, planned ignoring, and establishing conducive bedtime routines. Time was also allotted to discuss specific issues individual parents raised. Parents were given a booklet that was designed to be user-friendly to take with them for reference in the home. Most results of the intervention were nonsignificant, although children in the instruction group exhibited less overall sleep disturbance at the 6-month follow-up. Mothers who were trained showed greater understanding of behavioral principles at the 1-month follow-up only. A notable trend between treatment and control groups is that there was a gradual decrease across time in total sleep disturbance in the treatment group as well as a gradual increase in the control group over the 6 months of the study, culminating in the significant difference previously noted at the 6-month follow-up. Despite only one RCT study with mixed effects of the treatment, BPT is still proved to be an established practice for parents to tackle sleeping problems of their children with DD based on the evidence of eight SSD studies discussed in later section.

META-ANALYSIS: RANDOMIZED CONTROLLED TRIALS AND QUASI-EXPERIMENTAL DESIGN STUDIES

As introduced conceptually in chapter 1 and illustrated with several examples in chapter 2, meta-analysis is a way to put together the data from many different studies in order to characterize them as a group and is a useful tool for examining the efficacy or effectiveness of a variety of interventions (Singer, Ethridge, & Aldana, 2007).

Table 3.2 shows each of the 13 studies of BPT programs we have reviewed with a list of all of the different dependent measures used as outcomes in the studies with their corresponding *d* statistic shown on the last column: values range from the largest negative effect of -1.01, to the lowest positive effect size of 0 (meaning no effect), and then to the largest positive effect size of 2.27.

For example, the first study in Table 3.2 was conducted by Bagner and Eyberg (2007). In that study the researchers measured the treatment effect of BPT on both children and parents. For example, the effect size for the children's problem behavior was .97 (measured by the Child Behavior Checklist [CBCL, Total]), generally considered to be a high effect size indicating that by the end of the treatment the children with DD in the treatment group had much less severe behavior problems than those who did not receive treatment. It really makes sense that the *d* for this dependent variable of child's behavior problems was higher, because decrease of child's problem behaviors through parents' proper implementation of behavioral strategies was the main focus of the BPT treatment. The individual effect sizes on the last column of Table 3.2 are mostly a way of converting many different outcomes into the same unit, the *d* statistic. The most informative parts of meta-analysis happen after this step is completed.

Table 3.3 also summarizes the effect size results for each of the BPT studies. The second column indicates whether an outcome measure was used to study parents or children.

By following the same procedures of running a meta-analysis in chapter 2, we intended to group variables to ask questions that can give an overall picture of the data after calculating *d*'s for all of the different kinds of outcome measures. When we ask the question: "Overall what was the effect size for the children's outcomes when combined into an average *d*?," the answer can be found in the last column of Table 3.2: it is $d = 0.53$ in this case. This overall effect size for child outcomes was actually generated by averaging the effect sizes of two specific child outcomes reported in 13 studies: a moderate

TABLE 3.2 RESULTS OF META-ANALYSIS OF BEHAVIORAL PARENT TRAINING INTERVENTIONS

				Intervention			*Comparison*					
Study	*Measure*	*Group*	*Outcome*	*n*	*Pre M (SD)*	*Post M (SD)*	*n*	*Pre M (SD)*	*Post M (SD)*	*F*	*t*	*d*
Bagner & Eyberg (2007)	Child Behavior Checklist (CBCL; Total)	Child	Behavior	10	89.70 (29.45)	58.83 (27.87)	12	95.17 (16.41)	82.23 (20.44)	11.62		0.97
	Eyberg Child Behavior Inventory (ECBI)											
	Intensity	Child	Behavior	10	156.40 (34.30)	100.63 (26.22)	12	170.92 (19.47)	143.14 (30.33)	13.00		1.50
	Problem	Child	Behavior	10	21.40 (6.11)	9.31 (9.42)	12	18.67 (7.98)	15.33 (8.74)	2.68		0.66
	Parenting Stress Index—Short Form (PSI-SF)											
	Parental Distress	Parent	Stress/ Distress	10	30.60 (4.70)	29.18 (5.72)	12	30.17 (7.80)	29.35 (8.47)	0.19		0.02
	Parent-Child DI	Parent	Stress/ Distress	10	31.10 (10.10)	25.51 (8.93)	12	29.33 (6.75)	30.16 (8.82)	2.59		0.52
	Difficult Child	Parent	Stress/ Distress	10	42.60 (8.40)	33.97 (8.87)	12	43.67 (7.79)	38.61 (6.80)	4.80		0.59
	Dyadic Parent–Child Interaction (DPICS)											

	Do Skills	Family	Interaction	10	5.60 (2.63)	17.94 (8.90)	11	4.91 (2.66)	3.78 (4.86)	20.09	2.06
	Don't Skills	Family	Interaction	10	43.90 (14.45)	9.84 (9.94)	11	43.18 (16.78)	28.51 (18.29)	9.67	1.32
	% Compliance	Family	Interaction	10	63.88 (19.22)	85.90 (9.44)	11	68.89 (19.71)	59.10 (25.68)	9.68	1.53
	OVERALL										0.95
Baker & Brightman (1984)	Behavior Vignettes Test	Parent	Knowledge	10	7.80 (0.00)	12.10 (0.00)	8	7.60 (0.00)	8.50 (0.00)		1.58
	Teaching Proficiency Test	Parent	Performance	7	6.80 (0.00)	11.10 (0.00)	7	5.30 (0.00)	7.90 (0.00)		0.27
	OVERALL										0.91
Brightman et al. (1982)	Behavioral Vignettes Test	Parent	Knowledge	46			13			4.08	0.63
	Teaching Proficiency Test										
	Self-Help	Parent	Performance	46			13			6.23	0.78
	Play Skills	Parent	Performance	46			13			3.53	0.59
	Behavior problem checklist	Child	Behavior	46			13			2.41	0.49
	OVERALL										0.62
Chadwick et al. (2001)—Post	Disability Assessment Schedule (DAS)										

(continued)

TABLE 3.2 CONTINUED

				Intervention			*Comparison*					
Study	*Measure*	*Group*	*Outcome*	*n*	*Pre M (SD)*	*Post M (SD)*	*n*	*Pre M (SD)*	*Post M (SD)*	*F*	*t*	*d*
	Mean number of severe behavior Problems	Child	Behavior	38	3.45 (3.32)	2.97 (3.04)	24	1.90 (2.30)	2.90 (3.10)			0.48
	Mean number occurring more than once/week	Child	Behavior	38	4.25 (2.75)	4.96 (2.54)	24	3.20 (2.50)	4.10 (3.50)			-0.07
	Parenting Stress Index (PSI; Parental Distress)	Parent	Stress/ Distress	38	34.40 (8.96)	30.82 (9.78)	24	33.50 (9.50)	33.60 (11.20)			0.36
	OVERALL											0.26
Chadwick et al. (2001)—Follow-Up	Disability Assessment Schedule (DAS)											
	Mean number of severe behavior problems	Child	Behavior	38	2.97 (3.04)	2.26 (2.06)	24	2.90 (3.10)	2.60 (3.10)			0.16
	Mean number occurring more than once/week	Child	Behavior	38	4.96 (2.54)	4.02 (2.45)	24	4.10 (3.50)	4.10 (2.70)			0.37

	Parenting Stress Index (PSI)—Parental Distress	Parent	Stress/ Distress	38	30.82 (9.78)	31.36 (9.21)	24	33.60 (11.20)	31.10 (12.10)		-0.29
	OVERALL										0.08
Feldman & Werner (2002)	Child Behavior Management Survey										
	Problem Behavior	Child	Behavior	18		2.55 (1.08)	18		3.15 (0.91)		0.60
	Self-Efficacy	Parent	Self-Efficacy	18		4.71 (1.33)	18		3.73 (1.78)		0.62
	Questionnaire on Resources and Stress-Short Form (QRS-SF)										
	Limits on Family Opportunities	Parent	Stress/ Distress	18			18			1.84	0.61
	Child Physical Limitations	Parent	Stress/ Distress	18			18			1.82	0.61
	Beck Depression Inventory (BDI)	Parent	Stress/ Distress	18		7.17 (5.85)	18		8.33 (7.83)		0.17
	Family Quality of Life Questionnaire	Family	Functioning/ FQOL	18		30.94 (12.72)	18		47.53 (12.91)		1.30
	OVERALL										0.63

(continued)

TABLE 3.2 CONTINUED

				Intervention			Comparison					
Study	*Measure*	*Group*	*Outcome*	*n*	*Pre M (SD)*	*Post M (SD)*	*n*	*Pre M (SD)*	*Post M (SD)*	*F*	*t*	*d*
Griffin et al. (2010)	Strengths and Difficulties Questionnaire (SDQ)—Total Difficulties	Child	Behavior	46		14.71 (5.93)	35	18.13 (5.46)	17.17 (5.68)			0.52
	Parental Stress Scale (PSS)	Parent	Stress/ Distress	46	63.79 (11.84)	56.11 (12.50)	35	59.49 (11.57)	56.29 (13.32)			0.35
	OVERALL											0.43
Hand et al. (2012)	Strengths and Difficulties Questionnaire (SDQ)—Total Difficulties	Child	Behavior	16	20.56 (3.95)	16.44 (3.78)	13	15.62 (3.28)	16.15 (5.13)	8.610		0.07
	Parental Stress Index (PSI)—Total	Parent	Stress/ Distress	16	109.60 (33.54)	90.44 (28.24)	13	94.92 (16.11)	94.38 (23.85)	8.180		0.15
	OVERALL											0.11
Jang et al. (2012)	Researcher-developed ABA knowledge test	Parent	Knowledge	14	63.00 (0.00)	90.00 (0.00)	14	51.00 (0.00)	64.00 (0.00)		3.14	1.19
	OVERALL											1.19
Prieto-Bayard & Baker (1986)	Verbal Behavioral Vignettes Test	Parent	Knowledge	7	29.30	38.00 (0.00)	11	28.30 (0.00)	28.80 (0.00)	15.85		1.93

	Teaching Interview	Parent	Performance	7	15.60	18.00 (0.00)	11	14.10 (0.00)	12.70 (0.00)	4.90	1.07
	Child Behavior Checklist (CBCL)—Behavior Problems	Child	Behavior	7	27.90	15.30 (0.00)	11	27.80 (0.00)	26.90 (0.00)	4.85	1.07
	OVERALL										1.31
Quinn et al. (2006)—Post	Strengths and Difficulties Questionnaire (SDQ)—Total Difficulties	Child	Behavior	21	16.35 (4.47)	13.35 (3.88)	17	18.36 (3.73)	17.45 (6.08)		0.42
	Child Behavior Checklist (CBCL)—Total Problems	Child	Behavior	21	39.33 (21.26)	34.00 (20.33)	17	57.72 (24.16)	50.09 (30.51)		0.09
	General Health Questionnaire-12 (GHQ-12)—Parent adjustment	Parent	Stress/ Distress	21	21.40 (4.00)	18.85 (2.00)	17	28.18 (7.89)	25.63 (5.55)		0.00
	Family Assessment Device (FAD)—Family functioning	Family	Functioning/ FQOL	21	161.95 (12.91)	172.75 (15.85)	17	167.81 (24.28)	171.72 (25.42)		0.33
	Perceived Social Support Scale (PSSS)	Parent	Support	21	116.40 (16.52)	114.70 (18.71)	17	104.81 (22.35)	98.36 (23.70)		-0.23

(continued)

TABLE 3.2 CONTINUED

				Intervention			Comparison					
Study	*Measure*	*Group*	*Outcome*	*n*	*Pre M (SD)*	*Post M (SD)*	*n*	*Pre M (SD)*	*Post M (SD)*	*F*	*t*	*d*
	Family Inventory of Life Events and Changes (FILE)	Family	Functioning/ FQOL	21	256.35 (248.37)	194.40 (238.06)	17	385.90 (299.93)	314.90 (181.32)			0.04
	Parenting Stress Index (PSI)	Parent	Stress/ Distress	21	99.55 (26.00)	91.45 (20.63)	17	110.90 (17.06)	100.00 (24.20)			0.13
	Questionnaire on Resources and Stress (QRS)—Parenting stress	Parent	Stress/ Distress	21	26.30 (6.32)	27.90 (4.42)	17	34.00 (9.92)	32.90 (14.08)			-0.27
	OVERALL											0.06
Quinn et al. (2006)—Follow-Up	Strengths and Difficulties Questionnaire (SDQ)—Total Difficulties	Child	Behavior	19	13.35 (3.88)	12.95 (3.69)	11	17.45 (6.08)	13.09 (4.20)			1.02
	Child Behavior Checklist (CBCL)—Total Problems	Child	Behavior	19	34.00 (20.33)	36.27 (24.31)	11	50.09 (30.51)	50.00 (33.45)			-0.09
	General Health Questionnaire-12 (GHQ-12)—Parent adjustment	Parent	Stress/ Distress	19	18.85 (2.00)	23.10 (7.79)	11	25.63 (5.55)	19.27 (4.64)			1.55

	Family Assessment Device (FAD)—Family functioning	Family	Functioning/ FQOL	19	172.75 (15.85)	172.75 (43.05)	11	171.72 (25.42)	185.18 (19.19)	0.37
	Perceived Social Support Scale (PSSS)	Parent	Support	19	114.70 (18.71)	128.05 (75.78)	11	98.36 (23.70)	132.36 (39.60)	0.32
	Family Inventory of Life Events and Changes (FILE)	Family	Functioning/ FQOL	19	194.40 (238.06)	188.65 (243.95)	11	314.90 (181.32)	266.18 (148.32)	0.20
	Parenting Stress Index (PSI)	Parent	Stress/ Distress	19	91.45 (20.63)	90.35 (21.67)	11	100.00 (24.20)	93.54 (21.48)	0.25
	Questionnaire on Resources and Stress (QRS)—Parenting stress	Parent	Stress/ Distress	19	27.90 (4.42)	22.70 (8.44)	11	32.90 (14.08)	22.54 (9.30)	0.59
	OVERALL									0.49
Quinn et al. (2007)	Strengths and Difficulties Questionnaire (SDQ)—Total Difficulties	Child	Behavior	22	16.36 (4.58)	13.90 (4.34)	19	15.26 (3.34)	15.68 (3.60)	0.72
	Child Behavior Checklist (CBCL)—Total Problems	Child	Behavior	22	41.20 (21.80)	36.40 (20.81)	19	51.37 (32.82)	44.16 (26.48)	0.10

(continued)

TABLE 3.2 CONTINUED

				Intervention			Comparison					
Study	*Measure*	*Group*	*Outcome*	*n*	*Pre M (SD)*	*Post M (SD)*	*n*	*Pre M (SD)*	*Post M (SD)*	*F*	*t*	*d*
	General Health Questionnaire-12 (GHQ-12)—Parent adjustment	Parent	Stress/ Distress	22	21.59 (3.88)	19.04 (2.10)	19	20.05 (2.75)	19.63 (2.13)			-1.01
	Family Assessment Device (FAD)—Family functioning	Family	Functioning/ FQOL	22	170.04 (13.61)	171.36 (15.39)	19	178.63 (17.73)	176.05 (14.02)			0.26
	Perceived Social Support Scale (PSSS)	Parent	Support	22	112.41 (20.51)	113.45 (18.90)	19	117.00 (15.11)	120.89 (17.81)			0.16
	Family Inventory of Life Events and Changes (FILE)	Family	Functioning/ FQOL	22	268.95 (255.05)	191.63 (228.67)	19	135.00 (80.27)	129.00 (74.68)			0.41
	Parenting Stress Index (PSI)	Parent	Stress/ Distress	22	31.77 (7.70)	28.68 (7.80)	19	32.21 (7.54)	32.21 (7.87)			0.40
	Questionnaire on Resources and Stress (QRS)—Parenting stress	Parent	Stress/ Distress	22	9.86 (3.02)	9.77 (2.11)	19	10.92 (2.23)	9.64 (2.34)			0.54
	OVERALL											0.21

Solomon et al. (2008)	Eyberg Child Behavior Inventory (ECBI)										
	Intensity	Child	Behavior	10	67.00 (5.64)	59.70 (4.95)	9	65.67 (8.80)	62.22 (9.77)	0.75	0.51
	Problem	Child	Behavior	10	62.90 (6.30)	52.00 (6.52)	9	66.78 (8.51)	63.00 (7.31)	9.41	1.03
	Behavior Assessment System for Children (BASC)—Problem behavior										
	Aggression	Child	Behavior	10	63.90 (10.58)	59.00 (6.25)	9	70.33 (14.21)	67.78 (14.60)	0.44	0.21
	Hyperactivity	Child	Behavior	10	74.30 (8.29)	68.70 (11.68)	9	80.56 (13.95)	80.56 (8.31)	4.29	0.55
	Attention	Child	Behavior	10	72.80 (6.13)	65.80 (8.77)	9	70.89 (10.46)	70.67 (10.92)	4.01	0.69
	Conduct	Child	Behavior	10	67.40 (8.63)	59.90 (8.01)	9	67.00 (14.03)	66.00 (10.44)	4.14	0.70
	Behavior Assessment System for Children (BASC)—Social				0.00 (0.00)						
	Adaptability	Child	Skills	10	23.90 (7.91)	32.40 (10.23)	9	28.44 (6.48)	27.33 (10.38)	5.31	0.93

(*continued*)

TABLE 3.2 CONTINUED

				Intervention			Comparison					
Study	*Measure*	*Group*	*Outcome*	*n*	*Pre M (SD)*	*Post M (SD)*	*n*	*Pre M (SD)*	*Post M (SD)*	*F*	*t*	*d*
	Social Skills	Child	Skills	10	30.20 (3.77)	37.40 (5.80)	9	35.00 (10.52)	37.33 (6.91)	2.15		0.77
	Leadership	Child	Skills	10	36.20 (4.02)	38.10 (6.15)	9	33.89 (6.07)	37.56 (4.72)	0.08		0.32
	Depression	Child	Skills	10	60.00 (9.57)	53.60 (7.25)	9	72.33 (15.68)	65.11 (13.91)	3.28		0.08
	Atypicality	Child	Skills	10	75.50 (14.25)	69.10 (20.51)	9	72.33 (21.09)	78.33 (17.11)	4.59		0.65
	Parent Stress Index (PSI)	Parent	Stress/ Distress	10			9					0.63
	OVERALL											0.58
Tavormina (1975)	Hereford Parent Attitude Survey, Causation	Parent	Self-Efficacy	19			13				6.30	2.27
	Missouri Behavior Problem Checklist, Total	Child	Behavior	19			13				6.30	2.27
	Behavior observations of command play, Total	Family	Interaction	19			13				3.80	1.37
	Ratings of disruptiveness	Child	Behavior	19			13				2.50	0.90

	Ratings of parent emotional reaction to behavior	Family	Interaction	19	13	3.70	1.33
	OVERALL						1.54
All Studies		Parent					0.45
		Child					0.53
		Family					0.81
			Knowledge				1.20
			Performance				0.69
			Support				0.06
			Self-Efficacy				1.42
			Stress/ Distress				0.26
			Behavior				0.54
			Skills				0.54
			Interaction				1.48
			Functioning/ FQOL				0.40
	OVERALL BPT						0.58

TABLE 3.3 EFFECT SIZES OF BEHAVIORAL PARENT TRAINING GROUP COMPARISON STUDIES

Study	*Measures*	*d*	*95% CI*	*d and 95% CI*
Bagner & Eyberg (2007)	A + C + H	0.945	[0.645, 1.246]	
Baker & Brightman (1984)	D + E	0.914	[0.166, 1.661]	
Brightman et al. (1982)	A + D + E	0.623	[0.310, 0.936]	
Chadwick et al. (2001)—Post	A + H	0.256	[-0.042, 0.553]	
Chadwick et al. (2001)—Follow-up	A + H	0.080	[-0.217, 0.376]	
Feldman & Werner (2002)	A + B + F + H	0.663	[0.358, 0.908]	
Griffin et al. (2010)	A + H	0.433	[0.119, 0.748]	
Hand et al. (2012)	A + H	0.110	[-0.408, 0.628]	
Jang et al. (2012)	D	1.186	[0.383, 1.989]	
Prieto-Bayard & Baker (1986)	A + D + E	1.310	[0.705, 1.915]	
Quinn et al. (2006)—Post	A + B + H + I	0.064	[-0.163, 0.29]	
Quinn et al. (2006)—Follow-up	A + B + H + I	0.491	[0.221, 0.760]	
Quinn et al. (2007)	A + B + H + I	0.207	[-0.014, 0.427]	
Solomon et al. (2008)	A + G + H	0.580	[0.313, 0.846]	
Tavormina (1975)	A + C + F	1.541	[1.178, 1.903]	
Overall		0.579	[0.368, 0.790]	

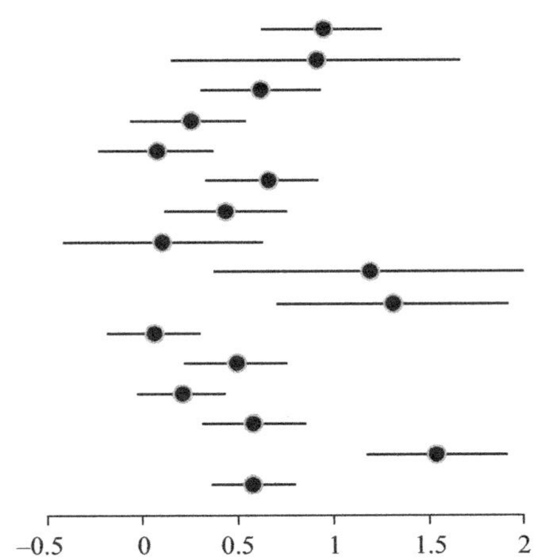

Note. A = Behavior; B = Functioning/Family Quality of Life; C = Interaction; D = Knowledge; E = Performance; F = Self-Efficacy; G = Skills; H = Stress/Distress; I = Support

treatment effect of BPT on child's problem behaviors ($d = 0.54$) and on child's learned skills ($d = 0.54$).

Likewise, the average effect sizes of all BPT programs on parent outcomes and family system outcomes were calculated, and Table 3.2 shows they are .45, and .81 respectively. The effect sizes corresponding to parent outcomes reveal small overall treatment effects of BPT for parents of children with DD, including the lowest treatment effect of BPT on parent's perceived support ($d = 0.06$), a small treatment effect of BPT on parent's reduced level of stress/distress ($d = 0.26$), a moderate treatment effect of BPT on parent's performance of learned skills ($d = 0.69$), a large treatment effect of BPT on parent's acquisition of knowledge ($d = 1.2$), and the largest treatment effect of BPT on parent's self-efficacy ($d = 1.42$). For the family system outcomes, the effect sizes of parent-implemented intervention programs suggest a small effect of family well-being (family functioning or family quality of life) ($d = 0.40$) and a large effect of parent and child interaction ($d = 1.48$). It indeed makes sense that a large effect of BPT on parent and child interaction suggests that BPT programs that focus on enhancing parents' capacity to implement proper behavioral techniques have made significant impacts on the ways that parents interact with their children with DD effectively.

In addition, we used another way of looking at the data to answer the question "Overall what is the effect size for the BPT programs?" The overall effect size of all BPT programs for children with DD is $d = 0.58$, suggesting a moderate treatment effect. This result is encouraging, and it suggests that BPT programs are effective for not only the treatment effect of proximal outcomes such as parent skill acquisition and parent self-efficacy, which the intervention programs directly target, but also collateral effect on distal outcomes such as improvement of both child outcomes (e.g., progress on skill learning and decrease of problem behaviors), parent reduced stress levels, and family well-being (e.g., family quality of life). However, the caveats to note are that BPT programs with a primary focus on acquisition and improvement of parents' skills do not necessarily eliminate caregiving stress despite a minimal collateral effect on parents' reduced stress level and have limited positive impact on family quality of life of families of children with DD.

EVIDENCE OF BEHAVIORAL PARENT TRAINING: SINGLE-SUBJECT DESIGN STUDIES

The core of BPT training for parents consists of the antecedent-behavior-consequence (ABC) model of ABA. Despite the diversity of behavior strategies training across different BPT programs, there are some common core topics and behavior strategies surrounding the ABC model. The behavior strategies are often organized as antecedent-based versus consequence-based strategies in the ABA literature. As a result of the literature search, we identified a total of 41 articles that meet the selection criteria. Table 3.4 summarizes these SSD studies. These articles report effects of parents' successful use of a variety of

TABLE 3.4 SUMMARY OF SINGLE-SUBJECT DESIGN STUDIES ON BEHAVIORAL PARENT TRAINING

Author(s)	*Design/Intervention components/Manual/ Fidelity*	*Participants (Sample, Age, Ethnicity)/Setting (Parent Training, Child Intervention)*	*DV Measures*	*Treatment Effect(s)*
Antecedents-Based Studies (23 studies)				
Adubato, Adams, & Budd (1981)	• SSD (multiple baseline across mother's and father's responses) • To train a parent child management skills and to teach procedures to spouse • Written and verbal directions and feedback for parents on using appropriate instruction, physical guidance, partial guidance, and reductions in parent preempts • No manual reported • No fidelity reported	• 6-year-old boy with multiple disabilities and his mother and father • No race/ethnicity information reported • Setting: clinic	PARENT • Appropriate instructions • Physical guidance, partial guidance • No parent preempts across training and generalization child behaviors CHILD • Sustained attending • Intermittent attending • Independent completion of steps • Noncompliance	Parenting behaviors improved in rate and stability when mother or father implemented procedures, except for physical guidance by mother (unstable baseline). With mother and father, child's target behaviors improved. Generalization to other child activities (eating and toy use) showed improvement in most parent responses and decreases in child noncompliance but inconsistent results for other child behaviors.

Derby et al. (1997)	• SSD (multiple baseline across subjects design) • To decrease child aberrant behavior (e.g., self-injury, aggression, destruction) • Parent training for implementing FCT treatment package; provision of report of the assessment results and a description of the treatment contingencies (positive reinforcement plus time-out or combination of negative reinforcement and positive reinforcement plus guided compliance), a 1-hour training session, feedback of the treatment contingencies, and daily 10- to 30-min training to the children • No manual reported • Child intervention fidelity (reinforcement integrity, punishment integrity) reported	• 4 children with aberrant behaviors and DD (3 boys and 1 girl, ages 2–5 years) and their mothers • No race/ethnicity information reported • Setting: PT and CI at home	PARENT • Reinforcement behavior • Mild punishment behavior CHILD • Target behavior • Mands • Appropriate behavior • Collateral responses	Short-term treatment effects showed immediate decreases in aberrant behavior for 3 of 4 children. Long-term effects revealed that all children showed not only reduction in aberrant behavior and increase in appropriate communication but also increases in the nontargeted social behaviors for all children.
Ducharme & Drain (2004)	• SSD (multiple baseline across subjects design) • To increase compliance to academic requests in children with autism • Parents training on errorless compliance training through two clinic-based group workshops (introduction and request delivery) and two individual sessions (treatment procedures) • No manual reported • No fidelity reported	• 4 children with autism (ages 42–80 months, 3 boys and 1 girl) • No race/ethnicity information reported • Setting: PT at clinic and CI at home	PARENT • Consumer satisfaction questionnaire • Compliance probability checklists (parental rating on child's compliance for level 1 or 2 request CHILD • Observations of child compliance	Errorless compliance training increased children's compliance on academic requests. Treatment showed generalization to nontreatment academic requests and nonacademic general request after intervention.

(*continued*)

TABLE 3.4 CONTINUED

Author(s)	*Design/Intervention components/Manual/ Fidelity*	*Participants (Sample, Age, Ethnicity)/Setting (Parent Training, Child Intervention)*	*DV Measures*	*Treatment Effect(s)*
Ducharme, Harris, Milligan, & Pontes (2003)	• SSD (multiple baseline across subjects design) • To increase children's compliance to parental requests • Parental instructions on using errorless compliance training (reinforcement for child compliance only and reinforcement compliance plus delivery of requests in a four-level hierarchy) • No manual reported • No fidelity reported	• 4 children at risk for DD (ages 4–7 years, 2 boys and 2 girls) and 4 mothers • No race/ethnicity information reported • Setting: PT and CI at home	CHILD • Compliance to parental requests	Increased child compliance to parental requests. Reinforcement compliance plus graduated request delivery is more effective than reinforcement compliance alone.
Ducharme et al. (1994)	• SSD (multiple baseline across subjects design) • To produce high percentages of compliance • Parental instructions using an abbreviated version errorless compliance training approach (reinforcement for child compliance and delivery of requests in a four-level hierarchy) • No manual reported • No fidelity reported	• 4 children with DD (ages 3–5 years, 3 boys and 1 girl) and 2 nondelayed siblings (age 3 years, 1 girl and 1 boy) and four mothers • No race/ethnicity information reported • Setting: PT and CI at home	PARENT • Consumer satisfaction questionnaire CHILD • Compliance to parental requests • Maladaptive behaviors	High levels of compliance and reductions in maladaptive behavior throughout treatment and follow-up sessions were reported.

Ducharme & Popynick (1993)	• SSD (multiple baseline across subjects design) • To produce high percentages of compliance of children • Parental instructions using an errorless compliance training approach (categorization of compliance probability, a technique of request presenting and reinforcement) • No manual reported • No fidelity reported	• 4 children with DD (ages 5–8, 3 boys and 1 girl) and their mothers • No race/ethnicity information reported • Setting: PT and CI at home	PARENT • Consumer satisfaction questionnaire CHILD • Compliance to parental requests • Maladaptive behaviors	High compliance levels were obtained. There was generalization to untrained requests. Maladaptive behavior decreased during compliance situations.
Ducharme, Popynick, Pontes, & Steele (1996)	• SSD (multiple baseline across-group design with simultaneous replication) • To increase child compliance to parental requests • A group format of parental instructions using an errorless compliance training approach (reinforcement for child compliance and delivery of requests in a four-level hierarchy) • No manual reported • No fidelity reported	• 5 children with DD (ages 4–5, 4 boys and 1 girl) and their parents (4 mothers and 1 father) • All Caucasian • Setting: PT at clinic and CI at home	PARENT • Consumer satisfaction questionnaire CHILD • Compliance to parental requests	Compliance of all children increased. The errorless compliance training can be trained in an efficient clinic-based group format.
Harrold, Lutzker, Campbell, & Touchette (1992)	• SSD (multiple probe design, two families received PAT followed by CMT, and the other two received PAT and CMT in a reverse order) • Parents training on Planned Activities Training (PAT, emphasis on antecedent control of behavior, activity planning, use of incidental teaching techniques, statement of the rules of each activity in advance) and Child Management Training (CMT, emphasis on consequences) • Manualized (Sanders, 1987; Sanders & Dadds, 1987, with modification) • No fidelity reported	• 4 children with DD (ages 3–8 years) and their mothers • No race/ethnicity information reported • Setting: PT and CI at home	PARENT • Leveling • Verbal response • Verbal instructions • Appropriate follow-up • Parenting stress index • Consumer satisfaction questionnaire CHILD • On-task behavior, • Cryig and aggre ssion	Both PAT and CMT increased the mothers' leveling, verbal response, instructions, and appropriate follow-up and the children's on-task behaviors, absence of crying or aggression. PAT was slightly preferred by mothers.

(continued)

TABLE 3.4 CONTINUED

Author(s)	*Design/Intervention components/Manual/Fidelity*	*Participants (Sample, Age, Ethnicity)/Setting (Parent Training, Child Intervention)*	*DV Measures*	*Treatment Effect(s)*
Humm, Blampied, Liberty (2005)	• SSD (multiple baseline across behaviors) • To increase child compliance • 2 training sessions and intervention manual on effective requests, descriptive praise, extinction, and high-*p* request procedure • Manualized (adapted from Ducharme & Worling, 1994) • No fidelity reported	• 3 children with DD (ages 6–10) • No race/ethnicity information reported • Setting: home	CHILD • Percentage of compliance across behaviors	Treatment associated with increases in compliance, with 2 of 3 participants maintaining compliance levels at follow-up.
Huynen, Lutzker, Bigelow, Touchette, & Campbell (1996)	• SSD (a multiple probe experimental design across two families with a replication across two more families) • To increase appropriate child behavior and parenting behavior • Individual parent training (five 90-minute sessions) on Planned Activities Training (PAT; planning and structuring activities to prevent challenging behaviors, emphasizing of the use of tangible reinforcers) using demonstration, discussion, role-playing, and feedback) • Manualized (Sanders & Dodds, 1987) • Child intervention fidelity (mother's implementation of skills) reported	• 4 children with a DD (ages 2–6 years) and their mothers • 3 Caucasian and 1 Hispanic • Setting: PT at home; CI at home or community	PARENT • Mother's use of the 18-item PAT skills • Mother's use of 7 parent skills CHILD • Appropriate child behavior (on task, following instructions, communication and physical contact) • Problem-setting questionnaire (PSQ) by mothers	Mothers' use of PAT procedures improved (more than doubled). Three mothers' appropriate behaviors increased from 25% to 40%. Child appropriate behaviors improved. Intervention gains were maintained at 1, 3, and 6 months.

Krantz, MacDuff, & McClannahan (1993)	• SSD (multiple baseline across participants) • To assess the effects of intensive, short-term, in-home assistance to teach parents to help their children follow photographic schedules • Parents training on the use of manual prompts and graduated guidance to teach following photographic schedules (for leisure, social interaction, self-care, and housekeeping tasks) using modeling, supervised practice, and feedback • No manual reported • No fidelity reported	• 3 children with autism (ages 6–8) and their families • No race/ethnicity information reported • Setting: home	CHILD • Engagement • Disruptive behavior • Social initiations	Increases in children's engagement and social initiations and decreases in disruptive behavior were found. Intervention gains were maintained for as long as 10 months.
Lerman, Swiezy, Perkins-Parks, & Roane (2000)	• SSD (multiple baseline across parent behaviors) • To increase child compliance • Written and verbal instructions and corrective feedback used to train parents on differential reinforcement, extinction, and prompting • No manual reported • Parents' fidelity reported	• 3 mothers and their children with ID (2 comorbid with autism, ages 5–12) • No race/ethnicity information reported • Setting: clinic or home	PARENT • Response to inappropriate behavior • Use of differential reinforcement • Use of instructional prompts • Response to compliance CHILD • Percentage of intervals with inappropriate behavior • Percentage of compliance	All parents reached criterion after instructions or instructions with feedback and maintained performance at follow-up. Increased child compliance for all 3 children and decreased inappropriate behavior for 2 children.
Matson & Francis (1994)	• SSD (multiple baseline design across behaviors) • To improve child's spontaneous verbalization • Caregiver training and implementation of a visual cue procedure (cueing, prompting, rewarding, and fading) • No manual reported • No fidelity reported	• 2 children with a DD (34 months and 4-years-old) and their caregivers (mother and aunt) • No race/ethnicity information reported • Setting: PT and CI at home	CHILD • Greeting response • Request for favored food	Increases in both children's greeting response and request for favored food

(*continued*)

TABLE 3.4 CONTINUED

Author(s)	*Design/Intervention components/Manual/ Fidelity*	*Participants (Sample, Age, Ethnicity)/Setting (Parent Training, Child Intervention)*	*DV Measures*	*Treatment Effect(s)*
Moes & Frea (2002)	• SSD (multiple baseline design across participants) • To reduce child problem behavior and increase functional communication • Individualized functional assessment and functional communication training (FCT) for the family use of FCT based on family context. Parent-implemented FCT. One to two days per week training sessions, with follow-up at 2-month intervals for 1 year after training completed • Manualized • No fidelity reported	• 3 children with autism (all age 3, 2 boys and 1 girl) and their mothers • No race/ethnicity information specified • Setting: PT and CI at home	PARENT • Index of the treatment package's fit with family context CHILD • Percent of 10-second intervals with problem behaviors • Percent of 10-second intervals with functional communication	Contextualized FCT decreased problem behavior and increased functional communication in both training routines and generalization probes. A larger increase was found in mothers' ratings of sustainability with training package than fathers'.
O'Reilly, Lancioni, & Taylor (1999)	• SSD (multielement) • To reduce high levels of aggression • Mother trained to assess two extinction interventions (extinction by omission and NCR) and both parents were trained to use NCR treatment at follow-up • No manual reported • No fidelity reported	• 10-year-old boy with mild ID and parents • No race/ethnicity information reported • Setting: home	CHILD • Percentage of intervals with aggression	With extinction by omission, aggression initially decreased to zero and reoccurred at end of phase. In NCR phase, aggression levels reached zero and occurred intermittently but did not reoccur at end of phase. Aggression occurred in less than 20% of observations at follow-up.

Powers, Singer, Stevens, & Sowers (1992)	• SSD (multiple probe across families design) • To confirm parents generalization of behavioral parent training techniques • Four 1-hour parent training sessions (implementing planned activities strategies and contingency management strategies using didactic instruction, demonstration, role-play) and ongoing biweekly coaching session (with one family's in vivo coaching) • Manualized (Sanders & Dadds, 1982) • Child intervention fidelity checked	• 3 children (ages 4–9) with a DD and disruptive behavior and their mothers • All Caucasian • Setting: PT at home; CI at home and community	PARENT • Parent accuracy of implementation of CMT and PAT CHILD • Percentage of intervals of disruptive behavior • Child management difficulty by mother's rating	Parents showed the accurate use of the techniques trained. Child disruptive behavior and mothers' rating of disruptive behavior decreased with intervention in both training and generalization settings. One parent required in situ training in generalization setting, suggesting a need for individualized BPT.
Russell & Matson (1998)	• SSD (multiple baseline across parent behaviors) • To train fathers to use behavior management skills while teaching child self-help skills • Using verbal and written directions, role-play, practice, and feedback, experimenters instructed fathers to give correct instructions, appropriate positive attention, and appropriate consequences • No manual reported • Child intervention fidelity checked	• 3 boys (ages 2–4) with DD or developmental delay and their fathers • Two children are White and one is Black • Setting: home	PARENT • Percentage of correct instructions • Percentage of correct positive attention • Percentage of correct consequences CHILD • Percentage of child compliance to commands • Parent's Consumer Satisfaction Questionnaire • Parenting Stress Index-Short Form	Compared with baseline, correct instructions, correct positive attention, and appropriate consequences increased. Two children made modest gains in compliance following fathers' correct instructions training. One child increased compliance following father's correct instructions training and made further gains following appropriate consequences training.

(*continued*)

TABLE 3.4 CONTINUED

Author(s)	*Design/Intervention components/Manual/Fidelity*	*Participants (Sample, Age, Ethnicity)/Setting (Parent Training, Child Intervention)*	*DV Measures*	*Treatment Effect(s)*
Sanders & Plant (1989)	• SSD (multiple baseline design across subjects including a non-treatment control subject) • To make improvements in the levels of deviant child behaviors • 9 weeks of parent training (4 weeks behavior management procedures and 5 weeks planned activities training) using instruction, discussion, modeling, rehearsal, and feedback • Manualized (Sanders & Dadds, 1982) • Child intervention fidelity checked	• 5 children with DD (4 boys and 1 girl, ages 3–5) • All Caucasian • Setting: home	PARENT • Percentage of intervals of parental aversive and nonaversive behavior • Percentage of intervals of correct implementation treatment procedures CHILD • Percentage of intervals of deviant behavior	Distinct reductions in children's deviant behaviors, changes in parental aversive and nonaversive behaviors, and increases in parental implementation procedure
Smith & Lerman (1999)	• SSD (multielement and multiple baseline across participants) • To train parents to increase children's compliance with low-probability (low-*p*) requests • Parents trained by written and verbal instruction, demonstration, role-play, and feedback to use guided compliance and high-*p* instructional sequences and praise • No manual reported • Child intervention fidelity checked	• 2 boys (ages 4 and 5) with autism/PDD and mild ID and their mothers • No race/ethnicity information reported • Setting: home	PARENT • Mean percentage of parents' correct treatment components CHILD • Percentage of intervals with compliance	While both guided compliance and high-*p* instructional sequence procedures increased compliance, compliance levels were higher when using guided compliance. Parents implemented procedures with high degree of accuracy that mostly maintained in final phase of treatment.

Van Hasselt, Sisson, & Aach (1987)	• SSD (multiple baseline across parent behaviors) • To increase child compliance and on-task behavior, decrease inappropriate behavior and stereotypic behavior • Individual training with direct instructions, role-playing, modeling, practice, and feedback on definitive commands and positive attention • No manual • Child intervention fidelity checked	• Mother of 4-year-old boy with DD and physical disability • Race/ethnicity: White • Setting: Clinic	CHILD • Percentage of intervals across child behaviors (compliance, oppositional behavior, on-task behavior, and stereotypic behavior) PARENT & CHILD • Percentage of intervals across parent behaviors (definitive commands, positive attention for child compliance, and persistence with command for child noncompliance)	Parent's appropriate parenting skills increased. Child compliance and on-task behavior increased while oppositional behavior decreased. No change in stereotypic responses.
Wacker et al. (1998)	• Single case analysis • To decrease child aberrant behavior • Individualized parent training on functional analysis (an extensive parent interview, observation, and functional analyses using a multielement design), functional communication treatment (reinforcement for appropriate behaviors, extinction or mild punishment) and child intervention (about 5–10 minutes per day) • Manualized • No fidelity reported	• 28 children with developmental disabilities and aberrant behavior, (ages 1–5, mean age 3 years 3 months) • Ethnicity/race not specified • Setting: PT and CI at home	PARENT • Treatment acceptability (average 6.35) CHILD • Percentage of intervals of aberrant behavior (87% decrease) • Percentage of intervals of appropriate social responding (69% increase)	Treatment resulted in decrease in aberrant behavior and increase in appropriate social responding, and the parent-rated treatment acceptability averaging 6.35 (ranging from 1 to 7).

(*continued*)

TABLE 3.4 CONTINUED

Author(s)	*Design/Intervention components/Manual/ Fidelity*	*Participants (Sample, Age, Ethnicity)/Setting (Parent Training, Child Intervention)*	*DV Measures*	*Treatment Effect(s)*
Wacker et al. (2005)	• SSD (nonconcurrent multiple baseline) • To decrease child aberrant behavior • Individualized parent training on functional analysis, function communication treatment (reinforcement for appropriate adaptive behaviors and communicative behaviors, and reductive procedures that were matched to the function of the behavior) • Manualized • No fidelity reported	• 25 children with DD (6 girls and 19 boys, ages 1–6, mean age 4 years 5 months) • No race/ethnicity information reported • Setting: PT and CI at home	PARENT • Treatment acceptability CHILD • Percentage of aberrant behavior (averaging 85% decrease) • Stimulus generalization (66.25% to 100% reduction)	Intervention resulted in pre/post decrease in problem behaviors averaging 85%. In addition, mean pre/post decreases showed across all stimulus conditions (persons, settings, and tasks). Study showed the package is effective in reduction of problem behavior and substantial stimulus generalization.
Wacker et al. (2013)	• SSD (nonconcurrent multiple base design across 6 participants) • To reduce child problem behavior and improve functional communication by delivering functional communication training (FCT) treatment via telehealth • Parents provided FCT program (FCT escape, FCT tangible, and FCT attention) at regional clinics (weekly 60-minute visits) by behavior consultants via telecommunication • Manualized • No fidelity reported	• 17 children with ASD who display problem behavior (1 girl and 16 boys, ages 29–80 months) and their parents (16 mothers and 2 fathers) • No race/ethnicity information reported • Setting: PT at clinic and teleconsultation center; CI at home	PARENT • Treatment acceptability (average 6.47 out of 7.00) CHILD • Percent of intervals of destructive behavior (93.5)	Child target problem behavior decreased over 90% for majority children (at least 68.7%). Parents perceived treatment highly acceptable averaging 6.47 out of 7.00.

Consequences-Based Studies (18 studies)				
Allen, Kuhn, DeHaai, & Wallace (2013)	• SSD (multiple baseline across participants) • To improve sleep-related behaviors • Parent training on creating a sleep-compatible environment, adjusting and regulating sleep-wake schedules and standard extinction • No manual reported • No fidelity reported	• 2 boys and 3 girls (ages 2–11) with Angelman syndrome • No race/ethnicity information reported • Setting: PT via video/ telephone connections	CHILD • Disruptive behavior • Independent sleep onset • Actigraphy measures	Decreased disruptive behaviors at bedtime, falling asleep independently, independent sleep onset, and increased length of sleep.
Anderson & McMillan (2001)	• SSD (reversal design) • To evaluate the efficacy of parental use of treatment for child food selectivity • Parent training on a treatment package including escape extinction and differential reinforcement using instruction, modeling, videotape review, and feedback • No manual reported • No fidelity reported	• 5-year-old boy with PDD and severe ID • No race/ethnicity information reported • Setting: Home	PARENT • Reinforcer delivery • Offering a bite of food CHILD • Bites accepted • Bites interrupted • Bites expelled • Bites presented during self-injury occurred	Parents were able to serve as change agents using escape extinction and DRA in a home setting. A child consumed age-appropriate portions of nonpreferred food.
Aurand, Sisson, Aach, & Van Hasselt (1989)	• SSD (multiple baseline across behaviors) • To reduce child's self-stimulating behaviors • Initial training conducted with classroom staff in DRI and physical interruption of nondesired behaviors • Mother trained to examine generalization and maintenance in home setting; booster training session initiated after increase of behaviors at home at follow-up • No manual reported • No fidelity reported	• 4-year-old boy with moderate DD, classroom staff, and mother • No race/ethnicity information reported • Setting: CI in classroom and home	CHILD • Percentage of intervals across behaviors (tongue chewing, hand flapping, hand weaving)	Self-stimulatory behaviors decreased and maintained at low levels compared with baseline. Probes conducted at home also showed reduction in behavior during treatment. Behaviors increased at follow-up at home. Following booster training session with mother, behaviors decreased.

(*continued*)

TABLE 3.4 CONTINUED

Author(s)	*Design/Intervention components/Manual/Fidelity*	*Participants (Sample, Age, Ethnicity)/Setting (Parent Training, Child Intervention)*	*DV Measures*	*Treatment Effect(s)*
Brehony, Benson, Solomon, & Luscomb (1980)	• SSD (multiple baseline across behaviors) • To reduce throwing and noncompliance and to increase compliance and time spent in chair • Parents trained in 12 daily 30-minute sessions; following baseline, sessions focused on verbal punishment for child's target behaviors and social reinforcement of positive behavior • No manual reported • No fidelity reported	• 7-year-old White male child with DD • Setting: PT and CI at clinic	CHILD • Frequency of throwing responses • Percentage of noncompliant responses • Duration of time spent in chair (in minutes)	Frequency of throwing responses and percentage of noncompliant responses decreased during treatment compared with baseline, while in-seat behavior increased in duration. Generalization to natural setting and maintenance of postintervention levels at 2-month follow-up occurred across behaviors.
Christopherson, Arnold, Hill, & Quilitch (1972)	• SSD (multiple baseline across social behaviors) • To increase some child behaviors (e.g., completion of chores) and decrease child inappropriate behaviors (e.g., bickering) • Parents trained using video, written directions, and therapist feedback to implement token economy system to reinforce desired behaviors and to use response cost to punish inappropriate target behaviors • Manualized (*Achievement Place*) • No fidelity reported	• Two families with one family having a child with ID (age 8) • No race/ethnic information reported • Setting: PT at clinic and home; CI at home	CHILD • Desired behaviors individualized per child • Inappropriate social behaviors individualized per child	For family with child with ID, all children completed desired behaviors consistently (100%) following implementation of home point system. For child with ID, introduction of 10-point fine substantially decreased problem behaviors (whining, bickering, and jumping on furniture).

Friman & Altman (1990)	• SSD (reversal) • To decrease disruptive behavior • Parents were instructed in DRI procedures to reinforce appropriate behavior and decrease inappropriate behavior (e.g., out-of-seat, throwing) • No manual reported • No fidelity reported	• 4-year-old boy with DD and low speech skills and few self-help skills; his parents • No race/ethnicity information reported • Setting: clinic	CHILD • Mean rate of child's out-of-seat behavior • Appropriate toy play • Mouthing occurrence rate • Throwing occurrence rate	Results indicated that DRI treatment was associated with gains in appropriate behavior and decreases in out-of-seat and mouthing of toy behaviors. Changes in toy throwing associated with treatment were less clear.
Friman, Barnard, Altman, & Wolf (1986)	• SSD (reversal and multiple baseline across settings) • To decrease child's aggressive behavior (pinching) • Parent and teacher trained using didactic presentations, modeling, written and verbal directions, and feedback • Parent implemented DRO, DRO plus time-out, DRO plus response interruption, and DRI (mealtime only) procedures • Teacher implemented DRO plus response interruption • No manual reported • No fidelity reported	• 10-year-old girl with DD, mother, and teacher • No race/ethnicity information reported • Setting: school and home	CHILD • Percent of intervals with pinching across settings (home play, school play, and mealtime)	During home play, pinching initially decreased but then increased to baseline levels in DRO, DRO plus time-out phases. Pinching decreased in DRO plus response interruption phases. During play at school, aggressive behaviors decreased after implementation of DRO plus response interruption. Pinching also decreased at mealtime following DRI implementation.
Handen, Parrish, McClung, Kerwin, & Evans (1992)	• SSD (ABAC design) • To increase child compliance • First phase, parents trained to implement differential reinforcement or guided compliance for error correction; second phase, parents implemented differential reinforcement or time-out. • No manual reported • No fidelity reported	• 5 boys (ages 3–6) with mild DD (ID, language delays, and nonspecific LD) • No race/ethnicity information reported • Setting: clinic	CHILD • Mean percentage of compliance	Child compliance increased for trained requests and generalized to untrained requests.

(*continued*)

TABLE 3.4 CONTINUED

Author(s)	*Design/Intervention components/Manual/Fidelity*	*Participants (Sample, Age, Ethnicity)/Setting (Parent Training, Child Intervention)*	*DV Measures*	*Treatment Effect(s)*
Hawkins, Peterson, Schweid, & Bijou (1966)	• SSD (reversal) • To reduce child's aggressive and noncompliant behaviors • Mother trained to tell child to stop behavior, to administer time-out, or to give attention and praise when experimenter provides specific signal contingent on child behavior • No manual reported • No fidelity reported	• 4-year-old boy with ID and mother • No race/ethnicity information reported • Setting: home	CHILD • Frequency (number of intervals) of problem behavior	Problem behaviors decreased slightly from baseline to first experimental phase. Problem behavior trended slightly downward during withdrawal phase and maintained in second experimental phase and during follow-up.
Lalli, Casey, & Kates (1997)	• SSD (reversal for 2 participants, multiple baseline across settings for 1 participant) • To reduce severe child problem behaviors • Parents were trained in the using written instructions, modeling, role-play, and feedback to implement NCR or NCR plus extinction in generalization phase • No manual reported • No fidelity reported	• 3 children (ages 3–9) with DD and their parents • No race/ethnicity information reported • Setting: clinic	CHILD • Rate (occurrence per minute) of child aggression or self-injurious behavior (and across settings for 1 participant)	Rates of aggression or self-injurious behaviors decreased during parent training for 1 child, initially spiked but decreased for 2 children.

Marcus, Swanson, & Vollmer (2001)	• SSD (multiple baseline across participants) • To decrease inappropriate and increase appropriate child behavior and improve parenting behavior • Individual training using role-play, modeling, immediate and delayed feedback, observation, and booster (as needed) on time-out procedures, as well as antecedents, differential negative reinforcement, and guided compliance or DRA and NCR • No manual reported • Child intervention fidelity checked	• 4 mother–child dyads with children with DD and speech delays (ages 3–5) • No race/ethnicity information reported • Setting: home or school	PARENT • Percentage of mother's correct and incorrect responses to child behaviors CHILD • Percentage of intervals with child compliance/tolerance and aggression	Increased child compliance and tolerance and decreased inappropriate behaviors. Parents improved appropriate responses to children's appropriate and inappropriate behaviors.
McDonald & Budd (1983)	• SSD (multiple baseline across behaviors for booster training) • To increase child compliance and improve parenting behavior • Individual training with didactic teaching, reading assignments, and discussion on defining target behavior, differential reinforcement with time-out, and follow-through techniques. Booster trainings with feedback and review of procedures were administered for correct follow-through and then for praise to compliance. • No manual reported • Child intervention fidelity checked	• Mother and 7-year-old boy with Down syndrome • No race/ethnicity information reported • Setting: home	PARENT • Percentage of instructional trials with parent's correct follow-through • Percentage of intervals with parental praise to child compliance CHILD • Percentage of intervals with child compliance	Increased parent follow-through at initial training and increased praise and child compliance at booster trainings.

(*continued*)

TABLE 3.4 CONTINUED

Author(s)	*Design/Intervention components/Manual/ Fidelity*	*Participants (Sample, Age, Ethnicity)/Setting (Parent Training, Child Intervention)*	*DV Measures*	*Treatment Effect(s)*
Najdowski, Wallace, Doney, & Ghezzi (2003)	• SSD (multiple baseline across settings) • To increase child food acceptance • Parent trained to implement functional analysis and treatment involving differential reinforcement, escape extinction, and demand fading • No manual reported • No fidelity reported	• 5-year-old boy with autism • No race/ethnicity information reported • Setting: home and community	CHILD • Bites of accepted and swallowed nonpreferred food	Parents were able to implement treatment package. Child showed increased food acceptance at home and in community.
Niemeyer & Fox (1990)	• SSD (reversal design) • To decrease child aggressive behavior in car-riding • Parents were trained to use DRO and token reinforcement with a formal training session, modeling by experimenter, and in vivo feedback in car ride • No manual reported • No fidelity reported	• 17-year old with ID and his parents • 5-year old with Down syndrome and his parents and sister • No race/ethnicity information reported • Setting: transportation	CHILD • Rate (occurrences per minute) of aggression (hitting or biting self or others, grabbing others, throwing objects) • Frequency of perseverative talk • Rate of seatbelt removal	For first child, aggressive behaviors reduced to zero and perseverative talk decreased during treatment phases. Levels increased or became more variable during reversal phases. Treatment was successfully faded and zero rates of aggression and perseverative talk were found during follow-up. For second child, aggression and seatbelt removal was reduced to zero at end of treatment phase, compared with variable aggression during reversal phase. Aggression and seatbelt removal remained low at follow-up.

Seiverling, Williams, Sturmey, & Hart (2012)	• SSD (multiple baseline across participants) • To improve parenting responses to children's food selectivity and to increase child food intake • Mothers trained by modeling, role-play, and feedback to implement DRA and escape extinction procedures • No manual reported • Child intervention fidelity checked	• 3 mother–child dyads with 3 boys (ages 4–8) with ASD • No race/ethnicity information reported • Setting: home	PARENT • Percentage of correct steps performed by parent CHILD • Percentage of accepted bites eaten within 30 seconds • Percentage of disruptive behavior	Mothers' correct implementation increased, compared with baseline, and maintained at follow-up. Children's food intake increased and disruptive behaviors decreased.
Thackeray & Richdale (2002)	• SSD (multiple baseline across participants) • To improve sleep related behaviors (settling, waking, cosleeping) • Parent trained on a treatment package including bedtime routines and standard extinction • Manualized (The 5 Step Sleep Programme) • No fidelity information reported	• 3 boys (ages 5–10) with ID • No race/ethnicity information reported • Setting: clinic and home and via phone	PARENT • Programme Evaluation Questionnaire CHILD • Actigraphy measures • Goal Achievement Scale • Developmental Behaviour Checklist • On-task classroom behavior observation checklist	Children fell asleep independently in their own bed and with reduced night waking for 2 of 3 subjects. Two of 3 children's daytime behaviors improved with increased alertness and on-task behavior and decreased disruptive behavior at home and school.
Weiskop, Matthews, & Richdale (2001)	• SSD (noncurrent multiple baseline across participants) • To fall asleep independently and in own bed for entire night • Parent training on setting bedtime, establishing bedtime routines, creating a sleep-compatible environment, reinforcement and standard extinction • No manual reported (written notes for each technique and checklists for each skill provided) • No fidelity reported	• One boy (age 5) with autism • No race/ethnicity information reported • Setting: PT at home and clinic	CHILD • Sleep diary • Falling asleep independently in own bed • Remaining in own bed all night • Time to fall asleep	Child fell asleep independently, in his own bed with reduced night waking and nighttime behavior problems.

(*continued*)

TABLE 3.4 CONTINUED

Author(s)	*Design/Intervention components/Manual/Fidelity*	*Participants (Sample, Age, Ethnicity)/Setting (Parent Training, Child Intervention)*	*DV Measures*	*Treatment Effect(s)*
Werle, Murphy, & Budd (1993)	• SSD (nonconcurrent multiple baseline design across participants) • To evaluate the effects of a BPT on parent and child feeding-related behaviors at home • Individual parent–child dyads training on contingent attention skills (specific prompts and positive reinforcement) and ignoring disruptive behaviors to increase a child's acceptance of nonpreferred foods • No manual reported • No fidelity reported	• 3 boys with DD (ages 21–54 months) and their mothers • No race/ethnicity information reported • Setting: Home	PARENT • Positive attention • Trained prompts CHILD • Acceptances of foods • Rejections of foods • Other negative behaviors	All mothers' increases in the use of trained prompts and offerings of target food. Two mothers' increases in the levels of positive attention. Children's increases in their acceptance of target foods and self-eating.

Note. BPT = behavioral parent training; CI = child intervention; CMT = Contingency Management Training; DD = developmental disability; DRA = differential reinforcement of alternative behavior; DRI = differential reinforcement of incompatible behavior; DRO = differential reinforcement of other behavior; LD = learning disability; NCR = noncontingent reinforcement; PAT = Planned Activities Training; PDD = Pervasive Developmental Disorders; PT = parent training; SSD = single subject design.

behavioral strategies encapsulated in the BPT programs and are categorized in two areas: Setting event and antecedent-based strategies and consequence-based strategies.

SETTING EVENTS AND ANTECEDENTS-BASED STRATEGIES

As described previously in this chapter, "antecedents" refers to things that occur (such as stimulus changes) or already exist in place (such as environmental conditions) before the behavior of interest and can occasion the behavior (Cooper et al., 2007). In contrast to antecedents, which are simple and discrete and have immediate proximity to the behavior, "setting events" refers to more complex and temporally distant occurrences in the environment that typically combine or interact with antecedents to influence the probability of behavior. In other words, for a child's behavior of concern, setting events alone do not trigger problem behavior (Carr et al., 1994), but affect the likelihood of an antecedent event to trigger the problem behavior (Horner, Albin, Sprague, & Todd, 1999; Lutzker & Steed, 1998). Setting event interventions typically focus on minimizing the effects of the setting events (i.e., setting the stage for problem behaviors to occur), neutralizing the setting events (intervening to reduce or eliminate the contribution of setting events to the likelihood that an antecedent will trigger a problem behavior), adding more prompts for desirable behavior, and increasing the value of reinforcement for desirable behavior (Kansas Institute for Positive Behavior Support [KIPBS], 2011). For example, when a child did not eat breakfast before school, his/her problem behaviors happened more frequently at school. After food was offered to the child before morning classes, his/her problem behaviors decreased. In this case, not eating breakfast was a setting event related to troublesome behaviors.

Antecedent interventions may include environmental modifications, modifying activities including curricular modification, changing task difficulty, changing an aspect of task presentation, providing opportunities to make choices between tasks, engaging children in a series of high-probability requests prior to requesting a more difficult request, modifying the length of a difficult task, and increasing the students' sense of predictability of upcoming events (KIPBS, 2011). Cooper et al. (2007) noted that there are three types of antecedent interventions recognized as effective with established experimental evidence: noncontingent reinforcement (NCR), a high-probability request sequence, and functional communication training (FCT). Moreover, use of a package of techniques for managing setting events/antecedents is not always in isolation but in conjunction with techniques for controlling consequences.

In order to increase children's sense of predictability of upcoming events, Krantz et al. (1993) taught three parents of children with autism to help their children follow photographic schedules that include various activities such as leisure, social interaction, self-care, and housekeeping tasks. The parents were provided 53, 74, and 90 hours of training delivered during in-home visits by a clinician. The training focused on teaching parents use of manual prompts and graduated guidance to teach their children to follow photographic schedules. The results of this multiple baseline across participants study showed that there were significant increases in children's engagement and social initiations and reduction of disruptive behavior as a collateral gain apart from the original outcome variables of the study.

Matson and Francis (1994) investigated the effectiveness of parents' implementation of a visual cues method at home using a multiple baseline across behaviors (greeting response and request for favored food) design. Two young boys with DD and their caregivers participated in the study. A behavioral therapist visited the children's homes and taught the parents how to give instructions, how to use the visual cue method, and how to elicit speech for about 1.5 hours via discussion and role-play. Both children's spontaneous verbalizations improved as treatment progressed. For instance, one child's greeting vocalization occurred in 77 treatment trials, whereas it had occurred zero times during baseline. However, one child had trouble generalizing, which is one of the most difficult skills for children with DD upon learning something new.

Antecedent strategies were also employed in Russell and Matson's (1998) SSD study with three fathers and their children with DD. This study is notable for its focus on fathers, a rarity in this body of literature. The parenting skills taught to the fathers are similar to central features of most BPT packages of techniques. The fathers were trained to teach their children everyday skills (e.g., putting on shoes and socks or brushing teeth), using three main treatment components: giving clear instructions, paying attention to appropriate behavior and ignoring inappropriate behavior, and giving their child appropriate consequences for their behavior. The interventionists examined the fathers' behaviors, seven of which were antecedent-related. In other words, they looked at parents' actions done before the occurrence of child behaviors, such the fathers' verbal prompts, gestural prompts, and physical guidance prompts. The researchers also recorded occurrences of incorrect parent commands and prompts. The results showed that the fathers made improvements in three areas of behavior training components and the children made positive changes in their behavior as a result. The fathers also reported a high sense of satisfaction with the program and the trainer.

Lerman et al. (2000) conducted a multiple baseline across parent behaviors design study to examine the effect of a BPT program on three mothers of children with DD who were trained to use instructional strategies of differential reinforcement, response to child compliance, and instructional prompts in response to their child's inappropriate behavior. The objectives of the BPT program were to help the parents learn how to reduce their child's misbehavior and promote their communication skills. Parenting skill training was individualized for each parent based on observations of their interaction with the child prior to the study. Lerman et al. (2000) kept track of parents' use of teaching skills and how the child responded to them. At baseline, the parents were asked to set up situations that trigger their child's problem behaviors and give their typical response. At the treatment phase, the parents were given both verbal and written instructions and received explicit feedback from the researchers about implementation. A follow-up session occurred a month after the final treatment session. Results showed that all three parents successfully applied effective parenting behaviors for at least one of the learned skills, showing the value of teaching parents to implement new parenting skills. Receiving specific feedback was reported as particularly helpful to the parents. Levels of proper application of their parenting skills maintained a month later following the treatment. It was also found that two of the three target children had decreased their inappropriate behaviors and that all three children were found to follow instructions after the treatment.

Adubato et al. (1981) conducted an SSD study with a 6-year-old boy with multiple disabilities and his parents to examine the effect of BPT on both father and mother in terms of acquisition of target parenting skills and changes of the child's behaviors. The mother was first trained by a professional to master child behavior management skills and was then asked to coach her spouse to learn the same skill set. The mother's training took place in both clinic and home settings that focused on the target parenting skills such as delivering appropriate task instructions, using physical guidance to correct child behaviors, using partial guidance to encourage child's independent compliance with task instructions, and minimizing parent prompts. The mother received 12 training sessions with written and verbal instructions as well as in vivo feedback. She was then prompted to teach her husband in a series of nine sessions without input from the trainer until the father successfully completed the procedures independently. After the mother successfully taught the procedures to her spouse, the couple had improved both rate and stability of their parenting behaviors. Moreover, they were able to generalize their parenting behaviors to some untrained activities. As a result of the BPT training and parents' implementation, the child significantly improved the target behaviors of sustained attending and independent dressing, and was able to generalize to other activities (e.g., eating and toy use skills). Data at the 2-year follow-up showed that both parents had retained the use of their trained skills. The finding of this study sheds light on the importance of BPT where mothers not only are trainees, but also become effective teachers of their husbands. As we will discuss barriers of implementation in chapter 7, this strategy could be used to facilitate the uptake of evidence-based practices in families when mothers are often the only ones who receive direct teaching by a therapist. In summary, the packages of antecedents-based techniques described in five SSD studies above only meet the criteria of promising practices for families of children with DD given the limited number of participants (total n =12).

Planned Activities Training

Planned activities training (PAT) is a collection of strategies to help parents to predict, plan, and have a positive effect on their children's behaviors. This approach involves teaching parents several components such as time management, choosing activities, explaining activities and rules, incidental teaching, and providing feedback and reinforcement. Planned activities training is a more natural approach than contingency management technique (CMT), which focuses on the use of consequences. So as an alternative to CMT, which is not effective in situations when parents can not apply contingencies, PAT helps parents to recognize risky settings and prepare their child for proper social behaviors in home and community settings by focusing on antecedent strategies (Lutzker & Steed, 1998).

Sanders and Plant (1989) examined the effect of PAT in conjunction with CMT for five young children with DD and their parents through a multiple baseline across participants design study including one no-treatment-control participant. The parents learned a combination of PAT and CMT strategies from a therapist. The study examined how the parents and their children responded to these strategies. As the parents were asked to identify home routines when children usually misbehave or have least problem behaviors, the effectiveness of PAT was examined even during very stressful home routines. In the first 4 weeks, child behavioral management procedures were taught to the parents through instruction, discussion, modeling, rehearsal, and feedback by the therapist. Then in the following 5 weeks the parents received PAT training focusing on strategies of stimulus control, environmental planning, and incidental teaching.

Planned activities training is designed to be an antecedent-based intervention to prevent predictable problem behaviors by changing the environment and encouraging appropriate play in its place before problem behaviors occur. But if any problem behavior occurred, parents might need to use CMT. At that point, parents were instructed to use PAT strategies in conjunction with CMT procedures. Without differentiating the effects of PAT and CMT in the analysis, Sanders and Plant (1989) reported that in three of the four families the children's noncompliant behaviors decreased while the parents increased the implementation of treatment procedures in both high- and low-risk settings, suggesting that PAT in conjunction with CMT affects both parent and child outcomes.

Another study, Powers et al. (1992), also investigated the effects of PAT and CMT on children's behaviors. Powers et al. (1992) examined the effect of BPT for three families who had a child with severe DD and disruptive behavior problems. For example, one child predictably misbehaved when his mother used the telephone and left him unattended. The purpose of the intervention in the study was to instruct three parents on PAT and CMT in the home setting and help the families generalize these practices to other areas in the home and community. First, families were trained in four 1-hour sessions consisting of (1) explaining the rationale for the training, and the child behaviors being observed during baseline; (2) discussing and role-playing PAT techniques; (3) learning CMT strategies; and (4) reviewing and practicing all strategies with the child. Again, without a separation of the effects of PAT and CMT strategies in the intervention, this study showed the result of generalization of PAT by the parents to difficult settings such as trips to a shopping mall and going to church for a service. For two of the parents the therapist was able to simply discuss how to use PAT in a specific place. Two of the three parents generalized PAT to community settings without any assistance from the therapist other than talking about the outings at home. One major finding from the study is that different mothers require different amounts of coaching. Two of the four families became gradually more competent and accurate in implementing PAT. They were able to use this method in new community settings by talking with the behavioral coach about the activity and using a card with the steps written out. Parents planned ahead before going to difficult places like stores and malls, bringing small toys with them for the child to play with instead of misbehaving. However, one family needed in situ training in the generalization setting. All target children showed decreases in disruptive behavior, as rated by their mothers, from baseline to intervention to follow-up in the generalization setting.

Similarly, Harrold et al. (1992) studied the effect of PAT and CMT to four children with DD and their mothers. Two mother–child pairs received PAT first, followed by CMT, and the other two pairs were provided the procedures in the reverse order. Both approaches were similarly effective in improving mothers' correct use of PAT steps and in the children's on-task behaviors, and absence of crying or aggression. In addition, four mothers in the study reported high levels of satisfaction with the services provided and slightly preferred PAT to CMT.

The effectiveness of applying PAT alone was studied by Huynen et al. (1996) using a multiple probe experimental design across two families with a replication across two more families. Four mothers of children with DD demonstrated an improvement in their use of PAT in the intervention and increase in the scope of positive interactions with their child in three generalization settings. The children demonstrated an improvement in their compliance and on-task behaviors ranging from 20% to more than 50% across home and community settings. Huynen et al. (1996) suggested that PAT is effective in its generalization across settings and over time because it is developed to increase generalization by using sufficient examples and naturally maintaining contingencies. In summary, four SSD studies identified in our review show the effectiveness of PAT used alone or in conjunction with CMT. Based on the criteria described in chapter 1, we conclude that the PAT program is a promising practice for supporting families of children with DD.

Errorless Compliance Training

Noncompliance with parental instructions is a common problem behavior in young children in general and, to greater extent, in children with DD. Apart from making daily routines more difficult, frequent noncompliance can also lead to a coercive escalation between the parent and child. Errorless compliance training (ECT) is another common BPT program similar to PAT that focuses on parents' control of antecedents to reduce the child's challenging behaviors. For ECT technique, a four-level hierarchy of commands is developed based on the probability of child compliance. Parents and therapists develop an individualized list of parental directives that typically trigger noncompliance. They assign each directive to a level from easy to hard. For example, level 1 comprises commands the child is most likely to follow, such as a request to go get a favorite toy, and level 4 comprises commands the child is least likely to comply with, such as a request to turn off a favorite TV show to help do a chore. Errorless compliance training starts with parents delivering instructions that have a high probability of eliciting child compliance (i.e., level 1).

Parents then gradually introduce instructions with low probability of eliciting compliance. Treatment ends with children's high compliance with level 4 commands (Ducharme & Popynick, 1993).

Ducharme and Popynick (1993) investigated the use of ECT by the mothers of four children with DD using a multiple baseline across subjects design. The children were given commands and demands with high probabilities of compliance and were praised for compliant responses by their mothers. Gradually, the mothers increased the level of commands and demands at lower probabilities of compliance. Results showed that the children achieved high compliance levels without use of punishment. In addition, these children exhibited reductions in their challenging behaviors and generalization of skills to untrained requests.

In a subsequent study, Ducharme et al. (1994) examined the effect of a short version of ECT intended to increase treatment efficiency and simplicity of the procedure. The investigators used fewer requests during the assessment of compliance probabilities, shorter treatment sessions with fewer requests issued in each session, and fewer sessions in each phase of treatment. Similar to the findings of previous study, the treatment resulted in generalization of high compliance for four children with DD and their two typically developing siblings. This study sheds light on the importance of increasing the effectiveness of an intervention by simplifying the procedures.

Ducharme et al.'s (2003) study examined the effect of adding reinforcement for child's compliance to the graduated request delivery. Using a multiple baseline across subject design, four children with DD and their parents were provided reinforced compliance alone and then reinforced compliance plus graduated request delivery to determine the individual contribution of two components to the treatment effects. When only reinforcement (e.g., hugs, pats, kisses) was provided for child's compliance, the children did not show consistent positive change over baseline levels. When graduated request delivery was provided with reinforcement, all children demonstrated consistent positive change. The results revealed that the use of reinforcement for compliance alone was not effective but simultaneous use of the graduate request hierarchy and reinforcement was effective to elicit child compliance. Through component analysis, this group of studies attempted to tease out the contribution different techniques made in a program. It can be useful to simplify an intervention to make it more readily effective.

The delivery format for ECT was then further studied (Ducharme et al., 1996). The group format for ECT was investigated in order to examine the efficiency, durability, and generalizability of treatment effects. Parents of five children with DD were provided with errorless compliance assessment and treatment procedures in a group format. Videotaped data on compliance to parental requests in all phases showed generalizability of effects. An intensive assessment done at 15 months follow-up indicated long-term maintenance of the training effect. Results suggest that ETC can be delivered to parents in a group format with generalization effects.

Errorless compliance training was then found to be applicable to academic request in children with autism (Ducharme & Drain, 2004). Four children with autism and their caregivers participated in the study. All children in the study exhibited behavioral concern in academic or everyday household requests by their parents. For instance, the child would not cooperate when asked to point to the letter B or to turn off the TV. Three mothers and one father of the children were trained through two clinic-based group workshops and two individual sessions. Similar to the procedures used in the studies discussed previously, the parents were asked to deliver a 4-level hierarchy of academic requests (level 1: the most likely to comply, level 4: the least likely to comply) to their children. Over the treatment session, all of the children demonstrated compliance to parent requests. Furthermore, treatment effects were manifest in children's generalization to nontreatment academic requests and nonacademic general request after intervention.

Guided Compliance

Similar to ECT, Smith and Lerman (1999) investigated the effectiveness of guided compliance versus high-probability (or high-*p*) instructional sequences in eliciting compliance with low-probability (or low-*p*) requests. With guided compliance, the therapist physically (usually in hand-over-hand action) guided the child to complete the requested action. With high-*p* instructional sequences, the procedure consisted of presenting a series of requests that have a high probability of compliance before presenting a low-*p* request. Praise for compliance is also given if the child completes a low-*p* request. Therefore, the high-*p* instructional sequence has both antecedent and consequence procedures. The rationale for high-probability instructional sequences is that a child will develop a momentum for compliance that increases the chance of obeying a comparatively nonpreferred demand. Singer, Singer, and Horner (1987) demonstrated the effect of giving a rapid series of high-*p* commands followed by praise. After four to five high-probability directions were given using rapid pacing and verbal enthusiasm, the low probability one was given while maintaining the pacing, the small timed interval between requests. This procedure was used to reduce problem behavior in transitions from activities the children preferred to ones they avoided.

Smith and Lerman's study (1999) tested the effect of a different version of ECT on two children with autism and IDs who exhibited no aggressive and disruptive behaviors other than noncompliance. Following the baseline phase, the parents were taught to implement both guided compliance and high-probability instructional sequences in two home visits. After giving the handout of procedures to parents, the researchers reviewed the steps and modeled and rehearsed the procedures with the parents. Subsequently, the parents were asked to practice the procedures with their children by following a practice flowchart in a worksheet and following researchers' feedback. Further feedback was provided to the parents after implementation. Using a multielement and multiple baseline across participants design, Smith and Lerman (1999) found that the rate of compliance grew higher in the intervention phase. However, surprisingly the guided compliance procedures were associated with greater rate of children's compliance to low-probability requests as compared with the high-*p* instructional sequence. The students did better with the consequence of guided compliance than with the procedure of high-*p* requests plus praise. In the reversal session, implemented to only one of the participants, low-*p* compliance dropped to baseline levels. At the follow-up when guided compliance was switched back, children's compliance once again increased. While being asked to evaluate the effect of two interventions, the parents rated both treatments as "moderately effective."

However, another study by Humm et al. (2005) found an association between high-*p* instructional sequences and differential reinforcement and increased rates of compliance post intervention. Replicating the procedures of Smith and Lerman's study (1999), Humm et al. (2005) found that across all three participants, gains in compliance from baseline to follow-up were evident in at least one targeted low-compliance response and levels of compliance maintained at follow-up for two children.

Van Hasselt et al. (1987) reported a SSD study where a mother of a 4-year-old with DD was trained in 15-minute sessions, twice weekly, for 3 months to increase positive mother–child interactions and child compliance via direct and explicit instructions, role-playing, modeling, behavioral rehearsal, and feedback. Definitive commands and differential reinforcement were a major focus of the training. The mother was taught to praise or to hug her child when he complied with her command. When the child did not follow her instruction, she restated her command or used guided compliance procedures. Despite no change in stereotypic responses, the child was found to display higher levels of compliance, decreased oppositional behavior, and increased percentage of on-task behavior.

This series of studies of ECT and its variation (guided compliance) provides evidence of an effective program for giving parents the skills they need to teach children with DD how to consistently follow directions without negative child and parent interactions. The attention to easy-to-hard sequencing of demands and the addition of physical prompting are ways to avoid setting off problem behavior. Regular noncompliance can make any parenting routine more difficult and risks increasing the escalating pattern of parent–child interactions (i.e., coercion). In summary, we have reviewed five SSD studies undertaken by the same research group of Ducharme and colleagues on ECT and three SSD studies conducted by three other independent researchers on guided compliance. Putting all these studies together, we conclude that errorless compliance training and guided compliance are established practices for supporting families of children with DD.

Noncontingent Reinforcement

Noncontingent reinforcement (NCR) refers to regularly delivering reinforcement such as a praise, a hug, or an affectionate comment, regardless of the child's behaviors, to decrease the child's motivation to engage in maladaptive behaviors (Cooper et al., 2007). O'Reilly et al. (1999) trained parents of a 10-year-old boy with mild intellectual disabilities to conduct a functional analysis and to compare an intervention using ignoring and NCR. The child in this study had high levels of aggressive behavior. One purpose of this study was to test whether parents could implement such procedures in the home environment, and so the therapists trained the mother to be a therapist in using NCR while they acted as observers. During the functional analysis, the mother enacted a series of conditions and found that attention was reinforcing the child's unwanted behaviors. In the NCR phase, the mother delivered attention to the child every 30 seconds. Once the aggression level decreased, the mother gradually increased the time between giving the child attention. In the ignoring phase that followed, the therapist sat away from the child and did not engage the child in any interaction during the session except to block aggression. In the follow-up phase that contained five sessions offered once a week, the parents implemented the NCR procedure with the child every 5 minutes, during periods when aggression levels were high. O'Reilly and colleagues found that NCR was the more effective intervention method for reducing aggression in this case. However, they conceded that neither strategy is universally applicable. The problem with using NCR or ignoring alone is that the child learns no new behavior to communicate his needs. Given that only one study was found in our targeted population, we caution against use of this method by parents as unproven practice until emergence of more proof of its efficacy.

Functional Communication Training

Functional communication training (FCT) is an appealing procedure, particularly for parents of children with autism and moderate or severe ID, because it aims to reduce problem behaviors by teaching individuals with DD to communicate their wants through means other than using problem behaviors. Originated by Carr and Durand (1985), it is a systematic intervention in which an appropriate communicative act is taught as a replacement for challenging behavior. For example, instead of throwing a tantrum in front of a refrigerator to communicate the need to eat, a child might learn to point to a picture of a person eating. Alternative communicative responses are expressed in various forms, such as vocalizations, gestures and signs, communication boards, graphic symbols, or vocal output systems (Cooper et al., 2007).

As one of the most common function-based treatments for difficult behavior (Tiger, Hanley, & Bruzek, 2008), FCT is associated with an extensive literature on the outcomes of addressing challenging behavior. Numerous empirical studies have reported successful outcomes of FCT for individuals with DD and several literature review papers have documented the results of studies on the outcomes of FCT for this population (Bambara et al., 1994; Mancil, 2006; Matson, Dixon, & Matson, 2005). However, only a few studies of sound quality have been reported with respect to parent-implemented FCT or parent involvement in FCT treatment.

Derby et al. (1997) evaluated the short- and long-term effects of FCT treatment packages that were implemented by parents in home settings using a multiple baseline across subjects design. After an assessment of the situations that led to problem behaviors at home, therapists carried out an FCT intervention with parents of four young children with DD and aberrant behavior. They found that it was very likely that the children used problem behavior to get their parents' attention or to avoid difficult tasks. Based on the assessment results, each parent was trained during a 1-hour session to implement FCT in teaching children ways to communicate instead of misbehaving. After the initial training, all parents were asked to conduct 10 to 30 minutes of the FCT treatment package with their child every day. Therapists made weekly to monthly home visits to give feedback regarding each parent's implementation of the treatment. The short- and long-term effects of treatment on reducing misbehavior and increasing communication were evaluated. Moreover, children's social and toy play behaviors (e.g., offering parents a toy) were measured to evaluate the collateral or side effects of long-term FCT. Immediate decreases in misbehavior for three of the four children suggest short-term treatment effects. The long-term (up to 27 months) treatment effects were evident in that all children used more communication and exhibited fewer problem behaviors and also presented better social behaviors. Results suggest that functional assessment and FCT treatment packages can be effectively carried out by parents in home settings not only to decrease the child's inappropriate behaviors but also to increase the child's communication and social skills.

Similar to the training procedures used in Derby et al.'s (1997) study, one intervention study involved contextualizing functional assessment and FCT in the home setting for young children with autism (Moes & Frea, 2002). Analysis was done to understand the daily routines and cultural values in the family's home to determine the cause of the children's problem behaviors. Based on functional analysis and functional level of each child, researchers discussed with parents appropriate forms of verbal or nonverbal communication to teach their children. Researchers then modeled FCT strategies, rehearsed these strategies with parents, and gave helpful feedback. In the next step, information about the family context, such as daily routines, resources, difficulties, cultural beliefs, and caregiving demands, was gathered. The existing FCT procedures were modified to incorporate family-chosen goals and patterns of family interaction. Results showed reductions in challenging behavior and increases in functional communication. For the contextualized FCT, challenging behaviors almost disappeared and communication continuously increased. Results from the self-report questionnaire completed by parents showed that the parents felt the program fit well with their home life and that they would keep using a set of practices after the end of the study.

Wacker and colleagues (1998, 2005, 2013) reported sequentially that parents can implement functional analysis and FCT treatment packages to children with DD who have challenging behaviors in their home settings. In a nonconcurrent multiple baseline across children design study (Wacker et al., 1998), 28 parents of young children with DD or multiple disabilities and aberrant behavior were trained to conduct a functional analysis of their child's aberrant behaviors and implement an FCT intervention. Based on the functional analysis results, each family implemented recommended FCT treatment packages to their child. The effectiveness of intervention was monitored at 3-month intervals for up to 12 months. On average, children's misbehavior was reduced by 87%, and the appropriate social responding increased 69%. In addition, parents rated the FCT procedures as highly acceptable. Similarly, Wacker et al. (2005) found comparable results with a second group of 25 young children who displayed destructive behavior. After FCT treatment, the average decrease in aberrant behavior for all participants was 85%, and similar results were gained for total destructive behavior. Furthermore, reductions in destructive behavior were also shown to generalize to other settings, tasks, and people. Results indicate that the children started using their communication skills as a general way to solve a problem and that such generalization is much more efficient than a typical treatment where every problem behavior or every home routine is targeted.

In a more recent nonconcurrent multiple baseline design study, Wacker and colleagues (2013) reported that FCT intervention could be conducted by parents through coaching by behavior consultants via telehealth, a long-distance, telecommunication service delivery system. Functional communication training was implemented by the parents of 17 children with autism. The parents received training on FCT procedures at regional clinics during 1-hour telehealth visits for an average of 13 weeks. Results showed that children's problem behaviors decreased by approximately 94%. In addition, it is noted that FCT training package can be implemented by parents dependent on coaching by a therapist, and the package was effective for reducing children's disruptive behavior and increasing adaptive behavior such as communicating requests and completing tasks. This study sheds light on the value of using new Internet-based media to teach BPT to parents who are far away. This can open new alternatives for providing this form of family support in rural areas where therapists may not be available to train in person.

Functional communication training has been evaluated extensively in the literature, and the quality of evidence is strong. It is noted that FCT treatment has several advantages as a way to support parents to prevent or replace problem behaviors that can bedevil families of children who have difficulty in learning normal appropriate ways to reach a goal in home and community settings. In summary, five SSD studies on FCT conducted by three different research groups provide strong evidence to suggest that functional communication training is an established practice for supporting families of children with DD.

CONSEQUENCES-BASED STRATEGIES

Eighteen SSD studies have been found to include consequence strategies as a major component in their BPT approach. These strategies include positive reinforcement, negative reinforcement, differential reinforcement and extinction, and mild punishment.

Positive Reinforcement

Parent training often involves teaching parents basic principles of behavior analysis, including the effect of consequences on changing children's problem behaviors and noncompliance. Many of these training programs focus on teaching parents behavioral principles related to systems of reinforcement. Reinforcement is when an event that occurs after a behavior has the effect of increasing that behavior (Cooper et al., 2007).

In many studies, parents are taught to use praise or positive attention as a form of reinforcement (see Adubato et al., 1981; Humm et al., 2005; Lerman et al., 2000; Moran & Whitman, 1985; Smith & Lerman, 1999), even if these programs do not explicitly count these types of positive reinforcement as a critical part of their behavioral parent training program. For instance, Adubato et al.'s (1981) intervention, discussed earlier, did not highlight praise and positive attention as a core child management skill discussed during training. Yet at the completion of the study, both the mother and the father noted that praise was a major component of giving task instructions and using physical guidance. Not only did this study show that one parent can be trained to teach the other behavioral management skills but also this intervention demonstrated that parent trainers may teach parents to praise their children along with other more perceivably important components of their intervention program. Although there is only one specific SSD study focusing on the use of positive reinforcement as a primary behavioral strategy identified in our review, the vast majority of SSD studies discussed in this chapter have used positive reinforcement as a consequence-based strategy in conjunction with other antecedent-based strategies or other consequence-based strategies. Therefore, without reservation we suggest that packages of BPT embedded with positive reinforcement are established practices for children with DD and their families.

Negative Reinforcement

By definition, negative reinforcement occurs when something is withdrawn and therefore causes the frequency of a behavior to increase (Cooper et al., 2007). For example, if a child tantrums during dinner because she dislikes eating vegetables and the parents remove the vegetables as a result of her misbehavior. If the tantrumming becomes more severe, we can conclude that removing the carrots is negatively reinforcing the inappropriate behavior. Negative reinforcement, in the form of allowing the child to avoid or escape doing nonpreferred activities, is sometimes used as treatment for children with DD to decrease problem behaviors (Vollmer, Marcus, & Ringdahl, 1995) and to increase compliance (Reed, Ringdahl, Wacker, Barretto, & Andelman, 2005) and appropriate communication (Mildon, Moore, & Dixon, 2004). However, rarely is negative reinforcement used in BPT programs.

Lalli, Casey, and Kates's (1997) intervention featured a parent training component that included both positive and negative reinforcement strategies. A functional analysis was conducted by therapists during the first phase of the study to determine why the participating children with DD engaged in aggressive behaviors toward others and themselves. Once they established that the children did these behaviors to obtain a preferred object or to avoid a particular unwanted activity, the therapist implemented the second phase. To reduce aggressive behaviors in this phase, therapists regularly reinforced the three participating children with DD by allowing them to obtain an object they wanted (e.g., a toy) or by allowing them to avoid an activity (e.g., by going for a walk). Permitting the child to escape from an activity is a form of negative reinforcement. Simultaneously, the therapists would ignore aggressive behaviors. At the point when the children displayed less aggression, the therapists trained the parents by providing written directions of the intervention procedures, modeling those strategies, role-playing the strategies, and giving feedback about parents' performance. Parents of two of the children implemented the reinforcement and ignoring procedures, while the parents and teacher of the third child learned to use only the reinforcement strategies. Results for the students showed that rates of aggression decreased during treatment, compared with the baseline condition(s). When parents implemented treatment procedures, low levels of aggression maintained for one child; for the other two children, aggression initially spiked but decreased and remained low for the rest of the study.

As explained previously, the problem with using noncontingent forms of reinforcement (intermittent reinforcement given whether or not a child performs the appropriate behavior) or with using ignoring alone is that the child does not learn to use positive behaviors to replace their misbehaviors. Therefore, noncontingent reinforcement and ignoring (when used by itself) are not recommended. Negative reinforcement was also used in a study by Marcus, Swanson, and Vollmer (2001), but in that study, reinforcement was contingent on appropriate behavior. Parents were asked to provide breaks for their child when their child followed directions. This one strategy, among other strategies used in that intervention, (see the next section, "Differential Reinforcement and Extinction," for more detail) was associated with positive results.

Differential Reinforcement and Extinction

Other studies discussed teaching specific reinforcement procedures, namely differential reinforcement. With differential reinforcement, children's desired behaviors are reinforced or increased with praise or with positive attention. Children are guided to follow directions or to learn more appropriate ways to get what they want (Van Hasselt et al., 1987). Typically, extinction is simultaneously implemented; that is, undesired behaviors are reduced through ignoring (Vollmer, Roane, Ringdahl, & Marcus, 1999). For instance, parents may be asked to use praise and positive attention when their children exhibit good behavior and are prompted to ignore incorrect behaviors.

Many of the behavioral training programs that teach children to better comply with directions employ differential reinforcement strategies. Van Hasselt and colleagues' (1987) aforementioned intervention, for instance, taught the mother to praise or to hug her child when the child complied with her command. When the child did not follow her instruction, she restated her command or guided her child to follow her directions (e.g., gently moving the child through the correct behaviors). Similar procedures are found in more recent child compliance studies (Humm et al., 2005; Lerman et al., 2000; Smith &

Lerman, 1999). Friman and Altman (1990) implemented a single-subject reversal design intervention specifically using differential reinforcement with a 4-year-old child with DD, who had no functional expressive speech, low receptive speech, and few self-help skills. The child had demonstrated great difficulty staying enrolled in a preschool program because of his disruptive behavior. With the help of the child's parents, the researchers sought to decrease his inappropriate behaviors (getting out of seat and throwing toys) and to increase appropriate toy play, so that the child will be more likely to be accepted into and remain in a preschool program. Since most studies only involve mothers, this study is important because both the mother and father were trained to work with the child and alternated between sessions. In the experimental condition, the parents were to implement differential reinforcement strategies to encourage the child to stay in his seat. Praise and food were delivered when the child stayed in his seat for a set amount of time. If the child did not stay in his seat, no reinforcers were given for that interval of time. The researchers observed that out-of-seat behavior decreased and appropriate toy play increased only during treatment phases, and not during baseline or when intervention procedures were withdrawn, although toy throwing did not follow the expected trend absolutely. The study ended when the child enrolled in the preschool. This study does provide evidence that, with differential reinforcement strategies, the child could be taught to engage in desired behaviors and that goals of the family (here, the goal was acceptance into preschool) were honored. However, Friman and Altman's study was not conducted in a naturalistic environment.

Scholars have also studied the use differential reinforcement strategies in the home and community setting. In one such study, Marcus and colleagues (2001) trained parents of four children, ages 3 to 5, to reward desired behaviors that replace their children's problem behaviors. For example, if the child followed parents' directions, they were given positive attention, praised (e.g., "good job"), or given a toy. For some of the children, their noncompliance was met with guided compliance or with a 5-second time-out (e.g., hands held down or removal of toy; time-out procedures are explored in the "Mild Punishment" section). Another study by Niemeyer and Fox (1990) employed differential reinforcement to reduce children's aggressive and dangerous behaviors during car-riding, when parents would transport the children to and from school and activities. Their participants were a 5-year-old boy with Down syndrome and a 17-year-old boy with ID. Niemeyer and Fox taught the parents to implement differential reinforcement strategies with a token economy system in which the parents would reward their children with praise and a token or sticker for not engaging in target behaviors (e.g., aggression or perseverative talk) for a predetermined amount of time (e.g., every 3 minutes). Such tokens could be exchanged for further praise and desired items (e.g., juice or a toy) or activities (e.g., special time with parents). Levels of children's misbehaviors substantially dropped during intervention for both studies, suggesting that differential reinforcement could have an effect on problem behaviors outside of the clinic setting.

Applications of Differential Reinforcement Extinction Techniques on Food Selectivity

Mealtime could be challenging for parents of children with DD who have narrow diets, but scholars have found consequence-based approaches to be particularly helpful. Differential reinforcement procedures were implemented in Anderson and McMillan's (2001) study, but with the addition of a strategy to decrease a child's avoidance behaviors, escape extinction. This study sought to encourage a 5-year-old boy with autism and severe ID to eat non-preferred foods (in his case, fruits). Using verbal and written directions, videotape review, and feedback during weekly home visits, the researchers trained the parents to praise the child and to provide a sip of milk (his preferred beverage) if he accepted a bite of fruit. All of the child's avoidance behaviors were disregarded; the boy's interruptions were ignored, and the meal only ended if he accepted a bite of fruit. In the last treatment phase, the child made immense gains. Compared with baseline, when he interrupted 55% of bites of fruit, the child accepted 100% of bites of fruit at the end of treatment. It is also important for parents to know how to generalize the strategies they learn in the home to other settings so that their child can demonstrate functional skills in the community. Whereas Anderson and McMillan's study to encourage food consumption was conducted only in the home, Najdowski et al. (2003) tested similar strategies in the home and in a community setting. As a result of intervention, the participating 5-year-old child with autism could eat a full meal of nonpreferred foods at home and learned to accept food at restaurants. More recently, Seiverling et al. (2012) took similar steps to treat children's food selectivity and came to find improvements in how parents implemented the intervention and in how much children reduced disruptive behavior and accepted different types of food. We have provided evidence that BPT can help parents reduce general noncompliance. What these food selectivity studies illustrate is that BPT can be adapted to target ever more specific behaviors across diverse environments, such as eating at restaurants.

Applications of Extinction Techniques on Sleep Disorders

Sleep difficulties are common in children with DD and can affect their ability to learn and increase the likelihood of having problem behaviors due to sleep deprivation (Wiggs, & Stores, 1996; Richdale, Francis, Gavidia-Payne, & Cotton, 2000). If a child is having disordered sleep, chances are that their parents and siblings are suffering as well, increasing the overall stress level in the household and possibly increasing the risk of marital discord (Davis & Carter, 2008; Meltzer & Mindell, 2007; Quine, 1991). As sleep issues in children with DD tend to be more common (Richdale et al., 2000), more severe, and longer lasting than those in the general population (Quine, 1991), effective interventions need to be made available to families sooner rather than later. Parents of children with DD have reported higher instances of children's sleep disorders such as difficulty falling asleep, night waking, and early waking (Richdale et al., 2000). Fortunately, when sleep is brought to an acceptably normal pattern through an individualized intervention, the functioning of the child and the entire family can improve (Wiggs, & Stores, 2001).

Sleep difficulties in children with DD can be treated pharmacologically, but behavioral interventions are particularly well suited for this population and have already been shown to improve child performance in school and home settings (Carr & Durand, 1985; Lovaas, 1977). One behavioral procedure is to ignore all behavior that is not desirable. In this so-called extinction procedure, the child's cries are ignored, and the child is returned to bed each time she gets up without being attended to. This practice has been found to be particularly effective in getting children to fall asleep on their own, but it can be difficult for parents to hear their children so upset and not intervene. Furthermore, children's negative behaviors sometimes become amplified (an "extinction burst") before they improve. Graduated extinction, when a plan is developed to systematically increase the amount of time between which the parent attends to their child until the child is able to fall asleep on his own has also been shown to be effective in children with DD, although this practice takes much longer to complete than standard extinction. Extinction and graduated extinction protocols have been rated positively by parents, exhibiting consistently high levels of social validity.

Thackeray and Richdale (2002) conducted a multiple baseline design study on three 5- to 10-year-old boys with ID and sleep problems in Australia. In the intervention phase, researchers trained parents individually on standard extinction procedures and establishing a bedtime routine in an intensive 2-week program at a local university. Parents were given manuals to take home for reference. Follow-up calls were made to parents by an investigator to be sure they understood the protocol and to clear up any misunderstandings. Results relating to sleep were measured by sleep diaries and a sensor worn to measure periods of rest and movement. Post-intervention, all three children were able to fall asleep independently in their own bed. One child continued to have issues with night-waking, but showed overall improved quality of sleep. Additional benefits of the intervention included increased length of sleep, decreased time to fall asleep, and delayed morning wake time. The parents reported that the program was "very appropriate" for their child, and that they would "strongly recommend" it to other parents. Similar results were reported by Allen, Kuhn, DeHaai, and Wallace (2013) and Weiskop, Matthews, and Richdale (2001) in sleep interventions using extinction approaches. Disruptive behavior for the children with Angelman syndrome in Allen et al.'s study immediately decreased at bedtime, and the participants were able to fall asleep independently. Improvements in daytime behaviors were also noted.

Whereas behaviors for the 5-year-old boy with autism in Weiskop and colleagues' (2001) intervention improved after a brief spike in disruptive behavior, the program quickly eliminated the child's difficulties in settling in to sleep alone, waking during the night, and cosleeping with the parent. The boy was able to fall asleep on his own and remain in his bed throughout the intervention and at the 3- and 12-month follow-up with nearly no subsequent presleep disturbances.

Although considered highly effective, individualized, and socially valid, these sleep interventions require a great commitment of time from parents and professionals, making them costly and difficult to apply for many families. Group trainings, such as the one implemented by Stores and Stores (2004) discussed previously, may be less expensive and time-intensive to administer. In summary, there are a dozen SSD studies conducted by numerous research groups that focus on the effectiveness of using differential reinforcement and extinction strategies. These studies provide strong evidence to support the claim for packages of BPT embedded with differential reinforcement and extinction strategies to be established practices.

Mild Punishment

Differential reinforcement, on its own, may not always be effective. Therefore, parents are rarely instructed to employ only reinforcement techniques in BPT programs. Much more likely, they are taught to use techniques to reduce misbehavior in conjunction with methods that reinforce good behavior. So far, we have discussed extinction, or planned ignoring, as a way to decrease the likelihood of a behavior from happening. However, parents oftentimes use mild punishment techniques to discipline their children, and scholars have examined the use of these procedures in reducing disruptiveness and noncompliance.

There are many forms of mild punishment. For instance, we found one study that taught parents to verbally punish the child (i.e., firm "no") for misbehaviors and to praise or offer gentle touches for compliant behaviors (Brehony et al., 1980). At times, BPT treatments involve multiple mild punishment strategies. The most common form of mild punishment technique taught in training programs is time-out. Children placed in time-out lose the privilege of getting positive attention and other rewards (Cooper et al., 2007). Another technique is response interruption, in which parents are taught to physically intervene to stop the child from performing an inappropriate behavior. In another study, by Friman et al. (1986), the mother of a 10-year-old girl with Batten's disease was taught how to use differential reinforcement, time-out, and response interruption. Prior to the study, the parent reported using corporal punishment, such as slapping to stop her child from pinching her. Hence, the investigators saw a great need to help the parent use less aversive strategies to reduce the child's problem behavior. The therapist demonstrated the steps of the treatment, provided written directions and verbal explanations, and gave feedback about how the parent and teacher followed the treatment steps. During play sessions at home, the mother praised her child and gave gentle touches if her child did not pinch for a certain amount of time. If the child pinched, the mother simply withdrew herself. In the second treatment phase, the mother placed the child away from the play area for a 5-minute time-out if the child pinched. For the third treatment phase, the parent gently held the child's hand if she pinched. Results for the at-home play sessions showed that only when the mother held the child's hand (i.e., response interruption) did pinching decrease. Here, the parent was able to adopt much more positive parenting strategies because of response interruption. Aurand et al.'s (1989) study also noted reductions in a child's stereotypical behaviors (e.g., hand flapping and tongue chewing) when the mother and school staff were trained to implement response interruption and differential reinforcement.

Even though child aggression did not seem responsive to time-out in Friman and colleagues' intervention, other studies have suggested the potential effectiveness of time-out procedures. One later SSD intervention by Handen et al. (1992) seemed to indicate that child compliance could be influenced by this form of mild punishment. Handen et al.'s study looked at whether the child complying with directions depended on whether the parent used planned ignoring, guided compliance, or time-out procedures. The findings indicate that, on average, compliance during the time-out condition was highest, followed by guided compliance, and then by the baseline condition.

The systematic use of antecedent strategies in conjunction with reinforcement and time-out has been found to be successful in multiple studies (e.g., Powers et al., 1992). An early study conducted by Hawkins et al. (1966) evaluated the response of a 4-year-old boy with ID to time-out, direct commands, and praise conducted by his mother in the home setting. Hawkins and colleagues found more positive parenting practices as well as slight positive changes in child behaviors. Another SSD study, by McDonald and Budd (1983), taught a mother of a 7-year-old boy with Down syndrome to give clearer directions, to use positive attention to increase appropriate behavior, and to ignore or use time-outs for inappropriate behaviors. The additional booster session trainings were associated with increased praise to child compliance, which remained after sessions. Time-out strategies have also been used with success in a food selectivity intervention (Werle et al., 1993) to help children who regularly refuse food to accept nonpreferred food. Additionally, time-out procedures can be implemented by parents of either gender. Russell and Matson's (1998) intervention, discussed briefly in the "Setting Events and Antecedents-Based Strategies" section, also employed time-out strategies in their training of fathers. While researchers of this study instructed the fathers to present clear instructions, they also stressed that the parents deliver correct positive attention and correct consequences, including planned ignoring, continuing with instructions, and giving time-outs when necessary. The children made gains in following directions, and the fathers also reported they were satisfied with the program. Fathers' stress levels did not dramatically decrease after training, however. This last result suggests that oftentimes stress management and coping skills, like those introduced in chapter 2, need to be directly taught in conjunction with BPT for parents to experience real changes in stress levels. We discuss interventions that combine cognitive-behavioral and behavioral management strategies in chapter 5.

Used to a lesser degree in parental training is response cost. Response cost occurs when, because of a child's problem behavior, rewards and reinforcement are taken away. In an early study, Christopherson, Arnold, Hill, and Quilitch (1972) evaluated the use of a token reinforcement system with two families, one of which had an 8-year-old girl who had mild cerebral palsy and ID. Researchers taught parents to implement a token economy system based on the achievement place model (Phillips, 1968) to be used at home. When children in the family completed a chore, parents would reward them with points, which would be exchanged for items or activities the children wanted. When they did not do a chore, parents would subtract points; this is the response cost. Any bickering or whining would also result in the loss of points. The findings were promising. Like her two siblings, the child with DD was able to complete desired tasks daily with the support of the point system, compared with the baseline condition. This study shows that if the behaviors are mild, a behavior management system could be put in place for the whole family, and not just between the parent and the child with DD.

In summary, eight SSD studies with a total of 13 participants were conducted by numerous research groups to examine the usefulness of mild and nonaversive punishment strategies for parents to deal with their child's problem behaviors. These studies provide evidence to suggest that packages of BPT mainly using mild punishment strategies when necessary are only promising practices for children with DD and their families. However, care must be taken when it comes to choice-making for parents applying mild punishment strategies. As suggested by Cooper et al. (2007) in the ABA literature, punishment should never be used alone as the sole behavioral technique, and it is recommended that punishment strategies be applied only when necessary and in conjunction with other behavioral techniques.

CONCERNS AND ISSUES SURROUNDING THE USE OF BEHAVIORAL PARENT TRAINING

According to Chronis, Chacko, Fabiano, Wymbs, and Pelham (2004), the field of BPT has moved in the direction of enhancing traditional BPT to maximize attendance, adherence, and outcomes for children and their families. Future work in this area is needed to examine which variations in format are most effective for families of children with ADHD in general, and specifically for families with different characteristics (e.g., less educated parents, single parents, parents with attention problems).

The format of BPT has changed considerably over the past two decades. Initially, BPT was a clinic-based treatment in which the therapist, parent, and sometimes the child attended individual family sessions. Recent research has attempted to understand how best to maximize gains experienced by families during and following BPT through modifications in the format, process, and procedures designed to enhance maintenance.

Individual BPT offers several advantages over group-based approaches, including increased flexibility on the part of the therapist and parent in terms of pace, content, individual attention provided to idiosyncratic problems of the child/parent, and potentially more active involvement by the parent. However, individual BPT is also costly, time-consuming, and inefficient. Alternatively, group-based BPT is far more cost-effective than individually based BPT, provides opportunities for social support with similar others, and most often produces equivalent effects to individually administered BPT.

There are two major limitations in BPT for parents of children with DD: (1) these treatments are insufficient to reduce high levels of parental stress, and (2) these interventions are minimally effective with a substantial percentage of these families.

Although parents can effectively modify their children's behavior and thereby improve the quality of family life, some parent training programs have suffered from high levels of attrition and/or and failure of some parents reach a criterion skill level (Singer et al, 2002). When BPT has been implemented with parents of nondisabled children or in treatments related to child mental health, attrition levels are high. Irvine, Biglan, Smolkowski, Metzler, and Ary (1999) reviewed literature suggesting that 50% of parents failed to complete training. Kazdin (1997) reported that 40%–60% of families who begin treatment for child mental health issues drop out before completion of the treatment. When parents do complete training, a sizable percentage fails to acquire knowledge and skills at a sufficient level of proficiency to accurately implement the procedures. Baker (1996) reported that approximately 45% of parents in his BPT program for parents of children with IDs failed to acquire sufficient knowledge of behavioral principles to implement them correctly. Webster-Stratton (1997) reported a rate of acquisition failure in 30% of parents served in her program for parents of young children with oppositional and noncompliance problems. Problems are further compounded by difficulties parents have in maintaining implementation of BPT methods over time. Baker, Heifetz, and Murphy (1980) found that 14 months after completion of their training program, 24% of parents had failed to teach at least one new skill to their children with mental retardation in the previous month. In a meta-analysis of the literature on maintenance of behavioral parent training for parents of children with conduct disorders, Serketich and Dumas (1996) concluded that BPT interventions were effective in the short term but that there was insufficient evidence to claim efficacy for durability of these effects.

Singer and colleagues reviewed the literature on barriers to BPT treatment and identified a set of specific problems that they posited as conditions that overshadowed parents' ability to take up the treatments. These obstacles to effective BPT were: (1) elevated parental depressive symptoms, (2) marital discord, (3) high levels of stress, and (4) daily hassles associated with low socioeconomic status and single parenthood (Singer et al., 2000). Other researchers in BPT have discussed these problems for many years, but there is little intervention research demonstrating that they can be effectively addressed (Bristol, Gallagher, & Holt, 1993; Harris, 1984). In a recent review of research needs in the field of autism, Schreibman (2002) noted the need for research on better approaches to serving parents who experience problems such as high levels of stress, depression, and marital discord in order to improve treatment outcomes based on BPT.

Researchers are often faced with difficulties in recruitment and attrition of participants. Baker (1996) examined a number of studies reporting on rates of recruitment. These studies assessed the participation of parents of children with intellectual impairment in BPT programs and found rates ranging from 11% to 54%. In determining why parents choose whether or not partake in BPT programs, studies have reported specific characteristics of parents who choose not to participate. These include lower socioeconomic status, lower education levels, less confidence in their ability to gain parenting skills, and a perception that their child is less troublesome than others who join (Baker, 1996). Researchers continue to make progress regarding these issues by combining multiple methods to improve on how BPT programs are marketed, designed, and implemented (Baker, 1996; Webster-Stratton, 1998).

It has been suggested that high attrition rates may be one of the most significant issues impacting the efficacy of BPT programs (Jensen & Grimes, 2010). Research conducted by Jensen and Grimes (2010) found that parents were more likely to attend BPT sessions if their child was receiving concurrent treatment. Specifically, during the concurrent child treatment phase families attended BPT sessions at a rate of 80%. When the child treatment phase ended, family attendance to parent-training sessions decreased to 26%. Methods for limiting attrition rates in BPT programs continue to be explored and researched.

CONCLUSION

Through a thorough review of current literature of BPT regarding its applications to children with DD, we have gathered empirical evidence from a few dozen studies employing either RCT or SSD methods. Adequate evidence has emerged from the research synthesis and meta-analysis of RCT studies suggesting that the BPT approach as a whole, albeit with diversification of BPT programs or models, has a medium treatment effect ($d = 0.58$) for children with DD and their families. When three major focus outcome areas are examined separately, BPT programs have a small treatment effect ($d = 0.45$) on parent outcomes (including parent's acquisition of knowledge and performance of learned skills, self-efficacy, perceived support, and reduced level of stress/distress), a medium effect ($d = 0.53$) on child outcomes (learned skills and problem behaviors), and a large treatment effect ($d = 0.81$) on family system outcomes (parent and child interaction and family well-being) for children with DD and their families. The effect size for the child outcomes ($d = 0.53$) is similar to moderate effect of BPT found for children with ADHD ($r = .34$; Lee et al., 2012) and is lower than a large effect size found for children with antisocial behaviors (Serketich & Dumas, 1996, $d = 0.80$). The moderate effect on parent outcomes, particularly on the reduced level of stress/distress ($d = 0.26$) is consistent with the previous findings on a meta-analysis study of BPT effect on parent stress level for parents of children with DD ($d = 0.25$; Singer et al., 2007). The effect of BPT on family system outcomes has not been reported in any published studies based on the result of our literature review. It is noted that BPT has a large treatment effect on parent and child interaction ($d = 1.48$) and a small effect ($d = 0.40$) on family well-being (family quality of life) for children with DD and their families. Therefore, we conclude that BPT is an established practice for supporting families of children with DD.

4

EVIDENCE-BASED PRACTICES FOR SUPPORTING FAMILIES OF CHILDREN WITH AUTISM

Mian Wang, Jiyeon Kim, Whitney Detar-Smith, and George H. S. Singer

Developmental disability comprises a wide array of disability conditions related to impairments in physical, learning, language, or behavior domains. As seen in the previous chapters, children with intellectual disabilities and autism have been the target population of treatment for evidence-based practices (EBPs). Despite lower prevalence as compared with intellectual disability, autism is the most rapidly growing disability under the umbrella term of developmental disability (Baio, 2012). In its full name by the American Psychiatric Association's definition, autism spectrum disorder (ASD) is a pervasive developmental disorder (PDD) increasing significantly in prevalence in recent decades and now affecting 1 in 50 children in the United States (Blumberg et al., 2013). Recent revision of the *Diagnostic and Statistical Manual for Mental Disorders* (DSM-5) has brought three core deficit areas in DSM-IV (social, communication, and restricted/repetitive behavior patterns) down to 2 (social communication and restricted/repetitive behavior patterns and interests) (American Psychiatric Association, 2013). Despite an ongoing debate on how this change in diagnostic criteria will affect the prevalence estimate, researchers suggested that approximately 20% of children who met the DSM-IV criteria will no longer meet the new DSM-5 criteria (Maenner et al., 2014).

Though the specific etiology of ASD remains unknown, several factors including both genetic and environmental ones have been found to play a role. Many parents report noticing symptoms in their children before their first birthday (Bolton, Golding, Emond, & Steer, 2012; Kozlowski, Matson, Horovitz, Worley, & Neal, 2011), and research has suggested that a reliable diagnosis can be made by 18 months (Zwaigenbaum et al., 2005). However, most children are still not diagnosed until 4+ years of age in the United States (Baio, 2012).

Autism is a condition with different levels of severity. At one end of the spectrum, children with autism may be highly intelligent and yet socially awkward with unusual levels of perseverative interests. At the other end of the spectrum, children may have intellectual disability and have only nonverbal communication. Children with severe symptoms of autism are at high risk of developing serious problem behaviors, which can limit their opportunities for inclusion as well as have negative impacts on their families.

Apart from medical costs, which are often 4–6 times greater for children with ASD than typically developing children, intensive behavioral intervention can cost parents $40,000–$60,000 per year (Amendah, Grosse, Peacock, & Mandell, 2011). Beyond the enormous financial burden on many families of children with ASD regarding choice of treatments, some families face tremendous challenges in receiving supports and adapting their family life to meet the needs of their child with ASD. Behavioral interventions for children with autism are not yet widely available, so that parents in many regions have difficulty finding helpful interventions.

The strains on families across the life course are evident in a recent survey of families of children with autism and individuals with autism in California (Autism Society of California, 2012). Of the 1,412 respondents, only half (51%) reported feeling completely accepted by extended family and 23% accepted in their own neighborhoods. Researching therapies and accessing services prove to be another obstacle; most parents and individuals rated the autism service system moderate to very difficult to navigate. Only 2% of the parents with transition age children (14 years and older) believed the available adult services would meet their children's needs. In addition, only a quarter of adults with autism were employed. It is also found in the National Longitudinal Transition Survey that only 19.3% of young adults with autism were employed in paying jobs after leaving high school compared with 46% of all youth with disabilities and 68% of nondisabled youth (ages 16–24) in 2007 (Wagner, Newman, Cameto, Levine, & Marder, 2007). Most of these young people live and spend their days at home. This pattern continues into middle and late adulthood. Thus families can realistically expect to be responsible for the day-to-day support of their children with autism for several decades. Severe problem behaviors, difficulty understanding communicative attempts, and limited social interaction can become a lifelong set of challenges for these families. Given these facts, it is not surprising that parents express high levels of anxiety about their children's futures (Haiman, 2002; Moes & Frea, 2002).

Effective interventions for families are critical, because children with autism pose long-term caregiving challenges for families and society. Even with the best of treatments, a person with autism continues to need some form of lifelong support, most often from the family. The extent of the support can range from occasional, intermittent help to intensive daily caregiving. In addition, in the process of pursuing effective treatments to ameliorate their child's conditions, parents are sometimes desperate to look for a magic cure. There is also evidence that for mothers caregiving increases the risk of elevated depression symptoms and stress-related physical illness (Singer, 2006). However, upon gaining appropriate supports, families can adapt successfully to living with their loved ones with autism. Many families perceive their children with autism as positive contributors to the family's quality of life and to parents and siblings' personal development (Hastings & Taunt, 2002; Hastings et al., 2005). As families seek supports, they often find themselves easily lost and confused in a plethora of autism treatment models and programs including even those snake-oil kinds. Considering the multitude of non-scientific-based treatments and unproven practices for autism, parents feel it challenging to judge trustworthiness of interventions. Thereby identifying EBPs in the field of autism intervention has critical implications for both researchers and families of children with ASD. In this chapter, we provide a brief overview of EBPs to treat children with ASD. We then present a research synthesis of both randomized controlled trials (RCT) and single-subject design (SSD) studies regarding family-based and parent-implemented interventions for children with ASD and report the meta-analysis results of RCT studies.

Despite the plethora of research literature on effective early intervention programs (Odom, Boyd, Hall, & Hume, 2010; Wong et al., 2013), we chose not to target early intervention literature in our search for the reasons explained in chapter 1. However, 10 studies (seven RCT and three SSD studies) regarding younger children with ASD emerged during our search on family-based and parent-implemented interventions for children with ASD, meeting all the selection criteria of our search except for the age screener. Although we exclude these studies from the research synthesis and meta-analysis, we provide a brief summary of these 10 studies in Table 4.1.

OVERVIEW OF EVIDENCE-BASED PRACTICES FOR CHILDREN WITH AUTISM

It is noted that two comprehensive literature review reports of evidence-based intervention practices for children with ASD were completed recently by the National Autism Center (NAC) and the National Professional Development Center (NPDC) on ASD (Odom et al., 2010; Wong et al., 2013). In the National Standards Project (NSP), a comprehensive review of educational and behavioral treatment literature between 1957 and 2007 was conducted. The NAC (2009) developed the Scientific Merit Rating Scale (SMRS) to evaluate the level of scientific merit (ratings of 0–5 representing the least to most rigor of a study) of all selected studies. The SMRS consists of five critical dimensions of experimental rigor: (1) research design, (2) measurement of the dependent variable, (3) measurement of the independent variable or procedural fidelity, (4) participant

TABLE 4.1 SUMMARY OF STUDIES OF PARENT TRAINING FOR YOUNG CHILDREN WITH AUTISM SPECTRUM DISORDERS AGES 0–3 YEARS (EXCLUDED FROM THE RESEARCH SYNTHESIS)

Authors	*Design/Intervention components/Manual/Fidelity*	*Participants (Sample, Age, Ethnicity)/ Setting/Country*	*DV Measures*	*Treatment Effect(s)*
Brookman-Frazee & Koegel (2004)	• SSD (repeated reversal design) • To compare two parent education models (Parent/Clinician Partnership vs. Clinician-Directed Model) using Pivotal Response Treatment strategies • Manualized (Koegel et al., 1989) • Clinician fidelity reported on type of parent education	• 3 boys with autism (age 2) and their mothers • Asian American: 1; Latino American: 1; European American: 1 • Setting: PT and CI in clinic and at home	PARENT • Parent stress • Parent confidence CHILD - Affect • Engagement Responding	All parents demonstrated decreased levels of parental stress and increased parent confidence in the partnership condition than in the clinician-directed condition. All children demonstrated more positive affect, and higher levels of engagement and responding in the partnership model.
Carter et al (2011)	• RCT • To investigate the effect of Hanen's "More Than Words" (HMTW) vs. treatment as usual. • HMTW: 8 weekly group sessions and 3 individual family sessions designed to teach parents to structure everyday routines and provide parental responses to children's communication. Individual sessions incorporated video feedback and involved parent implementation of HMTW strategies • Control: treatment as usual • Manualized • Parent training fidelity was reported (88% delivery of intended items at group sessions and 89.9% delivery of intended items at individual sessions)	• 62 toddlers with autism (diagnosis confirmed by the Screening Tool for Autism in Two-year-olds [STAT]; 32 in Intervention and 30 in Control) and their parent • Ages 15–25 months (mean age 20.25 months); 51 boys and 11 girls • 47.4% White, 38.6% Latino, 3.5% Black, and 5.3% Asian/White, 3.5% American Indian/Alaskan Native/White, 1.8% American Indian/Alaskan Native/ Hispanic • Setting: PT at clinic and CI at home	PARENT • Parental responsivity • Parent-Child Free Play Procedure (PCFP) CHILD • Nonverbal communication • Parent Interview for Autism-Clinical Version (PIS-CV) • Initiating joint attention and behavior requesting: the Early Social Communication Scales (ESCS) • Intentional communication: PCFP	PARENT • No main effects of the HMTW intervention parental responsivity (no statistical significance, but effect sizes medium to large (Glass's Δ = .71 at 5-month follow-up and .50 at 9-month follow-up) CHILD • No main treatment effects on children's communication (initiating joint attention, initiating behavioral requests, and nonverbal communication) • Intervention was effective for children with low object interest but not for children with high object interest

Dawson et al. (2010)	• RCT • To evaluate the efficacy of the Early Start Denver Model (ESDM) vs. a waitlist control (the community intervention) • Parent training: Parents received training on ESDM principles and specific techniques through semimonthly meetings with primary therapists • Child intervention: Parents used ESDM strategies during daily activities (average: 16.3 hours/week, SD: 6.2) in addition to the therapist-delivered intervention (average: 15.2 hours/week, SD: 1.4) • Manualized (Rogers & Dawson, 2009) • Child intervention hours reported	• 48 toddlers with autism (diagnosis confirmed by ADI-R, ADOS, and DSM-IV; 24 in intervention and 24 in control) and their parent • Ages 18–30 months (mean age 23.5 months); boys vs. girls (3.5:1) • Asian (12.5%), White (72.9%), Latino (12.5%), and Multi-racial (14.6%) • Setting: PT at clinic and CI at home	CHILD • Cognition: the Mullen Scales of Early Learning • Adaptive behavior: VABS • The severity of autism: AODS, the Repetitive Behaviour Scale (RBS)	CHILD • Mullen scales of Early Learning composite standard scores (ESDM > Control) • VABS composite standard scores (ESDM > Control) • ESDM more likely to change in diagnosis from autism to PDD than the control group
Drew et al. (2002)	• RCT • To compare "joint attention focused parent training" vs. routine care • Parent training: consultant model with parent acting as everyday therapist. A speech and language therapist visited parents every 6 weeks for a 3-hour session. Training session focused on social pragmatic approach for joint attention, nonverbal social communication, language, and behavior management. • Child intervention: Parents delivered activities 30–60 minutes daily incorporated into everyday routines and completed an activity checklist. • Control: ongoing local education and therapy provision • Manualized • No fidelity reported	• 24 toddlers with autism (diagnosis confirmed by ADI-R; 12 in intervention and 12 in control) and their parent • Mean age 22 months; 19 boys and 5 girls • No race/ethnicity information reported • Setting: PT and CI at home • United Kingdom	PARENT • Parental stress: PSI CHILD • Language: MCDI (words understood, words said, and total gestures produced) • Symptom severity: ADI (reciprocal social interaction, nonverbal communication, repetitive and stereotyped behavior, and overall language rating) • Nonverbal IQ: the Griffiths Scale of Mental Development-D and E subscales	PARENT • No difference between two groups on parental stress CHILD • Children in the training group showed marginal (statistically nonsignificant) improvement in language comprehension • No difference between groups on language expression and gesture production • More children in the intervention group moved from being nonverbal to having single-word or phrase speech • No difference on autism symptom severity

(continued)

TABLE 4.1 (CONTINUED)

Authors	*Design/Intervention components/Manual/Fidelity*	*Participants (Sample, Age, Ethnicity)/ Setting/Country*	*DV Measures*	*Treatment Effect(s)*
Oosterling et al. (2010)	• RCT • To compare "focused parent training" (including routine care) vs. routine care only • Parent training: consultant model with parent acting as the everyday therapist. A psychologist visited the parents every 6 weeks for a 3-hour session. Training session focused on social pragmatic approach for joint attention, nonverbal social communication, and language development • Child intervention: parents asked to deliver activities 30–60 minutes daily incorporated into everyday routines and completed an activity checklist • Control: ongoing local education and therapy provision • Manualized (Drew et al., 2002) • No fidelity reported	-75 toddlers with autism and PDD-NOS (diagnosis confirmed by ADOS and ADI-R; 36 in intervention and 31 in control) and their parent • Ages 12–42 months (mean age 34.5 months); 75% boys • Setting: PT and CI at home • Netherlands	PARENT • Parental skills (supportive presence, respect for autonomy, structure and limit setting, quality of instruction, nonhostility): Erickson scales CHILD • Language development (words understood, words said): MCDI • Engagement (compliance, nonnegativity, nonavoidance): Erickson scales • Early precursors of social communication (gestures produced): MCDI • Joint attention: ADOS • Social affect: ADOS	PARENT • No intervention effect on parental skills CHILD • No intervention effect on language development • No intervention effect on "clinical global improvement" • No intervention effect on mediating outcome variables (engagement, early precursors of social communication, and parental skills)

Kasari et al. (2010)	• RCT • To investigate an effect of a joint attention intervention for parent training vs. a waitlist control (routine care) • Parent training: focused on joint attention/ engagement skills development with individualized for each parent–child dyad. Eight weeks of interventions (3 sessions per week with each session about 40 minutes) • Child intervention: Parents completed the parent adherence to treatment and competence and the caregiver quality of involvement was measured • Control: ongoing local intervention services • Manualized • Both parent training fidelity and child intervention fidelity (adherence to treatment strategies) reported	• 38 toddlers with autism (diagnosis confirmed by ADI-R and DSM-IV; 19 in intervention and 19 in control) and their parent • Ages 24–71 months (mean age 34.4 months); 29 boys and 9 girls • 22 White and 16 children of color • Setting: PT at clinic CI at home	PARENT • Caregiver quality of involvement • Parental adherence to treatment • Parental competence CHILD • Engagement states: unengaged/other engaged, object engagement, joint engagement) • Joint attention: frequency of joint attention initiation, frequency of joint attention responses • Play acts: type of functional play acts, type of symbolic play acts	PARENT • Higher parental quality of involvement significantly predicted increased joint engagement CHILD • The intervention group showed significant increases in responsiveness to joint attention ($d = .74$), time jointly engaged ($d = .97$), decreases in object only engagement ($d = 1.09$) and diversity of functional play acts ($d = .88$) compared with the control group • No treatment effect on the initiation of joint attention and diversity of symbolic play

(*continued*)

TABLE 4.1 (CONTINUED)

Authors	*Design/Intervention components/Manual/Fidelity*	*Participants (Sample, Age, Ethnicity)/ Setting/Country*	*DV Measures*	*Treatment Effect(s)*
Rocha, Schreibman, & Stahmer (2007)	• SSD (multiple baseline design across participants) • To assess parent-implemented naturalistic behavioral intervention (DTT & PRT) targeting joint attention responding • Manualized (Koegel et al., 1989; Maurice, Green, & Luce, 1996) • Parent fidelity reported	• 3 children with autism (2 boys and 1 girl ages 2.2–3.6 years) and their parents (2 mothers and 1 father) • Typical comparison group of 4 children matched on developmental age (ages 1–2) • No race/ethnicity information reported • Setting: PT and CI in clinic, generalization probes at home	PARENT • Fidelity of implementation • Initiations of joint attention bids • Satisfaction questionnaire CHILD • Bayley Scales of Infant Development, 2nd edition • MacArthur Communicative Development Inventory Words and Gestures (CDI) • Unstructured joint attention assessment • Child joint attention responding	Parents were able to maintain a high level of fidelity of implementation in the clinic training setting (range 93%–100%) and at home (range 90%–100%). All parents increased in initiations of joint attention bids and a concomitant increase was observed in children's joint attention responding. Two of three parents demonstrated a generalized increase in joint attention bids at home through treatment and follow-up. All children improved on overall joint attention responding as measured by the unstructured joint attention assessment. Parents indicated they were satisfied with training program and felt children improved during course of training.

Rogers et al. (2012) Estes et al. (2014)	• RCT • To evaluate the efficacy of a parent-coaching intervention based on the Early Start Denver Model (P-ESDM) vs. a community intervention control • Parent training: After initial 1.5 hours treatment evaluation session, parents received training on P-ESDM principles and specific techniques (e.g., social attention and motivation, imitation, functional and symbolic play, behavioral management) through twelve 1-hour treatment sessions by a therapist. • Child intervention: Parents were encouraged to use P-ESDM strategies during daily activities at home with their child • Manualized (Rogers & Dawson, 2009) • Parent training fidelity (a measure of therapist fidelity of administration of the P-ESDM) and child intervention fidelity (ESDM Parent Fidelity Tool) and child intervention hours reported	• 36 children with autism (DSM-III diagnosis with autism; 16 in intervention and 19 in control) • Ages 24–72 months (mean 43 months; 34 boys and 1 girl) • White: 33; other: 2 • Setting: PT and CI at community center and home	PARENT • Parent–child interaction scores • Parental stress: the Questionnaire on Resources and Stress • Parental sense of competence: the Parent Sense of Competence Scale • Working alliance scale for interventions with children CHILD • Social affect: ADOS • Restrictive & repetitive behavior: ADOS • Development quotient: MSEL (verbal DQ and nonverbal DQ) • Words and gestures: MCDI • Adaptive behavior: VABS • Imitative sequences • Social orient/nonsocial orient/orient to joint attention	PARENT • P-ESDM reported no increases in parenting stress whereas the control showed increases • No group differences in parental sense of competence and parent–child interaction scores CHILD • No significant differences on any of the child outcomes (both groups of children showed progress) • P-ESDM reported a significantly stronger working alliance with their primary therapist than the control

(*continued*)

TABLE 4.1 (CONTINUED)

Authors	*Design/Intervention components/Manual/Fidelity*	*Participants (Sample, Age, Ethnicity)/ Setting/Country*	*DV Measures*	*Treatment Effect(s)*
Schretz & Odom (2007)	• SSD (mixed methods with multiple baseline design across behaviors and qualitative analysis) • To assess the effects of a parent implemented, developmental, joint attention mediated learning intervention • Manualized • No fidelity reported	• 3 children with autism (boys ages 22–33 months) and their mothers (ages 23–32) • No race/ethnicity information reported	PARENT • Social validity questionnaire CHILD • Focus on faces • Turn-taking • Responding to joint attention • Initiating joint attention	All 3 children improved on focus on faces and turn-taking. Two of the children improved on responding and initiating joint attention. All parents reported improved confidence in their own ability to support child's interactions and better long-term child competence. Two parents reported satisfaction with their child's improvement, while 1 parent (whose child did not improve on joint attention measures) reported dissatisfaction.
Wong & Kwan (2009)	• Randomized single-blind crossover design • To investigate the efficacy of "the autism 1-2-3 intervention" vs. no treatment (crossover trial) • Parent training: A short-term intensive training based on behavioral and social-pragmatic models focusing on the use of eye contact, gestures, and words (daily for 5 days per week over 2-week period) • Child intervention: Parents were encouraged to use home practice of taught methods 5–10 minutes every hour at home with child • Control: no treatment • Manualized • No fidelity reported	• 17 toddlers with (diagnosis confirmed by ADI-R, ADOS, and DSM-IV; 9 in intervention and 8 in control) and their parents (including two grandparents) • Ages 17–36 months (mean age 26.53 months); 16 boys and 1 girl • Setting: PT at clinic; CI at home • Hong Kong	PARENT • Parental stress: PSI/SF • Parent child interaction CHILD • Communication: ADOS communication subscale, Ritvo-Freeman Real Life Rating Scale (RFLS) • Social interaction: AODS reciprocal social interaction subscale, RFLS • Symbolic play: Symbolic Play Test	PARENT • Parents perceived significant improvement in their children's language and social interaction CHILD • Children in the training group showed improvement in language/communication, reciprocal social interaction and symbolic play * Results of combined analysis were not interest of this review

ascertainment, and (5) generalization (NAC, 2009). On the basis of these criteria, the NSP report has identified a total of 11 "Established" treatments, 22 "Emerging" treatments, and 5 "Unestablished" treatments (NAC, 2009).

Likewise, the NPDC on ASD undertook another literature review project for identifying EDPs for children with autism, and found 24 qualified studies published between 1997 and 2007 (Odom et al., 2010). The standards of EBP are specified as: (1) at least two experimental or quasi-experimental group design studies, (2) at least five single case design studies, or (3) a combination of at least one experimental/quasi-experimental study and three single case design studies. As a follow-up, the NPDC on ASD expanded their project to include studies published from 2007 to 2011 in the literature and identified 28 EBP studies. The review was restricted only to studies of focused interventions designed to address one or a few specific skills such as reinforcement, social skills training, discrete trial teaching, naturalistic interventions, or peer-mediated instruction and developmental outcomes for children with ASD. As a result, the comprehensive treatment models such as the Early Start Denver Model, UCLA Young Autism Project, and Treatment and Education of Autistic and related Communication-Handicapped Children (TEACHH) were excluded from the review. In the report, parent-implemented intervention, which is defined as "programs in which parents are responsible for carrying out some or all of the intervention(s) with their own child" (Wong et al., 2013, p. 68), is identified as one of the 28 types of EBPs. The results of 20 identified studies (8 group design and 12 SSD studies) suggested that parent-implemented intervention has yielded significant outcomes across a variety of areas such as social communication, behavior, and joint attention for young children to elementary school-age children. In contrast, the NSP report does not single out parent-implemented intervention as a category of EBPs. Yet, the NSP report has included 24 identified studies under "Other Intervention Categories" regarding interventions implemented by parents (Wong et al., 2013). Overall, the NSP and NPDC on ASD reports have not covered thoroughly EBPs of parent-implemented interventions, particularly those based on SSD studies given the primary focus of their review.

PARENT-IMPLEMENTED EBP FOR CHILDREN WITH ASD

We conducted a thorough search of the literature on parent training/education programs and parent-implemented interventions for children with autism in a number of educational, psychological, and biomedical databases (see chapter 1). Search terms used in either a single or combined term include: "autism" ("autism spectrum disorders," "autistic disorder," "Asperger syndrome," and "pervasive developmental disorders"), "parents" ("parents," "mothers," "caregivers," and "fathers") and "intervention models" ("parent training," "parent-mediated," "parent-implemented," and "homes-based"). Following the same search and screening procedures delineated in earlier chapters, we eventually identified 14 RCT studies and 19 SSD studies that meet the EBP standards defined in chapter 1.

RANDOMIZED CONTROLLED TRIAL STUDIES: RESEARCH SYNTHESIS

A total of 14 RCT studies emerged from our search regarding home-based and parent-implemented interventions for children with ASD (see Table 4.2). Following a research synthesis of these RCT studies we conducted a meta-analysis to examine the effect sizes of treatments reported in these studies. In the research synthesis, we report the 14 studies categorized into five focus areas: effect of combined home-based and center-based parent training programs (4 studies), naturalistic behavioral interventions (1 study), social communication and interaction interventions (2 studies), relationship and activity-based interventions (3 studies), and effect of variants of behavioral parent training and psycho-educational interventions (4 studies).

Effect of Combined Parent Training Programs

In this section, we summarize four studies that examine the effect of combined home-based and center-based parent training programs. In an RCT study, Jocelyn et al. (1998) evaluated a caregiver-based intervention program for children with autism at community day-care centers. Thirty-five preschool children with a DSM-III-R diagnosis of autism or PDD were randomly assigned to either the experimental or control group. The children in the experimental group attended a day-care center where their parents, together with day-care center professionals, participated in a series of educational seminars totaling 15 hours over a 12-week intervention period. The seminars were designed to help parents and day-care center professionals perform a functional analysis to understand behaviors of children with ASD and facilitate their communication, play, and social interactions. Supplemental on-site consultations were provided to the parents at the day-care centers 3 hours per week for 10 weeks. Additionally, a program social worker and an autism behavior specialist offered supports to the parents via home visits. The children in the control group received only regular service from childcare workers at the community day-care centers. Assessment data were taken before and after the 12-week intervention program (see Table 4.2 for more details about measures used in the assessment). As for the treatment effect on the child outcomes, the treatment group had significant gains in the language-development domain as compared with the control group ($d = 0.87$). For parental outcomes, the treatment group reported significant increases in caregivers' knowledge about autism, greater perception of control from mothers, and greater parental satisfaction. But there seems no treatment effect on the measures of parents' confidence and stress or arousal (e.g., the Stress Arousal Checklist).

In another RCT study that examined the effect of a combined program of home-based intervention program and center-based educational program (Rickards et al., 2007), 59 children with autism and other developmental disabilities, aged 3–5 years, were randomly assigned to a only center-based educational program ($n = 29$) as control group or to a combined center-based and home-based intervention program ($n = 30$)

TABLE 4.2 RANDOMIZED CONTROLLED STUDIES OF PARENT TRAINING FOR YOUNG CHILDREN WITH AUTISM SPECTRUM DISORDERS

Authors	*Design/Intervention components/Manual/Fidelity*	*Participants (Sample, Age, Ethnicity)/Setting/Country*	*DV Measures*	*Treatment Effect(s)*
Aldred, Green, & Adams (2004)	• RCT (randomization stratified for age and autism severity) • To compare social communication training (including routine care) vs. routine care. • Parent training: parent psychoeducational workshops based on a social communication model, then individual monthly clinic sessions for 6 months and bimonthly clinic session for a following 6 months • Child intervention: Parents used social communication strategies with their child 30 minutes daily at home • Control: routine care • Manualized (Aldred, Plooanrd, Phillips, & Adams, 2001) • No fidelity reported	• 28 children with autism (diagnosis confirmed by ADI and ADOS; 14 in intervention and 14 in control) and their parent • Ages 2:0–5:11 years (mean age 49.5 months), 25 boys and 3 girls • All Caucasian except two mothers (African-Caribbean), predominantly middle class with various educational and income levels • Setting: PT at a clinic CI at home • United Kingdom	PARENT • Parental stress: PSI • Parent–child interaction: communication acts, asynchronous parental communication, semantic contingency, and shared attention CHILD • Autism severity: ADOS total, subdomain of reciprocal social interaction, communication, and stereotyped and restricted behaviors • Adoptive functioning: VABS • Language: MCDI	PARENT • No significant difference between the groups on parental stress • Child communication acts (intervention > control), Parent synchrony (intervention > control), Shared attentions (ns) CHILD • ADOS social communication algorithm score improved (intervention > control) • MCDI words understood and words said (ns) • VSBS (ns)

(*continued*)

TABLE 4.2 (CONTINUED)

Authors	*Design/Intervention components/Manual/Fidelity*	*Participants (Sample, Age, Ethnicity)/Setting/Country*	*DV Measures*	*Treatment Effect(s)*
Casenhiser, Shanker, & Stieben (2013)	• Ongoing RCT (stratified by age and language skills) • To evaluate the effect of a DIR-based intervention vs. a community treatment control • Parent training: therapist' provision 2 hours per week sessions plus coaching every 8 weeks for 12 months based on a social-communication model aiming to improve social interaction and parent–child relationship • Control: community treatment (average 3.9 hours per week) while on the wait-list • Manualized • Child intervention fidelity (a brief version of the MEHRIT Fidelity Scale; Casenhiser et al., 2010) reported	• 51 children with autism (diagnosis confirmed by ADOS and ADI); 25 in intervention and 26 in control) and their parent • Ages 2–4 years (mean age 42.52 months) • No race/ethnicity information reported; English as mother's native language: 27/51 • Income less than Canadian $50,000: 12/51 • Setting: PT at a clinic CI at home • Canada	PARENT • Parental behaviors: coregulation, expression of enjoyment, sensory-motor, joining, reciprocity, independent thinking, use of affect CHILD • Social interaction skills: attention to activity, involvement, compliance, initiation of joint attention & enjoyment in interaction (A modified version of the Child Behavior Rating Scale) • Language: Preschool Language Scale IV (PLS) and Comprehensive Assessment of Spoken Language (CASL)	PARENT • Parents in the intervention group improved significantly on all of the items with the exception of the sensory-motor support item CHILD • Intervention group made significantly greater gains in social interaction skills (attention to activity, involvement, initiation of joint attention and enjoyment in interaction) compared with the control group • No between-group difference on language skills

Green et al. (2010)	- RCT • To investigate the efficacy of parent-mediated communication focused treatment (PACT) vs. routine care • Parent training: based on a social communication model and targeting communication skills development. Individual clinic sessions biweekly 2-hours for 6 months then followed by monthly booster sessions for 6 months • Child intervention: Parents were encouraged to use 30 minutes of home practice of taught methods at home with their child daily • Control: ongoing local intervention services • Manualized • Parent training fidelity reported	• 152 children with autism (diagnosis confirmed by ADI-R or ADOS-G, 77 in intervention and 75 in control) and their parent • Ages 2:0-4:11 years (mean age 45 months); 138 boys and 74 girls • Non-White: 34% (*n* = 51), at least one parent in professional or administrative occupation: 63% (*n* = 95) • Setting: PT at a clinic CI at home • United Kingdom	PARENT • Parent–child interaction CHILD • The severity of autism symptoms: AODS-G • Language and social communication: the Preschool Language Scales, MCDI, the communication and Symbolic Behavior Scales Developmental Profile (CSBS-DP) • Adaptive functioning: VABS	PARENT • Treatment effect of parental synchronous response was positive • Treatment effect of child initiation with parent and for parent–child shared attention was positive CHILD • Effect size of severity of autism symptoms: -0.24 • Treatment effect on directly assessed language and adaptive functioning in school were small. • Treatment effect of parent ratings of language and social communication was positive

(continued)

TABLE 4.2 (CONTINUED)

Authors	*Design/Intervention components/Manual/Fidelity*	*Participants (Sample, Age, Ethnicity)/Setting/Country*	*DV Measures*	*Treatment Effect(s)*
Jocelyn, Casiro, Beattie, Bow, & Kneisz (1998)	• RCT (randomization stratified for autism severity) • To evaluate the efficacy of a caregiver-based intervention program in community day-care center vs. a day-care center control • Educational seminar to parents and day-care staff involving introduction to autism, behavior analysis techniques, communication and social development, process of problem solving 15 hours over 12 weeks. Concurrent consultation to day-care center total 30 hours and home visit consultation and supportive work with the family • Control: standard community day-care with counseling from a social worker • No manual reported • No fidelity reported	• 35 children with autism (DSM-III diagnosis with autism, 16 in Intervention and 19 in Control) and their parent, a staff of community day-care centers • Ages 24–72 months (mean 43 months); 34 boys and 1 girl • White: 33, other: 2 • Setting: PT and CI at a community center and home • US	PARENT • Knowledge about autism: TRE-ADD autism quiz) • Parental stress: Stress Arousal checklist • Family Assessment Measure • Client satisfaction questionnaire CHILD • Development of perceptual/fine motor, cognition, language, social/emotional, self-care, and gross motor: the Early Intervention Developmental Profile (EIDP; 0–36 months)/the Preschool Developmental Profile (PSDP; 36–60 months)	PARENT • Caregivers in the intervention group made significant gains in knowledge about autism, greater perception of control on the part of mothers, and greater parent satisfaction • No difference reported in parents' confidence and stress or arousal CHILD • Significant increases in language development domain for the intervention children • Both groups' children improved on all developmental measures
Nefdt, Koegel, Singer, & Gerber (2010)	- RCT • To investigate an effect of a self-directed learning program (Pivotal Response Training: PRT) vs. a waitlist control • Parent training: a self-directed learning program that consisted of an interactive DVD with an accompanying manual covering the procedures used in PRT. DVD aimed to teach parents strategies to increase child motivation to engage in social communication • Control: waiting list control • Manualized • Parental implementation fidelity reported	• 27 children with autism (diagnosis confirmed by DSM-IV) and their parent (88% mothers) • Mean age 38.43 months (intervention); 38.92 months (control); 92.6% boys • 81% White • Setting: PT and CI at home • United States	PARENT • Fidelity of implementation of PRT procedures • Language opportunities • Observed parent confidence • Social validity evaluation • Understanding of PRT procedures CHILD • Functional verbal utterances	PARENT • Use of motivational procedures of pivotal response training (intervention > control) • Use of more language opportunities (intervention > control) • Parent confidence (intervention > control) CHILD • Children's functional utterance (intervention > control)

Rickards, Walstab, Wright-Rossi, Simpson, & Reddihough, (2007, 2009)	• RCT • To investigate the efficacy of a home-based intervention program plus center-based intervention vs. a center-based intervention only • Home-based intervention: a special education teacher visited family's home weekly over 12 months (total of 40 visits) discussing protocols developed in the center providing generalization skills and helping family's concern • Center-based intervention: formulated program designed by a multidisciplinary team, 5 hours spread over 2 session weekly over 1 year • No manual reported • No fidelity reported	• 59 children with autism (n = 39, diagnosis confirmed by DSM-IV or ADI-R, or ADOS); developmental delay (n = 9), and language delay (n = 11); 30 in intervention and 29 in control • Ages 3:0-5:11 years (mean age 43.8 months); 47 boys and 12 girls • Family with high social status scores: n = 20; low scores: n = 39 • Setting: PT and CI at home • US	PARENT • Parental stress: the short form of the Questionnaire of Resources and Stress (QRS-F) • The Family Empowerment Scale (FES) • The Family Support Scale (FSS) CHILDREN • Cognition: the Mental Development Index of the Bayley Scales of Infant Development-Second Edition, Wechsler Preschool and Primary Scale of Intelligence Revised (WPPSI-R) • Adaptive behavior: VABS • Behavior: Bayley Behavior Rating Scale, Behavior Screening Questionnaire, Preschool Behavior Checklist	PARENT • No difference in family measures between two groups CHILD • Cognitive development and adaptive behavior were higher in children who had the additional home-based intervention and sustained after 1 year (only cognitive development) • Child improvements were significantly associated with higher stress in the families

(continued)

TABLE 4.2 (CONTINUED)

Authors	*Design/Intervention components/Manual/Fidelity*	*Participants (Sample, Age, Ethnicity)/Setting/Country*	*DV Measures*	*Treatment Effect(s)*
Roberts et al. (2011)	• RCT • To compare the outcomes of an individualized home-based program (HB) vs. a small group center-based program for children combined with a parent training and support group (CB) vs. a nontreatment comparison group • Home-based program: a visit by a therapist 2 hour once every 2 weeks over a 40-week period • Center-based program: 40 weekly 2-hour sessions including 6 playgroups of 4–6 children with 6 concurrent parent support and training groups • Control: nontreatment • Manualized (the Building Blocks Manual) • Fidelity of the CB session was implemented (10% of the CB session) and a review of the CB and HB treatment fidelity was made by a member of the research team	• 77 children with autism (59 children's diagnosis of autism confirmed by ADOS; 28 in HB, 28 in CB, and 29 in control) • Ages 2.2–5.0 years (mean 3.5 years; 90.5% boys) • Language other than English spoken at home or in addition to English: 20 families • Setting: HB at home, CB at center • Australia	PARENT • Parental stress: PSI • Family quality of life: the Beach Family Quality of Life Questionnaire • Perception of competence in managing their child: the Parent Perception questionnaire CHILD • Communication: the Reynell Developmental Language Scales III, the Pragmatics Profile • Social skills: VABS • Adaptive functioning and psychopathology: the Developmental Behavior Checklist	PARENT • Parents in the CB reported greater gains in perception of competence and family quality of life CHILD • Children in the CB showed significant improvement for the Reynell developmental Language Scales and the social scale of VABS compared with HB and the control • No statistically significant differences between three groups for the Pragmatics Profiles and DBC

Siller, Hutman, Sigman (2013), Siller, Swanson, Gerber, Hutman, & Sigman (2014)	• Randomized clinical trial • To evaluate the efficacy of Focused Playtime Intervention (FPI) vs. a control • Parent training: 12 in-home training sessions (1 session per week for 12 weeks, 90 minutes per session) by a trained therapist aiming to improve responsive parental behaviors and children's communication • Control: four sessions of Parent Advocacy Coaching (FPI received three sessions of PAC) • Manualized • Parent training fidelity reported	• 60 children with autism (diagnosis confirmed by ADI-R, AODS-G; 36 in intervention and 34 in control) • Ages 32–82 months (mean 57 months; 64 boys and 6 girls) • Hispanic: 31, White: 14, Asian: 13, Black: 5, and Mixed: 7 • Annual household income below $20,000: 8 • Setting: PT and CI at home • United States	PARENT • Responsive parental communication: maternal verbal behaviors, maternal synchronization • The insightfulness assessment CHILD • Nonverbal cognitive and language abilities: MSEL • Response to bids for joint attention • Children's toy-directed attention • Attachment behaviors: Maternal Perception of Child Attachment questionnaire, Proximity/Contact Seeking Behavior Scale rated based on the separation-reunion episode	PARENT • FPI intervention effect on responsive parental behaviors, especially, moderated by baseline measures of maternal insightfulness CHILD • Conditional FPI effect on children's expressive language, indicating children with very low baseline language skills (below 12 months) benefited from FPI • FPI intervention effect on both attachment-related measures
Sofronoff, Leslie, & Brown (2004)	• RCT • To evaluate the efficacy of a short-term parent management training in 1-day workshop vs. individual sessions vs. waitlist control • Parent training included psychoeducation, Comic Strip Conversation, Social Stories, and management of behavior problems and anxiety. The training delivered in 1-day workshop or a 6 individual sessions (1 hour weekly) • Control: no intervention • Manualized • No fidelity reported	• 51 children with Asperger syndrome • Ages 6–12 years (mean age 9.4 years) • Setting: PT at clinic; CI at home • Australia	PARENT • The usefulness of the workshop (individual sessions) questionnaire CHILD • Number of problem behaviors and intensity of problem behaviors: the Eyberg Child Behavior Inventory (ECBI) • Social skills: the social Skills Questionnaire	PARENT • Parents reported the workshop to be useful CHILD • Both intervention groups reported significant fewer and lower intensity of problem behaviors compared with the control • Both intervention groups increased social interactions

(*continued*)

TABLE 4.2 (CONTINUED)

Authors	*Design/Intervention components/Manual/Fidelity*	*Participants (Sample, Age, Ethnicity)/Setting/Country*	*DV Measures*	*Treatment Effect(s)*
Tonge et al. (2006), Tonge, Brereton, Kiomall, Mackinnon, & Rinehart (2014)	• RCT • To evaluate the impact of parent education and behavior management intervention vs. parent education and counseling intervention vs. control group • Parent education and behavior management intervention (PEBM): manual-based education and behavior management skills training based on multiple early intervention and cognitive behavioral techniques. Ten 90-minute small-group sessions plus ten 60-minute individual family sessions • Parent education and counseling intervention (PEAC): all same training as the PEBM group except no skills training, no child present, and no homework tasks at individual sessions. Only discussion and counseling provided. • Control: treatment as usual • Manualized (Brereton & Tonge, 2005) • Parent training fidelity checked for a random 10% of sample of group therapy sessions.	• 105 children with autism (with DSM-IV diagnosis and confirmed by a screen observation by a independent clinician; 35 in PEBM, 35 in PEAC, and 30 in control) and their parent • Ages 2.5–5 years; 87 boys and 18 girls • Hispanic: 31, White: 14, Asian: 13, Black: 5, and Mixed: 7 • Annual household income below $20,000: 8 • Setting: PT and CI at home • Australia	PARENT • Parental mental health: the General Health Questionnaire (somatic symptoms, social dysfunction, anxiety and insomnia, and severe depression) • Parental stress: the Parenting Stress Thermometer • Family functioning: the McMaster Family Assessment Device CHILD • Adaptive behavior: VABS • Behavioral problems and autism symptoms: the Developmental Behavior Checklist • Cognition: the Psychoeducational Profile-Revised • Language: the Reynell Developmental Language Scales III	PARENT • Significant and progressive improvement in overall parental mental health for both treatment groups • PEBM was more effective in anxiety, insomnia, and family dysfunction than PEAC CHILD • PEBM showed significant improvement in adaptive behavior and symptoms of autism severity in comparison with PAEC • No significant effect on cognitive and language development

Whittingham, Sofronoff, Sheffield, & Sanders (2009)	• RCT (mixed within-between-subjects) • To investigate the efficacy of the parenting program Stepping Stones Triple P (SSTP) vs. a waitlist control • Parent training: partial group (4–5 parents) sessions involving parenting strategies and an individual sessions including observation, practice and feedback • Control: treatment as usual (waitlist) • Manualized (Stepping Stones Triple P; Whittingham, Sofronoff, & Sheffield, 2006) • No fidelity reported	• 59 children with ASD (diagnosis confirmed by DSM-IV; 29 in intervention and 30 in control) • Ages 2–9 years (mean age 5.91 months); 47 boys and 12 girls • No racial/ethnicity information reported • Setting: PT at a clinic CI at home • Australia	PARENT • Parenting style: Parenting Scale (laxness, overreactivity, and verbosity) • Parenting satisfaction and parental efficacy: Being a Parent Scale CHILD • Intensity and number of behavior problems: Eyberg Child Behavior Inventory	PARENT • Significant improvements in dysfunctional parenting styles (laxness, overreactivity, and verbosity) with the treatment effects of child behavior, parental overreactivity and verbosity being maintained at 6-month follow-up • Marginally significant improvements in parental satisfaction and conflict about parenting as well as a sleeper effect for parental efficacy CHILD • Significant improvements in parental reports of child behavior (the intensity and the number of problem behaviors)

as experimental group. The center-based program consisted of two sessions of 5 hours per week focusing on individualized education to children with autism over a school year. Families in the combined program were visited by a special education teacher weekly (1 to 1.5 hours per visit) over a period of 12 months. During the home visit, the special education teacher discussed with the parents the protocols developed in the center for home implementation, encouraged parents to help their children generalize skills learned at the center, and addressed other family concerns. Assessment data were taken before and after the 1-year program. In comparison with the only center-based program, the children with ASD in the combined program had obtained significantly larger improvements in cognitive development and adaptive behavior. In particular, children with ASD with greater gains seem to be significantly associated with those families with higher initial stress levels before the treatment. But no treatment effect was found on family outcome measures. Furthermore, after a 1-year follow-up of the intervention, Rickards et al. (2009) found that the children with ASD in the combined program had sustained improvement only on the cognitive development domain, but not on the adaptive behavior domain.

Yet another RCT study employed two treatment condition groups and a nontreatment control group to further investigate the treatment effect of parent training programs (Roberts et al., 2011). Apart from a nontreatment control group of 29 children with autism, 56 children with autism were randomly assigned to either a center-based treatment group with parent training and support program (n = 28) or an individual home-based program (n = 28). The center-based program offered 40 weekly 2-hour sessions to the participating children in six playgroups in conjunction with six concurrent parent support and training groups. The home-based program provided home visits (2 hours per visit) by therapists to the participating families once every other week over a 40-week period. Baseline and 12-month postintervention assessment data were taken on both child outcome measures (e.g., communication, social skills, adaptive functioning, and psychopathology) and parent outcome measures (e.g., parenting stress and family quality of life). The children with ASD in the center-based group outperformed over those in the home-based-only group and the control group on social and communication measures. While no difference was found between the parents in the home-based program and the control group on both child and family outcomes, the parents in the center-based group reported greater gains in perception of competence and family quality of life.

The results of the first three studies seem to favor the combined center-based and home-based programs over the only center-based program. But the findings of this fourth seem to suggest that the small-group center-based program along with concurrent parent training and support group is the most effective model. Given the mixed effect (2:1 ratio) of different types of parent training programs, we conclude that the combined center-based and home-based programs are promising practices for supporting families of children with ASD.

Naturalistic Behavioral Interventions

Nefdt et al. (2010) conducted an RCT study to examine a self-directed learning model of pivotal response treatment (PRT). Twenty-seven children with ASD who met DSM-IV criteria and had a language ability level of less than 20 functional words were randomly assigned to a treatment group ($n = 13$) or a waitlist control group ($n = 14$). Parents in both groups reported clinically significant levels of stress. The treatment group was involved in a self-directed learning program in which the parents received an interactive DVD along with a manual covering the PRT procedures to teach first words to children with ASD. The parents in the control group were on the waitlist for receiving PRT training later. Besides the primary outcome measure of expressive verbal language, the study included other measures such as language opportunities, observed parent confidence, and parental satisfaction. Results showed significant differences between the treatment and control groups at posttest on all the outcome measures with the treatment group consistently outperforming the waitlist control group. In particular, the children in the treatment group showed improvements in the use of functional utterances ($d = .953$). Parents in the treatment group gained significantly in their use of language opportunities ($d = 2.23$), in improvement in parent confidence ($d = 1.28$), and in fidelity of PRT implementation ($d = 4.12$). The unusually high effect size of treatment attests to a substantial gain in children's speech in the treatment group. Given the positive results of the PRT program at minimal cost and effort, it appears that the self-directed learning program may well serve as an initial step toward providing parent-education for families of children with ASD. We provide an evaluation of PRT as EBP in comjunction with the evidence of SSD studies in later section.

In addition, three studies emerged from our search with respect to the Early Start Denver Model (ESDM), which employs PRT as a major component of the program (Dawson et al., 2010; Estes et al., 2014; Rogers et al., 2012). These studies that examined the treatment effect of ESDM on young children with ASD (toddlers under the age of 3) were excluded from the research synthesis and meta-analysis because of the age screener of this book. A brief summary of the three studies is included in Table 4.1.

Social Communication and Interaction Interventions

An RCT study was conducted in the UK to examine the effect of intervention, focused on the development of parental abilities to understand and respond to their child's communication and facilitate the child's pragmatic intentions (Aldred et al., 2004). Twenty-eight children with autism were randomly assigned to the treatment group ($n = 14$) or the control ($n = 14$) group, and the randomization was stratified for participants' chronological age and severity of autism (e.g., Autism Diagnostic Observation Schedule [ADOS] scores). Parents in the treatment group received initial training via a workshop series and maintenance training via monthly individual sessions for 6 months and then bimonthly sessions for another 6 months at the clinic. The parent training primarily focused on shared engagement, parental sensitivity and responsiveness, adapted communication strategies, and consolidation and elaboration. Parents were recommended to apply their learned strategies for 30 minutes each day at home. After 12 months of the intervention, the assessment results showed significant improvements in the ADOS scores, particularly in the area of reciprocal social interaction, expressive language, communicative initiations and parent–child interaction for the treatment group. The study results reveal that a structured and individually tailored parent training program at relatively low intensity (once a month) is effective for improving children's social communication skills.

Following the previous trial (Aldred et al., 2004), a larger RCT study was conducted by the same research team in the UK involving 152 children with autism and their families (Green et al., 2010). Children were randomly assigned to a parent-mediated communication-focused intervention group (n = 77), referred to as PACT (Preschool Autism Communication Trial), or to a treatment-as-usual control group (n = 75). The PACT treatment targeted social interaction and communication skills of children based on a social communication development model. The PACT training was delivered individually to the parent–child dyad by the therapists in centers across the London, Manchester, and Newcastle areas. After an initial orientation session, the participants attended biweekly 2-hour sessions for 6 months and then monthly booster sessions for another 6 months. The trained parents were encouraged to engage in 30 minutes of daily home practice with their child applying the strategies they learned. The control group received only local intervention services as usual. Despite nonsignificant reduction in the ADOS scores, the PACT treatment group witnessed a positive treatment effect for parental synchronous response to child (effect size = 1.22) and child initiations with parent (effect size = 0.41), and for parent–child shared attention (effect size = 0.33). However, there seems to be no treatment effect on the standardized measures of child language and adaptive functioning in school which contradicts the parents' perceived improvements of their children's language and social communication in the PACT group. Despite mixed effect on the child outcomes, two well designed RCT studies provide us adequate evidence to conclude that the PACT program is an established practice of parents implemented social communication and interaction interventions.

In addition, one study by Kasari et al. (2010) offers strong evidence of the effect of a parent-mediated joint attention intervention for toddlers with autism. But because of the age range of children included in this book, we excluded this study in our research synthesis and meta-analysis. A brief summary of this study is included in Table 4.1.

Relationship and Activity-Based Interventions

Casenhiser et al. (2013) examined the effect of the Developmental, Individual Differences, and Relationship (DIR) program through a recent RCT study of 51 children with autism. Children were randomly assigned to either a (DIR)-based intervention or a community intervention (treatment as usual) group with stratification by age and baseline level of language function. The DIR-based intervention focuses on parent involvement in intervention to improve social interaction and communication skills of children with ASD and incorporates the use of sensory motor supports and coregulation. The parent training in the DIR-based intervention group was delivered by licensed speech and language pathologists (SLPs) or occupational therapists (OTs), and the families received 2 hours of therapy per week and coaching every other month for a period of 12 months. Parents were asked to spend at least 3 hours per day interacting with their child and applying the learned techniques. Children in the community intervention group received a variety of typical services available in the community, such as speech therapy, applied behavior analysis, occupational therapy, and social skills group averaging 4 hours per week. Casenhiser et al. (2013) found that children in the DIR-based intervention group made significantly greater gains in social interaction skills (e.g., attention to activity, involvement, initiation of joint attention, and enjoyment in interaction) in comparison with the community intervention group and that no differences were found between the two groups in the standardized measures of language. Additionally, regression analysis results reveal that variables of initiation of joint attention, involvement, and low level of language delay predict significantly children's improvement of language skills.

In two subsequent RCT studies, a research team evaluated the effect of a focused playtime intervention (FPI) on responsive parenting behaviors and communication of children with ASD (Siller et al., 2013; Siller et al., 2014). Seventy children were randomly assigned to either a FPI intervention group (n = 36) or a control group (n = 34). Both groups received an education program, Parent Advocacy Coaching, during the study, aiming at enhancing the parents' ability to participate in the planning of their children's intervention and educational programs. The FPI treatment group received another parent education program that consisted of 12 in-home training sessions (90 minutes per session per week for 12 weeks) in which parents received a standard treatment manual and training by therapists (Siller et al., 2013). Siller et al. (2013) found that the parents in the FPI intervention group made significantly greater gains in responsive parental behaviors and children's expressive language as compared with the control group. Interestingly, the intervention effect on responsive parental behaviors was moderated by baseline measures of maternal insightfulness, suggesting that only those parents classified as insightful at the baseline had effectively changed their communication behaviors in response to the FPI intervention. Likewise, the FPI effect on children's expressive language was moderated by the baseline language skills of children below 12 months. In the subsequent study, Siller et al. (2014) reported that the FPI intervention group also acquired significantly greater gains on children's attachment related outcomes as compared with the control group.

In summary, evidence from one RCT study on the DIR-based intervention only warrants it to be a promising practice regarding relationship- and activity-based interventions for children with ASD. In contrast, two RCT studies of the FPI program have provided strong evidence for us to conclude that it is an established practice.

Effect of Variants of Behavioral Parent Training and Psychoeducational Interventions

Two RCT studies were conducted subsequently by Tonge and colleagues to investigate the effect of a parent education and behavior management intervention (PEBM) on parents of children with ASD (Tonge et al., 2006; Tonge et al., 2014). In two rural and two metropolitan regions in Australia, children with ASD were randomly assigned to either the treatment condition ($n = 70$) or the control condition ($n = 30$). The children in the treatment condition were further assigned randomly to either a PEBM group ($n = 35$) or a parent education and counseling intervention (PECI) group ($n = 35$). Parents in the PEBM group received a manualized education and training on behavior management skills. The program consisted of 10 group sessions and 10 individual sessions. The 90-minute small group sessions focused on understanding autism, communication, social play and behavioral features of autism, principles of behavioral management, teaching new skills, improving social interaction and communication, and managing parental stress and mental health problems. The 60-minute individual family sessions over a period of 20 weeks focused on parent skills training using modeling, video, rehearsal, homework task, workbooks, and feedback. Parents in the PECI group also received a manualized education program through group sessions, like the PEBM group, and through different individual sessions focused on interactive discussion and counseling between parents and a therapist rather than skills training or homework tasks. The control group received no special intervention other than access to local services. Assessment data were collected at baseline, postintervention, and 6-month follow-up. Results showed that children in the PEBM group demonstrated significant improvement in adaptive behavior and autistic symptoms as compared with the PECI group. Further analysis reveal that the treatment effect of PEBM intervention is moderated by the children's pretest levels of communication skills, suggesting that children who have greater communication delays obtain greater gains from the PEBM intervention. In a subsequent study of the follow-up of the interventions, Tonge and colleagues (2014) found that both treatment groups achieved more significant and progressive improvements than the control group in overall parental mental health at follow-up. In particular, the parents who had the highest level of mental health problems demonstrated significant improvement. The PEBM program was also more effective than the PECI in alleviating a greater percentage of anxiety, insomnia, and somatic symptoms and family dysfunction.

Sofronoff et al. (2004) evaluated the efficacy of short-term parent management training on problem behaviors associated with Asperger syndrome in an RCT study. Fifty-one parents of children (aged 6–12 years) with Asperger syndrome were randomized to three conditions: a 1-day workshop, six individual lessons, or a waitlist control. The parent training program for the treatment groups focused on the nature of Asperger syndrome, Comic Strip Conversations, Social Stories, and management of behavior problems, routines, special interests, and anxiety. Child problem behaviors and social skills were measured at pretreatment, 1 month posttreatment and 3 month follow-up. Sofronoff et al. found (2004) that the parents in both treatment groups reported a significant decrease in the number and intensity of their child's behavior problems and significant increases in their child's social skills at 1-month and 3-month follow-up as compared with the waitlist control group. In addition, the individual session group reported significantly lower intensity of problem behaviors than the workshop and waiting list group at both 1-month and 3-month follow-up.

Moreover, this parent training program was further developed by the same research team to become a widely recognized multicomponent intervention program, the Stepping Stones Triple P program (SSTP) (Sanders et al., 2004). A detailed description about the SSTP program will be provided in Chapter 5 focus on multicomponent intervention programs. In a subsequent RCT study, Whittingham et al. (2009) reexamined the effect of this parent training program targeting problem behaviors of children with ASD. Treatment effect was found on both child outcomes (e.g., problem behaviors) and parent outcomes (e.g., parenting styles, parental satisfaction) in this study.

In summary, the results of two RCT studies of the PEBM program (as a variant of Behavioral Parent Training) and the PECI program have provided adequate evidence to conclude that both PEBM and PECI programs are established practices for supporting parents of children with ASD. Evidence of one RCT study of the SSTP program reviewed here in conjunction with other evidence about the SSTP program discussed in Chapter 5 warrants the SSPT program as established practices for supporting families of children with ASD.

META-ANALYSIS OF RANDOMIZED CONTROLLED TRIAL STUDIES

In addition to a research synthesis, a meta-analysis of 11 RCT studies was completed to calculate and examine the effect size of each individual intervention program, model, or package of techniques as well as an overall effect size of the home-based and parent-implemented interventions for children with ASD. As introduced in chapter 1 and illustrated with examples in chapters 2 and 3, meta-analysis is a way to put together the data from many different studies in order to characterize them as a group and is a useful tool for examining the efficacy or effectiveness of a variety of interventions (Singer, Ethridge, & Aldana, 2007). Effect sizes of intervention programs or models were first calculated using a computerized program, Comparative Meta-Analysis (2013). By following common procedures (Rosenthal et al., 2000), we calculated Cohen's *d* as an indicator of effect size on the basis of three types of statistical information: (1) reported effect sizes in the original studies (Casenhiser et al., 2013, and Nefdt et al., 2010), (2) F statistics or P values for difference in change scores (Roberts et al., 2011, and one dependent measure of Aldred et al., 2004), and (3) posttest means (means at posttest and follow-up) and standard deviations (for all other eight studies).

Table 4.3 presents the 11 parent-implemented autism intervention studies in columns. The second column denotes the type of outcome measures for either parents or children. The different outcome measures used in the studies are presented in the fourth column

TABLE 4.3 SUMMARY DATA FOR META-ANALYSIS OF RANDOMIZED CONTROLLED TRIAL STUDIES OF PARENT TRAINING PROGRAMS FOR CHILDREN WITH ASD

				Intervention				*Comparison*				
				n		*Mean (SD)*		*n*		*Mean (SD)*		*d*
Study	*Type*	*Outcome*	*Measure*	*Pre*	*Post*	*Pre*	*Post*	*Pre*	*Post*	*Pre*	*Post*	
Aldred et al. (2004)	Child	Adaptive behavior	VABS-C	14	14	22.6 (13.3)	36.9 (21.2)	14	14	20.0 (10.8)	28.7 (16.6)	0.29
	Child	Autism symptoms	ADOS	14	14	16.1 (4.5)	11.8 (6.4)	14	14	15.6 (4.9)	22.6 (13.3)	0.87
	Child	ESI (Attention)	Video Coding	14	14	72.0 (23.6)	77.6 (17.8)	14	14	62.8 (14.5)	62.6 (32.7)	0.22
	Parent	PCI (Synchrony)	Video Coding	14	14	57.8 (15.0)	65.1 (14.3)	14	14	57.1 (49.5)	49.5 (18.9)	0.89
	Parent	Parental Stress	PSI	14	14	$F = 0.290$		14	14			0.20
		Overall										0.48
Casenhiser et al. (2013)	Child	Behavior Problem	mCBRS	25	25	2.68 (0.75)	3.48 (0.96)	26	26	2.85 (0.78)	3.35 (0.80)	0.51
	Child	ESC (Joint attention)	mCBRS	25	25	1.28 (0.54)	1.84 (0.55)	26	26	1.31 (0.99)	1.23 (0.44)	0.69
	Child	Language	PLS/CASL	25	25	0.64 (0.32)	0.72 (0.39)	26	26	0.54 (0.26)	0.64 (0.32)	1.02
	Child	Social Interaction	mCBRS	25	25	2.56 (0.58)	3.20 (0.87)	26	26	2.62 (0.70)	2.69 (0.79)	0.23
	Child	ESC (Attention)	mCBRS	25	25	2.96 (0.74)	3.72 (0.61)	26	26	3.08 (0.80)	3.38 (0.75)	0.87
	Parent	PCI (Reciprocity)	mCBRS	25	25	1.12 (0.78)	1.76 (1.13)	26	26	0.85 (0.73)	0.65 (0.80)	0.86
		OVERALL										0.70
Green et al. (2010)	Child	Autism symptoms	ADOS	77	77	19.6 (4.2)	15.7 (6.0)	75	75	19.3 (4.0)	16.5 (5.7)	0.19
	Child	ESC (Initiation)	Observation	77	77	23.0 (17.4)	34.9 (19.7)	75	75	24.4 (18.5)	26.0 (17.5)	0.55
	Child	Language	MCDI-E	77	77	93.5 (114.8)	171.9 (150.7)	75	75	111.1 (128.6)	163.8 (144.3)	0.01
	Child	Language	MCDI-R	77	77	159.5 (114.4)	233.7 (129.6)	75	75	162.0 (122.4)	209.0 (131.3)	0.05
	Parent	PCI (Synchrony)	Observation	77	77	31.8 (14.8)	51.3 (19.6)	75	75	31.3 (14.6)	32.6 (14.0)	1.07
		OVERALL										0.37
Jocelyn et al. (1998)	Child	Autism symptoms	ABC	16	16	56.80 (21.71)	48.20 (23.33)	19	19	56.15 (26.41)	54.80 (23.63)	0.31
	Child	Cognition	EIDP/PSDP	16	16	25.90 (98.5)	27.20 (10.8)	19	19	25.10 (9.7)	27.00 (10.4)	0.03
	Child	Language	EIDP/PSDP	16	16	24.80 (13.6)	30.20 (15.0)	19	19	20.90 (10.6)	21.90 (9.6)	0.36
	Child	Social Interaction	EIDP/PSDP	16	16	30.90 (12.5)	31.90 (13.1)	19	19	28.40 (12.1)	31.90 (13.2)	0.19
	Family	Family Well-Being/ Functioning	FAM	16	16	45.30 (7.08)	46.10 (5.96)	19	19	45.44 (6.60)	46.75 (7.85)	0.07
	Parent	Knowledge/Skills	TAQ	16	16	18.45 (2.68)	20.4 (3.42)	19	19	19.8 (2.91)	20.1 (2.65)	0.55
	Parent	Stress	SAC	16	16	6.35 (5.67)	6.15 (5.60)	19	19	6.95 (4.96)	6.00 (5.08)	0.14
		OVERALL										0.25

Nefdt et al. (2010)	Child	Language	Observation	13	14	11.96 (-)	39.12 (31.45)	13	14	20.54 (-)	16.14 (16.77)	0.95
	Parent	PCI (Language Opportunity)	Observation	3	14	-	75 (21.31)	13	14	-	22.86 (25.46)	2.23
	Parent	Confidence	Observation	13	14	-	-	13	14	3.85 (1.14)	2.21 (1.42)	1.28
		OVERALL										1.41
Rickards et al. (2007, 2009)	Child	Adaptive behavior	VABS	30	28	63.14 (17.70)	66.21 (21.20)	28	23	56.52 (13.80)	60.70 (20.40)	0.05
	Child	Behavior Problem	BRS	29	24	99.67 (15.40)	103.67 (13.20)	28	23	97.35 (99.65)	99.65 (10.20)	0.14
	Child	Behavior Problem	BSQ	30	27	11.10 (5.10)	7.67 (5.20)	28	23	8.91 (4.10)	7.57 (3.60)	0.46
	Child	Behavior Problem	PCBL	27	26	17.87 (9.80)	11.83 (8.60)	26	23	16.87 (10.00)	17.17 (8.00)	0.76
	Child	Cognition	BSID/WPPSI	30	282	61.25 (19.10)	66.21 (22.30)	29	26	61.46 (21.50)	57.85 (22.80)	0.38
		OVERALL										0.35
Roberts et al. (2011)	Child	Adaptive behavior	VABS-C	29	29	66.9 (12.5)	76.1 (17.1)	28	28	68.5 (17.0)	74.2 (15.5)	0.27
	Child	Adaptive behavior	VABS-S	29	29	70.1 (7.3)	72.6 (11.2)	28	28	70.8 (9.9)	73.1 (10.8)	0.01
	Child	Behavior Problem	DBC	29	29	58.5 (20.4)	55.7 (19.5)	28	28	43.9 (21.9)	42.9 (24.3)	0.12
	Child	Language	RDL-E	29	29	6.9 (9.9)	11.4 (10.9)	2	28	5.8 (7.9)	11.1 (9.9)	0.11
	Child	Language	RDL-R	29	29	11.3 (13.8)	23.7 (19.9)	28	28	12.2 (14.9)	22.0 (17.8)	0.23
	Family	Family Well-Being/ Functioning	Beach Center FQOL Scale	29	29	3.5 (0.5)	3.7 (0.6)	28	28	3.7 (0.5)	3.8 (0.5)	0.21
	Parent	Knowledge/Skills	PSQ	29	29	3.5 (0.6)	4.2 (0.4)	28	28	3.7 (0.5)	4.1 (0.5)	0.89
	Parent	Confidence	PSQ	29	29	3.3 (0.7)	3.7 (0.7)	28	28	3.9 (0.6)	4.0 (0.7)	0.73
	Parent	Stress	PSI	29	29	103.4 (19.6)	98.2 (20.1)	28	28	97.1 (22.0)	90.4 (22.9)	0.08
		OVERALL										0.30
Siller et al. (2013) & Siller et al. (2014)	Child	ESC (Attachment)	Separation-reunion episode	28	31	3.47 (1.89)	3.83 (1.67)	31	28	3.83 (1.7)	3.1 (1.64)	0.66
	Child	Language	MSEL	36	34	3.70 (0.93)	4.02 (0.93)	34	30	3.75 (0.88)	3.90 (0.93)	0.38
	Parent	PCI (Synchrony)	Observation	36	34	0.57 (0.18)	0.72 (0.04)	34	30	0.63 (0.17)	0.61 (0.22)	0.11
		OVERALL										0.70
Sofronoff et al. (2004)	Child	Behavior Problem	ECBI-I	36	15	145.08 (26.43)	120.55 (22.70)	36	15	144.73 (26.39)	148.0 (31.75)	1.09
	Child	Behavior Problem	ECBI-B	36	15	17.17 (5.81)	10.59 (6.03)	36	15	18.13 (5.19	17.53 (5.65)	1.09
	Child	Social Interaction	SSQ	36	15	24.44 (9.481)	31.86 (7.998)	36	15	25.07 (6.64)	24.27 (8.57)	1.01
		OVERALL										1.06

(continued)

TABLE 4.3 (CONTINUED)

				Intervention				*Comparison*				
				n		*Mean (SD)*		*n*		*Mean (SD)*		*d*
Study	*Type*	*Outcome*	*Measure*	*Pre*	*Post*	*Pre*	*Post*	*Pre*	*Post*	*Pre*	*Post*	
Tonge et al. (2006) & Tonge et al. (2014)	Child	Adaptive behavior	VABS-C	35	35	64.74 (20.69)	71.71 (19.83)	35	35	63.24 (14.23)	69.53 (24.05)	0.11
	Child	Adaptive behavior	VABS-S	35	35	61.03 (9.84)	73.31 (16.59)	35	35	57.09 (6.33)	67.35 (16.70)	0.12
	Child	Autism symptoms		35	35	26.05 (9.14)	20.77 (8.05)	35	35	23. 80 (10.44)	22.89 (10.42)	0.45
	Child	Behavior Problem	DBC	35	35	64.91 (25.01)	53.29 (24.36)	35	35	73.77 (16.98)	63.83 (27.59)	0.07
	Family	Family Well-Being/ Functioning	MFAD	35	35	1.76 (0.46)	1.78 (0.32)	35	35	1.70 (0.64)	1.94 (0.52)	0.51
	Parent	Mental Health	GHQ	35	35	28.54 (13.43)	18.03 (13.56)	35	35	19.17 (7.61)	21.69 (10.20)	1.09
	Parent	Stress	PST	35	35	2.51 (0.82)	1.86 (0.94)	35	35	2.06 (0.87)	2.26 (1.09)	0.84
		OVERALL										0.44

Whittingham et al. (2009)	Child	Behavior Problem	ECBI-I	29	30	144.14 (31.32)	121.40 (25.28)	29	30	142.19 (31.73)	148.63 (30.33)	1.04
	Child	Behavior Problem	ECBI-B	29	30	18.06 (7.71)	11.21 (6.77)	29	30	19.72 (6.83)	18.82 (8.32)	0.78
	Parent	Confidence	BPS	29	30	29.28 (5.57)	29.1 (6.02)	29	30	29.10 (9.64)	29.26 (6.81)	0.05
		OVERALL										0.61

Note. ADI = Autism Diagnostic Interview-Revised (ADI - RSI = ADI Reciprocal Social Interaction subdomain, ADI - NVC = ADI Nonverbal Communication subdomain, ADI - SRB = ADI - RSB Repetitive and Stereotyped behavior); ADOS = Autism Diagnostic Observation Schedule (ADOS - RSI = ADOS Reciprocal Social Interaction subdomain, ADOS – NVC = ADOS Nonverbal Communication subdomain, ADOS - SRB = ADOS Stereotyped and Restricted Behavior, ADOS-G = Autism Diagnostic Observation Schedule-Generic, M-ADOS-S = Modified ADOS Social Affect); BPS = Being a Parent scale; BRS = Bayley Behavior Rating Scale; BSID = Bayley Scales of Infant Development; BSQ = Behavior Screening Questionnaire; CASL = Comprehensive Assessment of Spoken Language; ECBI = Eyberg Child Behavior Inventory (ECBI-I = ECBI Intensity scores, ECBI-P = ECBI Problem scores); DBC = Developmental Behavior Checklist; EIDP = Early Intervention Developmental Profile; ESCS = Early Social Communication Scales; ESI = Early Social - Communication; FAM = Family Assessment Measure; FQOL = Family Quality of Life; GHQ = General Health Questionnaire; GSMD = Griffiths Scale of Mental Development, D and E subscales; ADOS = Autism Diagnostic Observation Schedule; mCBRS = Modified version of the Child Behavior Rating Scale; MCDI = MacArthur Communicative Development Inventory (MCDI-C = MCDI Words understood, MCDI-E = MCDI Words said, MCDI-G = MCDI Gestures); MFAD = MacMaster Family Assessment Device; MSEL = Mullen Scales of Early Learning (MSEL-DQ = MSEL Developmental Quotient); PBCL = Preschool Behavior Checklist; PCI = Parent - Child Interaction; PCFP = Parent–Child Free Play procedure; PLS = Preschool Language Scale; PSDP = Preschool Developmental Profile; PSI = Parent Stress Inventory; PSOC = Parent Sense of Competence Scale; PSQ = Parent perception questionnaire; PST = Parenting Stress Thermometer; QRS = Questionnaire on Resources and Stress; RDL = Reynell Developmental Language (RDL-E = RDL Expressive, REL-R = RDL-Receptive); SAC = Stress Arousal Checklist; SSQ = Social Skills Questionnaire; TAQ = TRA-ADD Autism Quiz; VABS = Vineland Adaptive Behavior Scales (VABS-C, VABS Communication sub-domain, VABS-S, VABS Social skills subdomain); WPPSI = Wechsler Preschool and Primary Scale of Intelligence-Revised.

TABLE 4.4 EFFECT SIZES OF AUTISM STUDIES

Study	*Measure*	*d*	*95% CI*
Aldred et al. (2004)	A + B + E + J + L	0.48	[0.145, 0.821]
Casenhiser et al. (2013)	C + E + H + J + K	0.70	[0.455, 0.918]
Green et al. (2010)	B + E + H + J	0.37	[0.209, 0.498]
Jocelyn et al. (1998)	B + D + F + G + H + K + L	0.25	[-0.020, 0.485]
Nefdt et al. (2010)	H + I + J	1.41	[0.912, 1.898]
Rickards et al. (2007)	A + C + D	0.35	[0.098, 0.603]
Roberts et al. (2011)	A + C + F + G + H + I + L	0.30	[0.115, 0.481]
Siller et al. (2013)	E + H + J	0.70	[0.404, 0.999]
Sofronoff et al. (2004)	C + K	1.06	[0.694, 1.429]
Tonge et al. (2006)	A + B + C + F + L + M	0.44	[0.146, 0.533]
Whittingham et al. (2009)	C + I	0.61	[0.300, 0.909]
Overall		0.56	[0.385, 0.694]

d and 95% CI

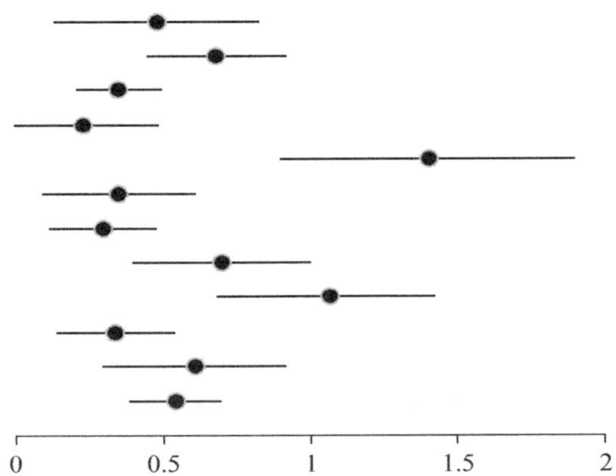

Note. A = Adaptive Behavior; B = Autism Symptoms; C = Behavior Problem; D = Cognition; E = Early Social Communication; F = Family Well-Being/Functioning; G = Knowledge/Skills; H = Language; I = Parental Confidence; J = Parental Interaction with Child; K = Social Interaction; L = Stress; M = Mental Health

TABLE 4.5 OVERALL META-ANALYSIS RESULTS OF PARENT TRAINING PROGRAMS FOR CHILDREN WITH AUTISM SPECTRUM DISORDER, PARENTS, AND FAMILIES

Subgroup	*Target Area (No. of studies included)*	*Effect Sizes (d)*
Child (Posttest)	Adaptive Behavior (4)	0.131
	Autism Symptoms (4)	0.329
	Language (6)	0.222
	Early Social-Communication (4)	0.591
	Social Interaction (3)	0.717
	Behavior Problems (6)	0.482
	Cognition (3)	0.241
	OVERALL	**0.434**
Child (Follow-up)	Adaptive Behavior (1)	0.001
	Language (1)	0.275
	Social Interaction (1)	1.180
	Behavior Problems (2)	1.134
	Cognition (1)	0.382
	OVERALL	**0.651**
Parent (Posttest)	Parental interaction with child (5)	1.095
	Knowledge/Skills (2)	0.658
	Parental Confidence (3)	0.584
	Stress (4)	0.401
	OVERALL	**0.797**
Family	Family Well-being/Functioning (3)	**0.312**
Parent training program for children with ASD		**0.561**

and their d statistic in the last column with values ranging from -.38 (negative small effect) to 2.23 (positive large effect). For example, the first study presented in Table 4.3 was the one conducted by Aldred et al. (2004). In this study they measured treatment effects on both children and on parents. For example, the effect size for the children's adaptive behavior was 0.29, generally thought of as a small effect, and the effect size for the children's reduced level of autism symptoms (measured by ADOS) was 0.87, a large effect size. Although both child outcomes are the indirect outcomes of parent training on social communication strategies, it appears that the parent-implemented social communication intervention has greater effect on improving the symptoms of children with autism (e.g., deficit on social communication) than on the improvement of child's adaptive behavior since improving child's social communication through parents' implemented intervention was the main focus of the treatment. Description of the confidence intervals for each study's effect size can be found in Table 4.4.

Like the meta-analysis summary in chapter 2, we grouped some variables together to ask overall picture questions of the data after the different kinds of outcomes were standardized into *d*'s. For example, if the question: "Overall what was the effect size for the children's outcomes when combined into an average *d*?" is asked, the answer can be found in the last column of Table 4.5: it is $d = 0.434$ in this case. This overall effect size for child outcomes was actually generated by averaging the effect sizes of seven specific child outcomes reported in 12 studies, varying from quite small effect of adaptive behavior ($d = 0.131$ of four studies), language development ($d = 0.222$ of six studies), cognitive ability ($d = 0.241$ of three studies), autism symptoms or severity ($d = 0.329$ of four studies), and behavioral problems ($d = 0.482$ of six studies) to medium effect of early social communication ($d = 0.591$ of four studies) and social interaction ($d = 0.717$ of three studies).

Likewise, the average effect size of all family-based and parent implemented intervention programs on parent outcomes and family system outcomes as calculated, and as shown in Table 4.5 under Cohen's *d* the average effect sizes of parent outcomes and family system outcomes are 0.797 and 0.312 respectively. The effect sizes corresponding to parent outcomes reveal stronger treatment effects of parent implemented intervention programs for children with ASD, including a small effect of parent stress levels ($d = 0.401$ of four studies) and a medium effect of parent confidence ($d = 0.584$ of three studies) and parent knowledge and skills ($d = 0.658$ of two studies). For the family system outcomes, the effect sizes of parent-implemented intervention programs suggest a small effect of family well-being (family functioning or family quality of life) ($d = 0.312$ of three studies) and a large effect of parent and child interaction ($d = 1.095$ of five studies).

More importantly, the field expects an answer for the fundamental question: Overall what is the effect size for the parent-implemented programs? The overall effect size of all family-based and parent-implemented intervention programs for children with ASD is $d = 0.561$, suggesting a moderate treatment effect. This is a quite encouraging result, because it seems to suggest that family-based and parent-implemented intervention programs are quite effective to not only affect the proximal outcomes such as parent skill acquisition and parent confidence often as the direct target of intervention programs but also bring collateral effect on distal outcomes such as improvement of various child outcomes (e.g., progress on adaptive behaviors, communication skills, social intervention, cognitive ability, and decrease of problem behaviors) and parent reduced stress levels. What can be further drawn from such encouraging result is that several short-term parent education programs seem to have achieved a meaningful positive effect on parents of children with autism. Yet in the meantime, these programs primarily focusing on improvement of parents' skills do not eliminate caregiving stress or remove the child's need for long-term caregiving and have limited positive impact on family quality of life.

SINGLE SUBJECT DESIGN STUDIES

As a result of the literature search, we identified a total of 19 SSD studies that met our selection criteria. These articles report effects of parent implementation of a variety of intervention strategies for children with ASD. Most of these studies employed multiple baseline designs, and mothers were the primary participants in the interventions while only a few studies involved fathers. ABA-based interventions were featured prominently in these studies (15 of 19 studies), with 7 studies particularly focusing on naturalistic intervention strategies. In the research synthesis (see Table 4.6), we organize these studies into two major focus areas: ABA-based interventions and communication-focused interventions. The ABA-based interventions consist of 15 studies further being organized in two subtopical areas: typical ABA approaches including traditional ABA (three studies), discrete trial training (DTT, three studies), and incidental teaching (two studies) and naturalistic behavioral interventions including natural language paradigm (NLP, three studies), pivotal response treatment (PRT, three studies), and milieu teaching (one study). The communication-focused interventions comprise the picture exchange communication system (PECS) (two studies) and the Improving Parents as Communication Teachers (ImPACT) program (two studies).

Typical Applied Behavior Analysis Approaches

As discussed in chapter 3, ABA-based interventions comprise many different techniques and approaches. In the context of supporting parents of children with ASD, all of these approaches focus on training parents skills to teach their child skills and change their child's behaviors via managing antecedents (what happens before a behavior occurs) and consequences (what happens after the behavior). Krantz, MacDuff, and McClannahan (1993) evaluated the effect of parent-implemented intervention on using manual prompts and graduated guidance to teach children with autism to use photographic activity schedules. This study used a multiple baseline across participants design across three boys with autism aged 6 to 8 who all had prior intervention in photographic activity schedules in the clinical setting. To help children generalize this skill to the home setting, parents were instructed to use modeling, supervised practice, and graduated guidance via home training across 17–22 sessions. After the parents' implementation, data showed marked decreases in children's disruptive behavior and increases in engagement. This study suggests that photographic activity schedules may have particular social significance for parent-implemented interventions (see a more detailed summary of this study in Table 3.4 of Chapter 3).

Reagon and Higee (2009) examined the effect of parent-implemented scripts and script fading to promote initiations during play given a concern about the lack of generalization of vocal initiations during play of traditional intensive language intervention programs. This multiple baseline across participants design study used the parents as both implementers and primary data collectors, with researchers conducting the reliability scoring. Parents were taught to use voice recorders, script development and preteaching procedures, and script-fading procedures (e.g., instructions, modeling, prompts, and feedback). Results showed that the parents were able to maintain high levels of procedural

TABLE 4.6 SINGLE SUBJECT DESIGN STUDIES OF PARENT TRAINING FOR YOUNG CHILDREN WITH AUTISM SPECTRUM DISORDERS

Author(s)	*Design/Intervention components/ Manual/Fidelity*	*Participants (Sample, Age, Ethnicity)/Setting (Parent Training, Child Intervention)*	*DV Measures*	*Treatment Effect(s)*
Ben Chaabane, Alber-Morgan, & DeBar (2009)	• SSD (multiple baseline design across behaviors comparing acquisition of mands across different symbol categories: colors, shapes, and functions) • To examine parent-implemented Picture Exchange Communication System (PECS) • Manualized • Parent intervention fidelity reported	• 2 boys with autism and their mothers (ages 5 and 6) • Caucasian • Setting: PT and CI at home	PARENT • Fidelity of implementation • Parent report measure of improvisations in untrained settings and items CHILD • Improvisations of colors, shapes, and functions • Errors	Both children demonstrated increased improvisations to untrained stimuli. Parents maintained a mean fidelity of implementation of 97%. Mothers reported use of improvisations outside of experimental session, procedures were easy to implement, and satisfaction with the results and plans to continue to implement procedures.
Charlop-Christy & Carpenter (2000)	• SSD (alternating treatments design comparing 3 treatment conditions and multiple baseline design across children) • To compare the efficacy and use of modified incidental teaching sessions (MITS), incidental teaching, and discrete trial • No manual reported • Parent fidelity reported	• 3 children with autism (ages 6–9, 3 boys and 1 girl) and their mothers • Caucasian, East-Indian American, and Hispanic • Setting: PT and CI at home	PARENT • Number of errors made by parents using each procedure • Parental satisfaction CHILD • Verbalization (imitation, spontaneous speech, incorrect verbal response)	Parents made relatively few errors during the treatment conditions (5%–10% of total trials in each condition). Parental satisfaction did not vary significantly for the parents. MITS led to a better acquisition and generalization than other interventions (incidental teaching and discrete trial). Study demonstrated that parents could use the MITS to teach and promote generalization of their children's spontaneous speech.

Coolican, Smith, & Bryson (2010)	• SSD (multiple baseline across participants design) • To evaluate a brief (three 2-hour sessions) parent training program in Pivotal Response Treatment • Manualized • Parent fidelity reported	• 8 children with autism (7 boys and 1 girl ages 2–5) and their parents (5 mothers and 3 fathers) • Setting: first 2 PT sessions conducted in clinic, with third at home; CI at home	PARENT • Fidelity of PRT Implementation • Self-efficacy • Satisfaction CHILD • Communication: functional verbal utterances • Language: The Preschool Language Scale & Peabody Picture Vocabulary test • Disruptive behavior	All eight children demonstrated an increase in functional verbal utterances, but no significant difference was observed in the standardized measures of language. Disruptive behavior, exhibited by two of the participants at pretreatment, decreased by follow-up. Overall, parent fidelity of implementation increased, with five of the eight parents meeting fidelity after the training. Low self-efficacy, shown by only two of the parents, increased following training. Parents reported high satisfaction with the training and intervention.
Crocket, Fleming, Doepke, & Stevens (2007)	• SSD (multiple baseline across behaviors design) • To examine the effects of an intensive parent training program on the acquisition and generalization of Discrete Trial Teaching to teach four different functional skills • Manualized • Parent fidelity reported	• 2 children with autism (boys age 4) and their mothers; 1 boy had a comorbid diagnosis of intellectual disability • Setting: PT and CI in clinic	PARENT • Correct discrete teaching for four skills • Number of errors made by the parents using each procedure CHILD • Correct/Incorrect/Prompted responding including verbal imitation, writing, labeling	Both parents showed acquisition and generalization of DTT procedures. Furthermore, they extended the use of DTT procedures across untrained and child skills. Correct responding in children increased while incorrect responding decreased.
Gillett & LeBlanc (2006)	• SSD (nonconcurrent multiple baseline design across participants) • To examine ability of parents to implement the Natural Language Paradigm (NLP) • No manual reported • Parent fidelity reported	• 3 children with autism (boys ages 4–5) and their parents • Caucasian: 1, Asian-American: 1, African American: 1 • Setting: PT and CI in clinic and at home	PARENT • Fidelity of implementation of NLP • Social validity questionnaire assessing difficulty and usefulness of LP and perceived effects of NLP on their children's language/play skills CHILD • Frequency of vocalizations • Mean length of utterance (MLU) • Appropriate and inappropriate play	All parents were able to implement NLP procedures, with an average of 96% fidelity. Prompted vocalizations increased for one child, and spontaneous vocalizations as well as MLU increased for the other two children. Appropriate play increased in two of three children, with the third exhibiting ceiling effects as he demonstrated appropriate play throughout baseline and intervention sessions. Two of the three parents returned the social validity questionnaire and rated NLP highly in usefulness, ease, and helpfulness for children's language and play skills.

(*continued*)

TABLE 4.6 (CONTINUED)

Author(s)	*Design/Intervention components/ Manual/Fidelity*	*Participants (Sample, Age, Ethnicity)/Setting (Parent Training, Child Intervention)*	*DV Measures*	*Treatment Effect(s)*
Hsieh, Wilder, & Abellon, (2011)	• SSD (concurrent multiple baseline design across participants) • To assess the effects of a parent education package of modeling, rehearsal, and feedback on learning to implement incidental teaching techniques. • No manual reported • Parent fidelity reported	• 3 children with autism (ages 8–10) and their parents. Two of the children had a comorbid diagnosis of intellectual disability and 1 had Phelan-McDermid syndrome • Setting: PT and CI at home	PARENT • Fidelity of implementation on five components of incidental teaching CHILD • Percentage of correct responses	Parents showed high levels of fidelity of implementation of incidental teaching components. All children increased percentage of correct responding by the feedback stage, but for two of the three children, improvement was slight.
Ingersoll & Gergans (2007)	• SSD (multiple baseline design across participants for three participants and a multiple baseline design across behaviors for one participant) • To assess the effectiveness of Reciprocal Imitation Training (RIT) • Manualized • Parent fidelity reported	• 3 children with autism (2 boys and 1 girl ages 31–42 months) and their mothers • No race/ethnicity information reported • Setting: PT and CI: clinic, generalization measured at homes	PARENT • The use of RIT strategies (modeling, prompting and reinforcement) CHILD • Spontaneous object and/or gesture imitation	All mothers showed an increase in their correct implementation of imitation training procedure. Mothers generalized their use of the imitation training procedure to their homes. All children increased their use of spontaneous imitation, maintained and generalized their imitation skills to their homes.
Ingersoll & Wainer (2013)	• SSD (multiple baseline design across participants) • To examine the efficacy of the project ImPACT (Improving parents as communication teachers) • Manualized • Parent fidelity reported	• 8 preschoolers with autism (7 boys, ages 44–80 months, mean age 53 months) and their mothers • Caucasian: 6, Black: 1, and Asian: 1 • Setting: PT and CI in clinic, generalization measured at home	PARENT • Parental fidelity CHILD • Child spontaneous language	The parents' average fidelity ratings were significantly higher during treatment. A multilevel model with fixed effects indicated a significant effect of treatment on the children's rate of spontaneous language.

Kaiser, Hancock, & Nietfeld (2000)	• SSD (A multiple baseline design across participants) • To examine the effects of parent-implemented enhanced milieu teaching (EMT) on social communication skills • No manual reported • Parent fidelity reported	• 6 children with autism (boys aged 2.5–5 years, Mean = 42 months) and their mothers • No race/ethnicity information reported • Setting: PT and CI in clinic, generalization measured at home	PARENT • 7 aspects of parent implementation of training CHILD • Social communication skills • Expressive and receptive communication • Linguistic complexity	All parents showed increases in correct use of milieu teaching. Parents learned EMT procedures and generalized and maintained their use across settings and time. All children showed increases in their total use of target behaviors (prompted plus unprompted). All children's spontaneous target use increased. Children demonstrated positive changed in social communication across settings and measures.
Kashinath, Woods, & Goldstein (2006)	• SSD (A multiple baseline design across behaviors) • To examine the effects of facilitating generalized use of teaching strategies by parents of children with autism within daily routines. • No manual reported • Parent fidelity reported	• 5 children with autism (4 boys and 1 girl aged 33–65 months) and their mothers • No race/ethnicity information reported • Setting: PT and CI at home	PARENT • Mother's teaching strategy use • Generalization of strategies CHILD • Frequency of child communication (gestures, single word use, multiword utterances)	All parents demonstrated proficient use of teaching strategies and generalized their use across routines. All parents perceived the intervention to be beneficial. The intervention had positive effects on individualized child communication outcomes.
R. L. Koegel, Symon, & Koegel (2002)	• SSD (A nonconcurrent multiple baseline across participants design) • To evaluate the effects of an intensive, week-long, center-based parent education program using Pivotal Response Training (PRT) • Manualized • Parent fidelity reported	• 5 children with autism (2 boys and 3 girls ages 3–5) and their parents (4 mothers and 1 father) • No race/ethnicity information reported • Setting: PT and CI at clinic	PARENT • Parents' implementation of PRT techniques • Affect during parent child interaction CHILD • Child's functional verbal responses	The parents' use of PRT procedures and affect improved. Child's functional expressive verbal language improved and confirmed at follow-up assessment.

(*continued*)

TABLE 4.6 (CONTINUED)

Author(s)	*Design/Intervention components/ Manual/Fidelity*	*Participants (Sample, Age, Ethnicity)/Setting (Parent Training, Child Intervention)*	*DV Measures*	*Treatment Effect(s)*
Lafaskis & Sturmey (2007)	• SSD (multiple baseline across participants design) • To examine the effects of parent training of use of discrete-trial teaching and its generalization • No manual reported • Parent fidelity reported	• 3 children with developmental disabilities (boys age 4; 1 with Autism, 1 with Down's syndrome, and 1 with intellectual disability) and their mothers • Two were born in Nigeria • Setting: PT and CI in clinic	PARENT • Parents' correct use of discrete trials of gross motor imitation (GMI) • Parent's correct use of discrete trials of vocal imitation (VIM) CHILD • Child's GMI • Child's VIM responses	The parents' percentage of correct use of 10 components during 10 consecutive discrete trials of GMI improved, and VIM improved (their skills generalized to novel programs). Children's correct responding of GMI and VIM increased
Laski, Charlop, & Schreibman (1988)	• SSD (multiple baseline design across participants with a typical comparison group) • To examine the effects of parent-implemented Natural Language Paradigm • Manualized • Parent fidelity reported	• 8 children with autism (7 boys and 1 girl ages 5–9.6) and their parents • 6 typically developing children as a comparison group • No race/ethnicity information reported • Setting: PT and CI in clinic	PARENT • Parent verbalizations in the free play setting • Parent verbalizations in the breakroom setting CHILD • Child vocalizations (combined imitations, answers, and spontaneous speech) in the free play setting • Child vocalizations in the break-room setting • Echolalia	All parents increased verbalizations, where they presented a discriminative stimulus for vocalizations to their child, in the free play setting and two of the three increased in the breakroom setting. All children increased in vocalizations in both the free-play and break-room setting. With typical comparison group, slight increases in parent verbalizations to their children and child vocalizations were observed following NLP training but of a smaller magnitude than the experimental group.
Reagon & Higbee (2009)	• SSD (multiple baseline design across participants) • To assess the effects of parent-implemented scripts and script fading • No manual reported • Parent fidelity reported	• 3 children with autism (boys ages 2–6) and their mothers • No race/ethnicity information reported • Setting: PT and CI at home	PARENT • Fidelity of implementation CHILD • Scripted initiations • Unscripted initiations	Parents were able to meet high levels of fidelity of implementation (mean range: 83%–96%). Scripted and unscripted initiations increased for all participants.

T. Smith, Buch, & Gamby (2000)	• SSD (multiple baseline design across participants) • To assess the effects of a parent-implemented ABA intervention (UCLA treatment model) • Manualized (Lovaas et al., 1981) • Parent fidelity reported	• 6 children with autism or PDD-NOS (boys ages 31–45 months) and their parents (6 mothers and 4 fathers) • No race/ethnicity information reported • Setting: PT and CI at home and in clinic	PARENT • Parent report of number of therapy hours the child received • Correct 1-1 discrete trial procedures • Parenting Stress Index • Parent Satisfaction Questionnaire (PSQ) CHILD • Early Learning Measure (ELM) • IQ • Reynell Developmental Language Scales • Vineland Adaptive Behavior Scales	Parents reported that children received a mean of 26.2 therapy hours per week. Parents were able to use correct discrete-trial techniques most of the time. Five of the six children increased their correct responding to receptive actions, nonverbal imitation, and verbal imitation as measured by the ELM. Two of the children improved on expressive labels to a maximum of 30% correct. Two of the boys showed large increases on all standardized measures. Mothers decreased in their measure of parental stress from 3 months into therapy to follow-up. Four of the mothers returned their PSQ and reported children as "greatly improved." All indicated treatment had positive effects on the family, bolstered their optimism about child's future, and increased their confidence in handling child's problem behaviors.
Stiebel (1999)	• SSD (multiple baseline design across behaviors) • To assess the effects of teaching parents a problem-solving technique for using augmentative communication (taught using NLP procedures) in daily routines • No manual reported • No fidelity reported	• 3 children with autism (ages 4–6) and their parents • No race/ethnicity information reported • Setting: PT and CI at home	PARENT • Communication opportunities provided • Perception of parent and child skill CHILD • Spontaneous picture card use	All 3 parents increased in their communication opportunities provided. All children improved on spontaneous picture card use for communication during three different routines. Effects were maintained at follow-up. All parents reported an increase in their perception of their own skills to encourage child to communicate. Further, all three reported improvements in their perceptions of their child's communication skills following training.

(*continued*)

TABLE 4.6 (CONTINUED)

Author(s)	*Design/Intervention components/ Manual/Fidelity*	*Participants (Sample, Age, Ethnicity)/Setting (Parent Training, Child Intervention)*	*DV Measures*	*Treatment Effect(s)*
Symon (2005)	• SSD (nonconcurrent multiple baseline design across participants • To evaluate the generalized effects of a weeklong intensive parent education program (Pivotal Response Training) to new caregivers • Manualized (Koegel et al., 1989) • Fidelity reported	• 3 children with autism (boys ages 2–5) and their parents (3 mothers, 1 father, and 2 significant caregivers) • Caucasian: 2, Asian: 1 • Setting: PT and CI in clinic and at home	PARENT • Fidelity of implementation for primary and significant caregivers CHILD • Functional verbal utterances and appropriate behaviors	All parents showed mastery of the PRT skills, and generalized their skills into home settings. The skills spread from primary caregivers to significant caregivers. The children's functional verbal language and appropriate behaviors improved during interaction with their primary caregivers, and these gains transferred to interactions with significant caregivers.
Tarbox, Wallace, & Tarbox (2002)	• SSD (multiple treatment reversal design) • To compare parent-implemented schedule thinning and response blocking with prompting for appropriate toy play to reduce automatically reinforced object mouthing. • No manual reported • Parent fidelity reported	• 1 child (boy, age 4) and his parents • No race/ethnicity information reported • Setting: PT in clinic and CI at home	PARENT • Fidelity of implementation CHILD • Functional analysis • Frequency of Mouthing	Schedule thinning was initially successful in maintaining low rates of mouthing, but effects did not maintain past 1-minute reinforcement intervals and so was discontinued. Parents were able to display 100% accuracy in fidelity of implementation for response blocking. Response blocking, with prompted toy play, was effective in decreasing mouthing to low rates across several sessions in the home.

fidelity (mean range = 83%–96%) and that scripted and unscripted initiations increased during play for all participants. (see Table 4.6 for detail).

Problem behaviors maintained by automatic reinforcement can be one of the most troublesome behaviors for parents. Tarbox et al. (2002) compared parent-implemented schedule thinning to response blocking with prompting for appropriate toy play on levels of automatically reinforced object mouthing. As shown in Table 4.6, this multiple treatment reversal design SSD study of one child with autism revealed that response blocking brought object mouthing down to low rates across several sessions in the home setting even though schedule thinning resulted in limited gains. Despite a caveat needed for the generalization of this study finding, it sheds light on the effect of parents' use of response blocking to reduce significant problem behaviors that are maintained through sensory stimulation.

Discrete Trial Training

Discrete trial training is a traditional ABA approach that is typically implemented by trained clinicians. However, parental involvement in therapy has multiple benefits, including child performance, parent satisfaction, and freeing up therapist time to serve more clients and keep costs down. T. Smith et al. (2000) evaluated the effect of parent-implemented DTT on their preschoolers in home settings. Immediately following six one-day workshops (6 hours each) in their homes, the parents implemented DTT to their child at home and were monitored by the professionals longitudinally for 2–3 years. In this multiple baseline design across participants study, all the parents were able to achieve a high level of accuracy in using discriminative stimuli, discrete trials, and consequences correctly. However, the child outcomes of six participating children varied on the adaptive behavior and IQ measures possibly due to small degrees of fidelity of parent implementation (see Table 4.6 for detail). The most highlighted study result is that by the follow-up time, five out of six children had made the transition from home to school in a general education classroom. In addition, it is noted that the parents' stress level was associated with their implementation of intervention. For example, at 3 months into therapy, all participating mothers had high levels of stress (in the 90th percentile). By the follow-up time, their stress levels decreased to the 25th–35th percentile, possibly related to the perceived improvements of their children.

Crockett et al. (2007) evaluated the effect of an intensive DTT parent training program on four different functional skills using a multiple baseline across behaviors design. Two parents of 4-year-old children participated in the training and were able to demonstrate appropriate use of DTT to teach four skills to their children: attending, writing, counting, and choosing. It was noted that some carryover effects across skills might exist given the increasing baselines of the second, third, and fourth behaviors. Despite a potential design concern, it is evident that the training has enabled the parents to generalize DTT skills and that differing numbers of exemplars may be needed for each parent (e.g., one parent improving almost immediately after training and the other taking approximately three exemplars to reach high levels). These data suggest that it may be important to measure generalization throughout training programs, as training on all specific skills may not be needed if generalization occurs.

Lafasakis and Sturmey (2007) also evaluated the effect of parent-implemented DTT using a multiple baseline across participants design. During baseline, parents were provided with a list of the definitions of 10 components of DTT and instructed to do DTT "to the best of your ability" (Lafasakis & Sturmey, 2007, p. 687). During this baseline, parents demonstrated a low-to-moderate success rate in implementing DTT procedures, with child behaviors remaining low. Dependent measures included measures of DTT trials of gross motor imitation (i.e., clapping hands, arms up, and touch nose) and vocal motor imitation (i.e., saying "ah," "mm" and "mmaa"). Following the training, which included review of their performance graph, modeling, and feedback along with the list of 10 components of DTT, all parents immediately increased their correct performance on gross motor imitation and vocal imitation trials. The children concomitantly improved on their correct gross motor imitation and vocal imitation.

Incidental Teaching

Incidental teaching is a behavioral intervention with a focus on teaching skills in the natural environment, where a child can learn real-life meaning to skills and then apply them naturally. Hsieh et al. (2011) used a brief training package of modeling, rehearsal, and feedback to teach parents to implement IT techniques in a multiple baseline across participants design study. Parents were taught the following components of incidental teaching: arranging the environment to promote learning, getting the child's attention, providing a discriminative stimulus, waiting for the child's response, and one of two last options: (1) if the child emits the response, deliver the natural consequence immediately along with verbal praise; or (2) if the child does not emit the target response, use a least-to-most prompting sequence. All parents demonstrated high fidelity of implementation during the training phases, and all three children increased in correct responding following training.

Charlop-Christy and Carpenter (2000) compared parent-implemented traditional IT, modified incidental teaching (MITS), and DTT on the acquisition of target verbalizations using both an alternating treatments design and a multiple baseline across participants design. The MITS condition differed from traditional IT in that it had increased training trials in naturally occurring settings and other modifications to maximize effectiveness of the procedures (i.e., using adult-initiated trials in the child's area of interest instead of waiting for the child to initiate). Modified incidental teaching led to acquisition of target verbalizations for all three children, whereas only one acquired these in traditional IT and only two in the DDT condition. Further, MITS led to generalization of the target verbalizations, whereas the traditional IT and DDT did not.

In summary, a collection of eight studies of typical ABA interventions (with total number of participants >20) renders solid empirical evidence to warrant a conclusion that typical ABA intervention approaches are established practices for supporting families of children with ASD.

Naturalistic Behavioral Interventions

Naturalistic behavioral interventions seek to incorporate learning techniques within typical environments and activities to promote motivation and generalization of skills. Children with autism typically are much more difficult to motivate to communicate or interact socially with others. They also often have a great deal of difficulty in learning to use a new skill outside of the place where it was first taught or with new people. Kashinath et al. (2006) evaluated the parents' generalized use of naturalistic behavioral teaching strategies during daily routines in the parents' homes for five children ages 33–65 months in a study using a multiple baseline design across participating children's target behaviors. The researchers worked with the participating parents collaboratively to identify family routines that they wanted to target in the study. The parents identified common caregiving routines such as snack time, dressing, and hand washing, along with a variety of family- and child-preferred play routines. The naturalistic behavioral strategies were taught using a parent-focused intervention that included arranging the environment to promote interaction, using natural reinforcement, using time delay, imitating contingently, modeling, and gestural/verbal cueing. During the training, the parents received a family-friendly written handout, a review and discussion of a video model of another parent implementing the strategies, in vivo clinician modeling, supervised practice with feedback, and discussions of how to incorporate the strategies into other routines. All parents demonstrated proficient use of the teaching strategies in the training environment as well as generalized use across other routines (except for one parent). Further, all parents reported that the intervention was beneficial. Communication goals varied for each child (e.g., frequency of single word use, use of multiword utterances), yet all five children improved on their target communication goals, with one exception where the child improved on use of single words during indoor play, but not in the caregiving routine.

Natural Language Paradigm and Pivotal Response Treatment

Pivotal response treatment is a naturalistic intervention based on the principles of ABA. Originally termed NLP, which focused exclusively on verbal communication, PRT focuses on key pivotal areas that produce collateral gains in untargeted areas. Laski et al. (1988) evaluated generalization of behaviors and settings after parent training in NLP, which included discussion of the NLP procedures, modeling, in vivo training, and feedback. The study employed a multiple baseline across participants design and compared the results with a typically developing comparison group. Four parents of nonverbal children and four parents of echolalic children received five to nine training sessions until they reached criteria on four strategies: direct reinforcement of verbal attempts, turn-taking with the stimulus material, task variation and multiple exemplars, and shared control. Increases in parental intervention behaviors were accompanied by increases in the children's successful communicative attempts. Though the parents of nonverbal children all reported consistent implementation of NLP sessions at home, only one of the parents of the echolalic children reported doing so. These parents reported that they incorporated the principles in their daily routine, but did not conduct regular NLP sessions, suggesting the need for therapists to teach parents to use NLP techniques throughout daily routines.

Gillett and LeBlanc (2007) replicated the study of Laski et al. (1988) using a multiple baseline across participants design to evaluate parent-implemented NLP on both verbal communication and appropriate play. They found that parents were able to implement NLP with a high degree of fidelity. The most difficult component of parents' implementation was the provision of a sufficient delay after modeling to allow for spontaneous vocalizations. However, parents did not report any particular trouble with any of the steps of NLP. Results showed that two of the three children had increased spontaneous vocalizations and mean length of utterance as well as appropriate play. Further, in the returned social validity questionnaire, two parents rated their participation as "very useful" and the intervention as "very easy" and very or somewhat helpful. Coolican et al. (2010) evaluated the effect of parent-implemented PRT after a brief training of just three 2-hour sessions. A multiple baseline across participants design was used across eight children with autism and their parents, and both visual and statistical analyses were used. Overall, parents were able to implement PRT following the training, with five of the eight meeting fidelity of implementation. Further, they reported high satisfaction with the training and intervention. The children increased their functional verbal utterances, but such increase did not exhibit on standardized measures, suggesting possible lack of sensitivity of standardized measures to the small gains made after a short training.

Parent education models are an important consideration when studying parent implemented interventions. R. L. Koegel et al. (2002) and Symon (2005) evaluated an intensive, week-long PRT parent training program using multiple baseline across participants designs. The training consisted of 5 hours per day for 5 consecutive days (for a total of 25 hours), where parents were taught to use PRT procedures. Results of the first study (R. L. Koegel et al., 2002) demonstrated that parents were able to incorporate PT techniques into their daily interactions and generalize their use from the center to their home environments. Further, four of the five children gained in social communication skills in a 1-week period, and all five children improved by follow-up. The second study (Symon, 2005) sought to expand on this by evaluating parents' ability to teach the PRT strategies to other significant caregivers who were not part of the clinic-based intensive intervention program. In this program, parents were seen as collaborative partners, not just trainees who serve as the experts themselves. All parents met fidelity of implementation of PRT by the end of the 1-week training program and maintained and generalized their skills to the home environment. Further, all additional significant caregivers met fidelity by 1-month follow-up after the training program, suggesting that the trained parent was effective in training their identified caregiver without clinician intervention. Further, the children improved in their social communicative behaviors with the significant caregivers.

Traditional milieu teaching, viewed as a naturalistic intervention approach, involves modeling (e.g., narrating activities), mand-modeling, time delay between prompts to allow for a response, and some incidental teaching techniques (e.g., environmental arrangement to promote interaction, following the child's lead, etc.). Kaiser et al. (2000) used a multiple baseline across participants design to evaluate parent-implemented enhanced milieu teaching (EMT). Enhanced milieu teaching includes three components: (1) environmental arrangement, (2) responsive interaction techniques, and (3) milieu teaching techniques. Five of the six parents reached the criterion of EMT learning during 24 training and practice sessions in a clinic and demonstrated generalization to the home setting. All six children demonstrated varying levels of increases in social communication targets, and only three showed improvements in mean length of utterance and diversity of word roots, respectively. The parents reported satisfaction with the training and very positive experience of intervention.

In summary, a collection of seven studies of naturalistic behavioral interventions (total number of participants > 20) provides strong evidence to conclude that naturalistic intervention approaches are established practices for supporting families of children with ASD. In addition, PRT (with three SDD studies reviewed here and one RCT study discussed earlier) qualifies as an established practice.

Communication-Focused Interventions

Regarding parent implementation of augmentative communication systems, Ben Chaabane et al. (2009) examined parent implemented PECS in a systematic replication of a clinician implemented study by Marckel, Neef, and Ferreri (2006) using a multiple baseline design across behaviors. The PECS uses picture cards that children are taught to exchange for access to preferred items. In this study, the parents implemented improvisation training with their children, who were expected to pick a similar card (either similar in color, shape, or function) when the specific card was unavailable, thereby making the PECS communication system more efficient for the child. Two mothers participated in the study with their male children, aged 5 and 6. The parents were able to maintain a high level of fidelity of implementation, and both witnessed increased improvisations in their children. However, consistent use of augmentative communication systems may encounter some barriers in generalization across daily routines. Stiebel (1999) assessed the effect of teaching parents a problem-solving technique to increase opportunities of using a naturalistic intervention to teach their children's use of an augmentative communication device upon considering contextual fit of the intervention in families' lives. This problem-solving process engaged the parents to identify the problematic routine where children were not using their picture cards and brainstorm solutions to increase picture card use in that particular routine. Results of this multiple baseline design across behaviors study demonstrated that the parents increased the opportunities they provided for communication throughout daily routines and generalized their skills to new routines. All three children increased their spontaneous picture card use for communication across three different routines during intervention, and the high rates maintained at follow-up. Further, the parents reported that they felt more confident in their own skills to encourage their children to communicate and reported improvements in their children's communication.

Reciprocal Imitation Training and Project ImPACT

Ingersoll and Gergans (2007) examined the effectiveness of parent-implemented reciprocal imitation training (RIT), which is considered to be a variation on other naturalistic behavioral interventions such as IT, PRT, and the ESDM targeting teaching imitation skills through play. Reciprocal imitation training includes contingent imitation, where the parent imitates the child's actions and describes the objects and actions of the child's play in simplified language (called "linguistic mapping"). Then, the parent would model the play action with an object and prompt the child to imitate using physical guidance, verbal commands, or gestural prompts. A multiple baseline across participants design for three children as well as across behaviors design was used to look more closely into one mother's acquisition of both object and gesture imitation. All three parents were taught object imitation, and one was also taught gesture imitation. All three mothers increased in their correct use of imitation training strategies and generalized the procedure to their homes. It was noted that all three mothers increased their use of linguistic mapping and contingent imitation during training and that at follow-up two parents maintained these rates for linguistic mapping and only one mother maintained her rate of contingent imitation. Results of parent implementation of object and gesture imitation trials were highly variable, but higher than baseline. Results of child gains in object and gesture imitation paralleled those of the parent's implementation of the trials.

The Project ImPACT program trains parents to implement naturalistic teaching strategies through play and daily routines, including making play interactive, modeling and expanding language, providing opportunities for initiations, helping increase the complexity of initiations, and pacing the interaction to keep the child engaged. Ingersoll and Wainer (2013) used a multiple baseline across participants design to evaluate the acquisition of these skills and their effect on children's spontaneous language. All mothers increased their use of the intervention techniques, and six of the eight children showed improvements in spontaneous use of language. The results showed a significant association between parents' implementation of the intervention strategies and their child's spontaneous language use.

Despite the empirical evidence of two good SSD studies for the PECS and ImPACT programs respectively, communication-focused interventions for children with ASD still fall short to qualify as promising practices and thus remain as unproven practices at present. Future research is required to further strengthen the evidence of such interventions.

SUMMARY AND CONCLUSIONS

Despite a growing body of research that recommends a myriad of EBPs for children with ASD (Wong et al., 2013), home-based and parent-implemented EBPs remain in paucity. Through our 2-year literature search, we were able to identify a total of 30 studies (12 RCT studies and 18 SSD studies) that met our selection criteria. This search result reflects a body of research literature that resembles the one identified in the most recent comprehensive review report by the NPDC on ASD (Wong et al., 2013).

On the basis of a research synthesis of the SSD studies for children with ASD, we conclude that ABA-based interventions (including general ABA approaches and other ramifications such as DTT and IT) have very strong empirical evidence to support the effectiveness of those programs. Likewise, naturalistic behavioral interventions with a strong root in ABA such as PRT and NLP also garner very strong empirical evidence to bolster the claim of established EBPs. Other intervention programs with a major orientation to communication, such as Project ImPACT and the PECS, will retain the status of unproven practice until more research is conducted to bring new evidence augmentatively. In addition, the research synthesis of RCT studies informs us that home-based intervention programs outperform center-based intervention programs on all major outcome areas (child outcomes, parent outcomes, and family system outcomes). Such results have important policy and practice implications. Autism is a lifelong condition of disability and often requires long-term care and a sustainable support system from the family of the individual with autism as well as from professionals. Therefore, strengthening family support toward families of children with ASD should be promoted as a disability service policy and should be prioritized in social and disability service practices. The research evidence generated from the literature review in this chapter appears to support such a position. Moreover, the research synthesis brings out evidence to support the efficacy of several specific intervention programs or models. There are more than two good quality RCT studies on the combined models of behavioral parent training and psychoeducational interventions and on joint attention and early social communication interventions, suggesting these programs or models are established practices that deserve more policy attention and promotion of use in practice. The meta-analysis results are encouraging in terms of adding support to the evidence of effectiveness of home-based and parent-implemented interventions. The overall effect size of such interventions, 0.561, albeit a medium effect, gives a strong indication of effectiveness of home-based and parent-implemented interventions, considering that many evidence-based special education programs usually have an average effect size around 0.30 (Singer et al., 2007). Although the effect sizes of different outcomes vary (e.g., child posttest outcomes of 0.434, child follow-up outcomes of 0.651, parent outcomes of 0.797, and family system outcomes of 0.312), it is evident that home-based and parent-implemented interventions can make important impacts on the lives of families of children with ASD on both proximal outcomes (e.g., primary parent outcomes—knowledge and skill acquisition) and distal outcomes (e.g., child outcomes and secondary parent outcome—reduced stress level).

5

MULTICOMPONENT INTERVENTIONS AS EVIDENCE-BASED PRACTICES FOR FAMILIES OF CHILDREN WITH DEVELOPMENTAL DISABILITIES

Mian Wang, Yeana W. Lam, George H. S. Singer, and Kelsey Oliver

Efficacious family support is often a complex endeavor in which no single technique or program will suffice. Part of the complexity comes from the uncountable ways that families can differ. They vary in their structure (e.g., one parent, two parent opposite sex, two parent same sex, multigenerational, grandparent headed, remarried, remarried with combined family). They can differ on any and all demographic variables (e.g., age, ethnicity, education, socioeconomic status [SES], place of residence, number of children). Their daily routines are multiply determined by parents' work hours, cultural values, transportation, distance to and from school and work, social class, living conditions, and routines from families of origin. It is complicated additionally when there are more than one major purpose of support. These include strengthening families' long-term capacity to give assistance, promoting family cohesion, reducing sources of stress and reactions to stress, and treating the many kinds of distress families can experience. Add to this mix the way intellectual disabilities (IDs) and autism are expressed in a wide range of severity and, for all practical purposes, the permutations are countless. Given such complexity and diversity, families need to be treated as unique, with support plans formulated family by family based on careful assessment, interventions tailored and evaluations ongoing. One implication of this complexity is that no single intervention is likely to meet the needs of all families. Families under the greatest internal and external stress may have need for multiple forms of support. There is in addition a small percentage of families with very extreme problems often confounded by poverty and severe social problems including substance abuse, child or elder mistreatment, mental illness, imprisonment, undocumented immigration status, and chronic or acute illness. Lutzker, Campbell, Harrold, and Huynen (1992) explained the rationale for Project Ecosystems, a comprehensive multicomponent program for families of children with severe disabilities:

> Ecobehavioral approaches to family problems represent a comprehensive set of strategies to tackle the complex issues impinging upon families . . . who suffer the stresses associated with developmental disabilities. Simple, narrow approaches focusing on singular or a few variables are not likely to produce durable change with these families (Lutzker et al. p. 12).

These researchers described a package of programs consisting of several different components including stress management training, behavioral parent training, problem-solving training, basic caregiving instruction, and behavioral pediatrics—12 different behaviorally based interventions matched to the needs of multiproblem families. Thus, complex problems may require complex solutions. In this chapter we review the evidence from multicomponent interventions. These are combinations of two or more packages of techniques. Many of these interventions are primarily designed to address the intensified challenges that arise when individuals with developmental disabilities are gripped by severe, longstanding and multiple problem behaviors. Although this is a small percentage of individuals with ID and autism, they represent one of the biggest challenges facing families and an underfunded, often ill equipped, service system.

The approaches to supporting families in this chapter represent some of the most recent research. Several of the changes in the design of support programs are creative and consequential; they represent second-generation studies, which build on previous work but include innovative treatment components. Table 5.1 presents the studies with brief descriptions of their components, subjects, and outcomes. One set of published studies are SSD evaluations of Positive Behavior Support (PBS) treatments which combine treatment elements (Binnendyk & Lucyshyn, 2009; Buschbacher, Fox, & Clarke, 2004; Cheremshynski, Lucyshyn, & Olson, 2012; Duda, Clarke, Fox, & Dunlap, 2008; Feldman, Condillac, Tough, Hunt, & Griffiths 2002; Lucyshyn, Albin, & Nixon, 1997; Lucyshyn et al., 2015; Lucyshyn, Albin, Horner, Mann, Mann, & Wadsworth, 2007; Phaneuf & McIntyre, 2011; Vaughn, Clarke, & Dunlap, 1997). As a group, the PBS studies include

TABLE 5.1 RESEARCH SYNTHESIS OF MULTICOMPONENT INTERVENTIONS

Author(s)	*Design*	*Participants*	*Intervention*	*Results*
Binnendyk & Lucyshyn (2009)	Multiple-probe design with five phases: baseline, training with therapist, parent training, generalization, and follow-up.	6-year-old boy with autism and severe food refusal and his parents	Multicomponent intervention combined interview-based assessment of family ecology with functional assessment of child's feeding behaviors. Also conducted food preference assessments and the *Behavioral Feeding Assessment Parent Interview.* Escape-extinction procedure implemented first by the researcher then by the mother with coaching and feedback. Researcher then coached the mother to train the father. Training included setting event/antecedent/consequence strategies and occurred 1–2 times per week for a total of 15 sessions in 8 weeks.	Significant increase in total food consumption from 0% at baseline to 64% after intervention and 56% at follow-up. Significant increase in number of steps of the mealtime routine that the child completed (0% at baseline to 97% at follow-up). Increase in the duration of mealtime routine to within mother's ideal range. Additional quality of life ratings showed increases related to the domains of family interaction, parenting, health and safety, family resource, and supports for persons with disability.
Blair, Lee, Cho, & Dunlap (2011)	Multiple baseline design across three children and home and school settings with follow-up at 3 months. Generalization across nontargeted behaviors also reported.	4.5-year-old girl with autism and ID with self-injury and aggression; 4.5-year-old boy with autism and cerebral palsy and spitting, tantrums, and screaming; 5.5-year-old boy with autism and ID with head banging, aggression, and stereotypy	Intervention included team building with joint training of parents and teachers, person-centered planning, functional analysis, multicomponent treatment plan, including preventive strategies such as choice making, embedding preferences in activities, using visual schedules. Instruction included teaching following home and school routines; requesting attention, items and activities; waiting for reinforcements; and responding to social initiations.	All children showed substantial increases in appropriate and reduction of inappropriate behaviors at home and school. Gains generalized to appropriate classroom and playground behaviors without direct training, mothers' and teachers' positive interactions with children increased substantially and negative interactions decreased. Effects maintained at 3 months after treatment.

(*continued*)

TABLE 5.1 (CONTINUED)

Author(s)	*Design*	*Participants*	*Intervention*	*Results*
Buschbacher et al. (2004)	Concurrent multiple baseline design across three daily family routines	7-year-old boy with autism and Landau-Kleffner syndrome and his parents	Multicomponent intervention combined interview-based assessment of family members, teachers, and grandmother with observational functional analysis. Training included in vivo coaching with feedback in prevention strategies, replacement behaviors, and consequence procedures for three daily routines: dinnertime, family television watching, and bedtime.	Significant decrease in disruptive behaviors during dinnertime routine from 41% at baseline to 12% during intervention and 8% at follow-up. Increase in engagement during dinnertime from 77% at baseline to 97% during intervention and 100% at follow-up. For family television routine, disruptive behavior decreased from 55% during baseline to 18% during intervention and 7% at follow-up. Engagement during this routine significantly increased from 18% at baseline to 89% during intervention and 100% at follow-up.
Carr et al. (1999)	Concurrent multiple baseline probe design across two individuals in several settings and task conditions.	A 14-year-old girl with cerebral palsy and ID, a 17-year-old adolescent with autism. (a third adult not include d in our analysis).	A multiple component intervention combined extensive assessment, building rapport, functional communication training, building tolerance for reinforcement delay, providing choices, and embedding stimuli for socially appropriate behavior in conditions in which problem behavior was likely and programming generalization.	Tantrums, aggression, and property destruction went from 243 in baseline to 3.4 during intervention and 1.0 during maintenance for the girl, the male's went from 110 to 9.5 to 1.7. Engagement in appropriate activities increased dramatically and maintained for both.
Cheremshynski et al. (2012)	Single-subject withdrawal with five phases: baseline, intervention, withdrawal, reimplementation of intervention, and follow-up	5-year-old boy with autism and his mother	Multicomponent intervention combined cultural assessment tool in the form of semistructured interviews with mother with functional behavior assessments of child's disruptive behaviors. Parent training occurred one to three times per week for a total of seven sessions in five weeks and lasted from 15 to 30 minutes. It included setting event/antecedent/consequence strategies and self-management and problem-solving training. The PBS plan for the targeted routine of mealtime included implementation checklist for the mother and picture schedule for the child.	Significant effects for disruptive behaviors during dinner routine (average of 87% at baseline, 16.7% during intervention, 45.3% during withdrawal, 2% on reimplementation of intervention, and 2% at follow-up). Significant effects for independent completion of dinner routine steps, with 0% of steps completed at baseline, 78% during intervention, 40% during withdrawal, 95% during reimplementation, and 100% at follow-up. Latency of routine completion increased from 3.1 minutes at baseline to an average of 9.2 minutes during intervention and 6.8 minutes at follow-up.

Clarke, Dunlap, & Vaughn (1999)	Single-subject reversal design	10-year-old boy with Asperger's and his mother	Multicomponent intervention combined functional analysis with assessment interviews with each family member. The morning routine was targeted for intervention. The mother was taught to implement three components of intervention for the morning time routine: visual chart of routine, modifications to clothing, and choice chart for reinforcement.	Child engagement in morning routine increased from average of 25% of intervals at baseline and withdrawal to average of 80% during intervention phases. Disruptive behaviors during routine decreased from an average of 68% across baseline and withdrawal phases to an average of 13% during intervention. Duration of the routine decreased from average of 27 min 5 sec during baseline and withdrawal to average of 10 min 50 sec during intervention. Mother described intervention as being easy to implement and applicable to other family routines.
Coughlin, Sharry, Fitzpatrick, Geurin, & Drumm (2009)	Sequential block design with control	74 parents of children (aged 6–11 years) with significant behavioral, emotional, and developmental difficulties	Comprised 9 weekly group sessions of *Parents Plus Children's Programme* (PPCP). Trainers used videos, discussion, role-play, and weekly planning to train parents in positive parenting and parent–child interactions. Ninth session added to cover family problem-solving and parent self-care.	Significant differences in total difficulties, conduct problems, impact of difficulties, behavior problems, goal attainment, parent stress reduction, parenting confidence, in favor of intervention group. Further analysis showed that PPCP was more helpful for children with behavior problems than for children with developmental problems in total difficulties and child peer problems.
Duda, Clarke, Fox, & Dunlap (2008)	Multiple baseline designs across four family routines and three siblings.	5-year-old girl and 32-month-old fraternal twins with high rates of triadic and dyadic fighting. One twin with DD and serious problem behaviors.	After conducting a functional analysis and collaborative planning with parents, researchers coached parents to use a multicomponent PBS treatment including stating clear expectations, providing choices, prompting appropriate play, warning signals, and pairing commands with preferred stimuli.	When observations of three children were aggregated across four routines, there were substantial reductions in problem behavior. Individual direct observations using multiple baseline designs across routines showed substantial reductions in problem behavior and gains in appropriate targeted behaviors in all three children.

(continued)

TABLE 5.1 (CONTINUED)

Author(s)	*Design*	*Participants*	*Intervention*	*Results*
Durand, Hieneman, Clarke, Wang, & Rinaldi (2013)	Randomized, controlled trial design	54 families of children (aged 3–6 years) with DD	Trainers implemented a combination of positive behavior support (PBS) and the cognitive-behavior-based positive family intervention (PFI) for the intervention group, whereas the control group only received PBS training. Through the eight weekly 90-minute training sessions, intervention families were exposed instruction and practice on an adapted version of Seligman's (2002) optimism training.	Both groups significantly decreased their levels of parent pessimism, but the PFI group attained significant parent-reported behavioral improvements compared with the PBS-only group. Observations of child behaviors indicated reliable changes for more children in the PFI group, but behavioral changes were not significantly greater for the overall PFI group than for the PBS group.
Erbas (2010)	Alternating treatment design across three children in Turkey	4.5-year-old boy with developmental delays, serious aggression; 5-year-2-month-old boy with DD and aggression against peers; 5-year-4-month-old boy with DD and tantrumming and aggression in community settings.	Compared two methods of implementation, consultation meetings alone versus consultation meetings plus feedback based on videos of mother's implementing procedures.	Parents correct implementation of treatment practices improved under both conditions, but more so with video-based feedback plus consultation. Children's problem behavior reduced under both conditions, but more when mothers received feedback.
Feldman, Condillac, Tough, Hunt, & Griffiths (2002)	Multiple baseline across 10 children with developmental delays, autism, and ID. Seven subjects included for our evaluation.	Subjects ranged in age from 1 year to 26 years. Problem behaviors included disruption, self injury, and aggression.	Intervention included prevention by changing setting events, offering choices, teaching replacement skills, errorless compliance training, FCT, extinction and response interruption, addition of preferred activities.	Significant decreases in problem behaviors ranging from 100% to 76% reductions with concurrent increases in replacement skills. Functional effect established for seven participants according to our analysis.

Hudson et al. (2003)	Quasi-experimental, controlled design	Mothers of 115 children with ID	Parents in *Signposts for Building Better Behavior* program assigned or self-selected into three intervention conditions (group support, telephone support, and self-directed). Self-directed parents receive core instructional manuals and videos on measuring, replacing, planning, and teaching behaviors and adjunctive manuals and videos on dealing with stress and family team work. Telephone support parents received additional assistance from therapists via phone, and group support parents received support through six in-person, 2-hour trainings.	Significant improvements in parents stress, parenting competence, and feelings of parent needs being met at post-intervention and maintained at follow-up for treatment parents, compared with control group. No child outcome differences were found between intervention and control groups.
Hudson, Cameron, & Matthews (2008)	Noncontrolled, matched group, repeated measures design	1,790 families of children with ID and difficulty behavior	Wide-scale *Signposts* implementation evaluation with additional intervention group (individual support). See Hudson et al. (2003) for general procedures including several established individual treatments from applied behavior analysis combined into a treatment package.	Medium to large effects found in mothers in individual and telephone support groups, smaller effects for group support, and nonsignificant effects for self-directed group. Both mothers and fathers improved in parenting efficacy, parent satisfaction, and parenting hassles. Mothers, but not fathers, reported decreased depression and anxiety.
L. K. Koegel, Stiebel, & Koegel (1998)	Multiple baseline design across three sibling dyads.	Three young children with autism and their infant or toddler siblings.	Functional behavior assessment (FBA) identified antecedent stimuli for aggression against infants. Antecedent environmental stimuli were removed, FCT and teaching of replacement play skills, and contingent attention.	For three dyads, large reductions in aggression which maintained at 1 year for first child, 4 months for the second, and not measured for third. Measures of happiness indicated positive affective changes in children with autism. Appropriate alternative behaviors increased substantially.
Lucyshyn, Albin, & Nixon (1997)	Multiple baseline across family routines	14-year-old girl with severe ID, functional blindness, and severe forefoot pronation and her parents	Multicomponent intervention combined functional analysis training with an ethnographic assessment of the family. Individualized PBS plan was collaboratively developed to improve on behaviors in four routines valued by the family. Researchers trained family using direct coaching, modeling, and teaching self-monitoring and self-evaluation skills. Training sessions occurred one to three times per week, ranging in length from 20 to 75 minutes.	Significant decreases in child's total disruptive behaviors after intervention. Self-injurious behaviors and aggression decreased to near-zero levels in three of four family routines with significant decreases in fourth routine. Follow-up at 3 and 9 months post-intervention showed maintenance of decreased disruptive behavior. Additional collateral benefits observed in family quality of life and maternal anxiety levels.

(*continued*)

TABLE 5.1 (CONTINUED)

Author(s)	*Design*	*Participants*	*Intervention*	*Results*
Lucyshyn, Albin, Horner, Mann, & Wadsworth (2007)	Longitudinal SSD	Female with severe ID and autism (began study at 5 years old and completed study at age 10) and her parents	Multicomponent intervention combined functional behavior assessment training with interview-based assessment of family ecology. Collaboratively developed PBS plan for four daily family routines. Training consisted of implementation checklists for parents, modeling skills, coaching with feedback, self-monitoring training, and training in setting event/antecedent/consequence strategies.	Decreases in problem behavior demonstrated at each follow-up probe at 6, 18, 36, 67, and 86 months following intervention. Overall decrease of problem behavior of 94% from baseline to final follow-up. Significant increase in number of community activities the child participated in.
Lucyshyn et al. (2015)	Multiple baseline across family routines and within subject statistical comparison of coercive and constructive processes as measured by sequential coding of dyadic interactions.	Ten children with autism and or ID between 3 and 8 years old with severe problem behaviors.	Cooperative planning to reflect parental culture and family routines were designed, including preventive interventions for setting and trigger events, use of picture prompts, warning cues for changes of activities, embedding of preferred items in routines, direct and systematic instruction of prosocial replacement skills, praise, contingent access to attention and preferred items, planned ignoring, and redirection were used to modify long-standing severe problem behaviors.	Multiple baseline across activities designs found clear functional effects for seven of 10 children and their families. Statistical analysis of coercive and constructive family routines found significant reductions in the former and gains in the latter.
McIntyre (2008b)	Randomized controlled trial design	44 families of children (aged 2–5 years) with DD	Adaptation of Webster-Stratton's (1984) *Incredible Years Parent Training* program for DD population. Twelve weekly sessions consisting of group discussions, videos, role-play, lectures, and homework to teach parenting strategies (e.g., parent–child play, praise and reward, limit setting, behavior management).	Negative parenting behaviors, child behavioral problems, and child internalizing behaviors reduced in treatment group compared with control group. No differences found in child-directed praise between groups.

Phaneuf & McIntyre (2011)	Single-subject changing conditions design	Eight mother–child dyads (children aged 2–4 years)	Adapted *Incredible Years Parent Training* program within response-to-intervention model. In Tier I, parents read or listened to self-directed training materials. Parents needing more guided support participated in the 11-week group training (for procedures, see McIntyre, 2008b) of Tier 2. Parents needing intensive intervention received individualized video feedback training in Tier 3.	Rates of observed negative parenting strategies decreased from baseline to post-intervention across all parents. Child behavior problems decreased across all but two parents. At 3-month follow-up, six of six participating dyads maintained or reduced negative parenting.
Plant & Sanders (2007)	Randomized, controlled trial design	74 families of preschool-aged children (< 6 years) with DD	Treatment parents assigned to Standard *Stepping Stones Triple P* (*SSTP*) program or Enhanced *SSTP* program. Standard *SSTP* trained parents in 25 core child management strategies (e.g., activity schedules, rewards, incidental teaching, rule-setting, direct commands, time-out) in 10 sessions, using modeling, practice, therapist feedback, and parent homework assignments. Enhanced *SSTP* provides Standard *SSTP* training and training on copings strategies and partner- and family-support skills.	Child problem behaviors and problem caregiving tasks significantly decreased in treatment groups, compared with control group. Parenting skills and parent competence also improved for treatment groups. Mothers in enhanced group reported less difficult child behavior in caregiving, and standard treatment group mothers reported less disruptive child behavior at postintervention. Overall child disruptive behavior was significantly different between enhanced and control groups at 1-year follow-up, in favor of enhanced group.
Roberts, Mazzuchelli, Studman, & Sanders (2006)	Randomized, controlled trial design	44 families of 47 children (aged 2–7 years) with DD	Standard *STTP* were compared to Enhanced *SSTP*. See Plant & Sanders (2007) for general procedures.	Significant reductions in oppositional behavior reported by treatment parents, compared with control group. Decreases in child problem behaviors at post-intervention and at 6-month follow-up found for treatment mothers, but not for treatment fathers. Treatment fathers exhibited less negative parenting, and mothers exhibited less overreactive parenting. Treatment parents provided more positive social attention to children.

(*continued*)

TABLE 5.1 (CONTINUED)

Author(s)	*Design*	*Participants*	*Intervention*	*Results*
Singer, Irvin, Irvine, Hawkins, & Cooley (1989)	Randomized controlled trial design	27 mothers and 14 fathers of children with moderate to severe ID and/or autism	Stress management training, behavioral parent training, volunteers took children to community activities, individual marital or personal short-term behavioral counseling when requested	Statistically significant reductions in depressive symptoms and anxiety symptoms in mothers. Statistically significant reductions in anxiety symptoms in fathers. Depressive symptoms in fathers reduced to near significance level. Children combined participated in over 300 community activities. Highly positive social validity scores. Lower symptoms levels maintained at 1-year follow-up.
Sofronoff, Jahnel, & Sanders (2011)	Randomized controlled trial design	53 parents of children with DD (including ID, ASD, multiple disabilities, SLD, etc.)	Standard *SSTP* with some Enhanced strategies were condensed into two 2-hour seminars, with handouts provided at the end of each seminar.	Number of perceived child problem behaviors significantly reduced for treatment group, compared with control group. Dysfunctional parenting also decreased for treatment group. Differences maintained at 3-month follow-up. No significant differences found in parent relationship quality, parental adjustment, and family functioning between groups.
Vaughn, Clarke, & Dunlap (1997)	Multiple baseline design across two settings	8-year-old boy with multiple severe disabilities including agenesis of the corpus callosum and his mother	Multicomponent intervention combined interview-based assessment of family with functional behavior analysis. Training occurred twice per week. The mother was taught to use visual schedules and supports during bathroom routine and fast food dining routine. She was also taught to use visuals of child's preferred reinforcers when presenting demands related to these tasks.	Significant decrease in child disruptive behaviors during both bathroom routine and fast food dining routine after intervention. These results maintained at follow-up. After intervention, engagement increased during both bathroom routine and fast food dining routine and remained high at follow-up. Further, results generalized to a novel restaurant setting.

several innovative contributions to the family-based support programs research literature. The creative development of new practices under the PBS category represents some of the most important innovation in family support programs for families whose offspring with developmental disabilities (DDs) have serious problem behaviors.

The group comparison studies reviewed in this chapter include several new contributions to the family support literature. These include an evaluation of distance learning delivery of behavioral parent training (e.g., Hudson et al., 2003) using videos, manuals, and phone calls. Phaneuf and McIntyre (2011) studied a service design that is innovative in this literature. They organized treatment into tiered stages in which each successive stage required more intensive intervention and more commitment of time and effort by parents. A first tier provided parents with manuals and audiotapes, the second consisted of 11 weeks of behavioral parent training. A third tier for parents who needed further assistance with interacting successfully with their young children with autism consisted of giving parents individualized feedback on videos of parent–child interchanges.

The study by Durand, Hieneman, Clarke, Wang, and Rinaldi (2013) is a good example of a second-generation research study using a randomized group comparison design. As described in what follows, they combined a PBS intervention with optimism training. The package of components was designed to help parents who were unlikely candidates for successfully taking up and using positive behavioral interventions because they were assessed as unusually pessimistic about their abilities to benefit from parent training and doubtful of success in changing their children's behavior problems. The focus on a resistant subgroup of parents is important because, as discussed earlier, there is considerable room for improving the outcomes of parent training programs. This dual component program echoes earlier work by Singer, Irvin, Irvine, Hawkins, and Cooley (1989), which demonstrated the positive impact of a four-component intervention on mothers and fathers of children with moderate/severe intellectual disabilities (IDs) or severe autism.

GOING TO SCALE

One intervention reviewed in this chapter has been replicated on a large scale and demonstrates the way multicomponent behavioral parent training can be delivered using a public health model potentially benefiting large numbers of families. The Stepping Stones Triple P (SSTP; Sanders, Mazzucchelli, & Studman, 2004) was developed as a specialized version of a program of behavioral parent training aimed at preventing and treating problem behavior in nondisabled children with behavior problems. This parent program is currently being replicated in several nations across cultures and languages. While it has not yet been replicated at this scale, the offshoot Stepping Stones program has demonstrated efficacy with relatively large numbers of families. It has also successfully integrated many behavioral techniques in one behavioral parent training program. A study by Plant and Sanders (2007) is notable because parents in one group were taught as many as 25 skills, which the researchers garnered from previous BPT research. This is a more comprehensive curriculum than seen in other studies in the DD field. They compared one group that received the multiple skills training with an enhanced program. In the enhanced treatment, in addition to the curriculum of parenting techniques, they also provided training on coping with stress and on building more cooperation between partners. At a 1-year follow-up, the enhanced treatment group had better child outcomes. In keeping with the emerging focus on the family context, this study supports the value of addressing other key parts of the family system. Several randomized control treatment (RCT) studies also evaluate more complex combined treatment components and open new ground.

AN ECOBEHAVIORAL MODEL

Singer et al. (1989) first developed and tested individual components for supporting families of children with severe disabilities and subsequently combined them into a multiple component intervention for families of children with severe DDs. They conceptualized their practices as ecobehavioral and, as such, had four forms of intervention combined into a model.

Influenced by Lutzker and colleague's ecobehavioral work (Lutzker, Campbell, Harrold, & Huynen, 1992), Singer et al. (1989) evaluated a multicomponent model for supporting families of school-age children with severe DDs. Their intervention package is the most comprehensive set of combined programs that we have found in the literature evaluated that used RCT designs. The components of their model were: (1) case management, (2) respite care, (3) family involvement with community volunteers as companions to their children for community outings, (4) behavioral parent training, (5) cognitive-behavioral stress management training, and (6) short-term behavioral couples or individual counseling when needed. They randomly assigned parents to one of two groups. The intervention group received all of the components, and a comparison group received case management and respite care. The comparison group was designed as a demonstration of the generally available services for families in the town where the study was implemented. That is, it was a "business as usual" comparison group and largely consisted of little or no external assistance from community agencies. The treatment group classes followed treatment manuals developed by Hawkins and Singer (1988).

The treatment outcomes that were measured were depressive symptoms and anxiety symptoms and a social validation measure of parents' satisfaction with the components of the program separately and together. The researchers also gathered process data to document the implementation of respite care, community volunteers' activities with the children, and goals addressed via case management services.

Depressive symptoms were measured with the Beck Depression Inventory (BDI) (Beck, Ward, & Mendelson, 1961) and the State Trait Anxiety Inventory-Trait Scale (STAI-T) (Spielberger, Gorsuch, Lushene, Vagg, & Jacobs, 1983). Data was collected a pretest, posttest, and a 1-year follow-up. Outcomes were reported separately for fathers

TABLE 5.2 CLASS TOPICS FOR A MULTIPLE COMPONENT TREATMENT

Parent-Focused Stress Management Skills

1. Identifying stressors and stress reactions with self-monitoring
2. Progressive muscle relaxation—long form
3. Progressive muscle relaxation—short form
4. Self-monitoring and brief relaxation in home and community
5. Modification of negative thoughts through self-coaching
6. Covert rehearsal for difficult social situations
7. Techniques for managing worries and obsessive thoughts
8. Strengthening social support networks, utilizing respite, and advocacy

Child-Focused Behavioral Parenting Skills

9. Describing child behavior as antecedents, responses, and consequences
10. Strengthening valued behavior with praise and attention
11. Using back-up rewards and simple token systems
12. Responding to the child's initiations and giving opportunities for choice
13. Partial participation as a way to increase the child's involvement in home and community activities
14. Teaching children to follow clear directions and redirecting the child to appropriate behaviors when problem behaviors occur
15. Using brief nonexclusionary time-out for severe problem behavior
16. Participating in community activities with the child

Source: Singer, Irvin, Irvine, Hawkins, and Cooley (1989)

and mothers. Parents in the model treatment group attended two series of 8-week-long classes for 2 hours each week. One class taught behavioral parent training skills and the other cognitive-behavioral therapy (CBT) stress management skills. Table 5.2 presents the topics presented each week. Parents listened to brief lectures, discussed their experience each week with implementing treatments, and practiced them as homework. A midweek phone call from one of the therapists was meant to encourage parents to do the homework and to address any obstacles parents encountered in using the techniques. Both interventions made use of interventions that were well studied in the literature in the late 1980s.

The outcomes were as follows: The measure of depressive symptoms and on anxiety symptoms between groups of mothers at posttest was significantly different with $F(3, 27) = 10.9$, $p = .00$, and $d = 0.82$ on the BDI and $F(3, 27) = 6.00$, $p = .003$, and $d = 0.56$ on the STAI-T. For the fathers, the differences on the BDI approached significance, $F(1, 12) = 3.95$, $p = .07$ and were significant for the STAI, $F(1, 12) = 7.35$, $p = .019$. The fathers had relatively low scores at pretest on the outcome measures, so there was less room for improvement at the posttest and follow-up. These are among the higher effect sizes found in the group comparison studies in this volume.

At a 1-year follow-up, the scores for the intensive treatment group were not significantly different from the posttest scores, indicating the effects had maintained over a 1-year period. Effect sizes appear in a table later in the chapter. The researchers also reported on the number of parents whose depression and anxiety scores moved out of the clinical range in both groups with outcomes strongly favoring the intensive treatment group. Social validation measures indicated that parents viewed the goals of the program as moderately to highly important and the program successful in achieving these goals.

Process data showed that the volunteer component accounted for over 300 community activities with the 30 volunteers accompanying the children to community activities an average of 10 times each. The parents were particularly appreciative of this component of the program, because at the time access to inclusive community settings and programs was a relatively new development for children with this level of disability.

The outcomes of this multicomponent study indicated that a comparatively complex program was effective in supporting parents of children with severe cognitive disabilities. It was efficacious for mothers and fathers. This multicomponent intervention is promising but awaits replication by a third party. We evaluate this program as promising. Treatment manuals are available core components of the program, but it has not been replicated in published research studies.

OPTIMISM AND POSITIVE BEHAVIOR SUPPORT TRAINING

The Positive Family Intervention (PFI) program (Durand & Hieneman, 2008) is a second-generation multicomponent intervention that has been tested with parents of children with autism and other DDs (Durand et al., 2013). The intervention combines positive behavior support (PBS) and CBT for pessimism. It consists of eight sessions led by a human service professional and includes homework assignments for practicing skills presented in sessions. At each class meeting, the presenter teaches parents using a description of a treatment component, a vignette illustrating it, and the rationale for it. PBS differs from the more established applied behavior analysis in stressing the importance of molding the design of the intervention to fit the ecocultural niche and unique characteristics of a family. It treats the context of home, school, and community not just as the places where problem behaviors occur with antecedents and consequences but also as key to the design of the program and the process of implementation. Positive behavior support practitioners strive for a goodness-of-fit of the treatment program with the family's patterns of living, values, and strengths. Finally, PBS aims to go beyond helping to prevent, reduce, and replace problem behavior to promote a better quality of life for the child and family. One way this is done is by helping families with goal setting and by addressing other family issues that might get in the way of uptake and implementation of the treatment.

The positive family intervention (PFI) program aimed to directly treat parents who had elevated levels of pessimism when they entered parent training. Traditional CBT methods were integrated into the PBS sessions. The cognitive behavioral components of the combined PBS and CBT treatment included (1) teaching parents to self-monitor their thoughts, (2) identify problematic thinking that often is part of an overall pessimistic outlook, (3) challenge this thinking rather than automatically believing it, and (4) replace it with more positive thoughts or beliefs. These are standard CBT treatment components. Previously, we explained how this sequence was used in Singer et al.'s (Singer, Irvin, & Hawkins, 1988; Singer, Irvin, Irvine, Hawkins, & Cooley, 1989) sets of randomized intervention studies and in Nixon and Singer's (1993) intervention to help parents with excessive self-blame. Durand and colleagues' intervention differs from Singer and colleagues' in that it combines PBS classes with CBT as part of each session. Singer et al. (1988), on the other hand, first provided eight classes of BPT followed by eight additional sessions on cognitive-behavioral stress management.

Durand's research is particularly valuable for the field because it represents a second-generation study in which interventions are fashioned for specific subgroups of parents. In Durand et al.'s study, the selection criteria for participating parents included assessments indicating the parents had elevated levels of stress and pessimism. Out of 257 families initially assessed, 203 did not meet these criteria, suggesting that the eventual participants represented a smaller and more difficult to treat subgroup of families. These difficult-to-treat families are important because there is evidence that behavioral parent training is ineffective for a substantial percentage of parents who do not take it up readily.

The PFI program has been evaluated in a randomized trial (Durand et al., 2013). The PFI research meets high standards for evaluating clinical programs. It has a published facilitator's guide (Durand & Hieneman, 2008). Of the CBT and multiple component interventions reviewed here, it is one of only two manualized interventions along with Singer et al.'s work (1989) on stress management and multiple component treatments. This randomized trial was one of the few comparing a new intervention (PBS plus optimism training) with one that was previously evaluated and effective. The authors compared a PFI group of randomly assigned pessimistic parents of children with DDs and behavior problems to a similar group of pessimistic parents who received PBS alone without the optimism training. Positive family intervention has two major components, PBS and CBT; consequently, the study serves as a component analysis, in that it is possible to ask what CBT adds to the behavioral parent training program. The study is also notable for combining direct observation of parent–child interaction and parent self-report data to measured outcomes. Because PBS has substantial evidence supporting its efficacy, both groups were expected to show improvements on measures of children's problem behavior, parent optimism/pessimism, and satisfaction with the intervention. Based on direct observation measures, both groups of children showed statistically significant reductions in problem behaviors. There was no winner on this variable when the extent of changes from pre- to posttest was analyzed. The groups did differ on a statistic called the *reliable change index* (RCI). It takes into account the error in the measures and contributes to evaluating how confident one can be that the observed changes in children's behaviors were due to the treatment rather than measurement error. Twice as many children in the PFI group showed reliable changes compared with the PBS-only group. In the BFI group, 56% of the children showed reliable changes compared with 29% in the PBS group. In addition to direct observation, the researchers gathered data based on parents responses to a standardized measure of problem behavior. When looked at in this way, the PFI group showed changes in this parent report measure significantly greater than the changes from before the study began (pretest) and after it ended (posttest) in the PBS group. Again, when the RCI was calculated, 72% of the children in the PFI group showed reliable change compared with 35% in the PBS only group. Durand et al.'s research is also notable for publishing attrition data; both groups lost a third of the participants. On the measure of pessimism, both groups improved significantly from pretest to posttest, but there was no significant difference between the two groups. That is, both treatments lowered pessimism in the parents. The study adds to the research showing positive benefits of PBS in changing children's problem behavior and it establishes the PFI as a promising practice for working with parents who may be resistant to change.

HOME-BASED POSITIVE BEHAVIOR SUPPORT

There is a growing body of research suggesting that training and supporting families within the context of their homes with multiple component PBS can lead to a variety of positive outcomes. Home-based parent training founded on principles of PBS has been implemented to increase appropriate behaviors and decrease maladaptive or disruptive behaviors and to help parents develop effective parenting skills, thus contributing to a family's quality of life. In the following review of a set of notable PBS studies, we have benefited from a review of the literature on home-based, family-focused PBS (Lucyshyn et al., 2015), although we have conducted our own evaluation of these studies to confirm that they meet acceptable standards for categorizing the status of the evidence supporting them. Home-based PBS poses a definitional challenge for a reviewer, because it is a general approach that is consistent at a molar level but varies at a more molecular level in the specific techniques used for individual families. It does constitute a definable set of practices that are consistent enough to warrant recognition as a distinctive intervention for families. In order to be included in this review, PBS studies had to include five core intervention practices that together constitute in-home PBS.

First, there is a major emphasis on collaborative planning and implementation between interventionists and the family so that there is a goodness of fit of treatment plans and implementation with family routines and family values (Lucyshyn, Blumberg, & Kayser, 2000). A study by Moes and Frea (2002) compared a more traditional approach to planning with one that emphasized contextual fit. In a multiple baseline study across three families, they demonstrated improved outcomes when interventions were more carefully customized than when a standardized top-down approach to planning was used. Contextual fit involves taking into account environmental variables as well as characteristics of the individual with disruptive behavior and other family members involved (Albin, Lucyshyn, Horner, & Flannery, 1996; Lucyshyn & Albin, 1993). Creating contextual fit requires extensive collaboration with the family members who implement the treatment practices. Fettig, Schultz, and Sreckovic (2015) described the collaborative nature of the planning process in the assessment and planning phases of the treatment:

> Through out the training, parents were encouraged to share their parenting philosophies and values and experiences of strategies they tried before the study. Together, the researchers and parents brainstormed ideas of what might be helpful for the child based on the child's strengths and the parents own home/parenting philosophies and values. In addition, videos of other parents implementing the FA-based strategies and sample visual supports were also shared with the parents. Based on this discussion the researchers provided parents with choices of intervention strategies and visual supports. The researchers took notes on parents choices, and at the end of the training each parent was given the collaboratively created behavior support plan with a description of target behaviors, functions of the behaviors, and strategies to try during the routine. (Fettig et al., 2015, p. 173)

A second core feature of in-home PBS is it incorporates intensive assessment to identify the functions of problem behaviors and to understand the family's ecobehavioral niche, consisting of home and community routines that powerfully influence parent–child interactions and, when considered together, make up the architecture of family life with its customary ways in which family members organize and make sense of their daily lives.

A primary goal of the assessment process is to determine what conditions occasion and motivate problem behaviors, a process known as a functional behavior assessment (FBA). These are usually conducted in homes via interviews and direct observation and sometimes are followed by directly manipulating hypothesized antecedent conditions to verify the cause (or function) of a problem behavior. This later step, functional analysis, is more common as a procedure in research studies and may not be necessary or suitable in applied work with families. Considerable time and attention is put into the assessment process, because the design of treatment is greatly dependent on what it reveals. In long-term PBS studies, assessment is an ongoing process, because stimulus conditions can change dramatically over the course of years and new problem behaviors emerge in these new contexts or old ones can resurface. Carr et al. (1999) conducted a multiple component treatment study of three individuals with severe problem behaviors, two who lived at home with their parents. The study lasted for 6 years and involved repeated assessments as needed. The researchers interviewed parents and others who were present when problem behaviors occurred in order to obtain a description of the antecedents of the problem behaviors and the consequent changes in the environment after these occurred. Interviewees were also asked to speculate about whether the behaviors seemed to be motivated by attempts to gain attention, to escape from a demand or nonpreferred activity, or to obtain a desired item or activity. Following interviews, the interventionists went into the environments where problems happened and directly observed them. Assessments required approximately 36 hours for each of the three participants and produced over 100 direct observations of problematic incidents per client. Observers wrote brief descriptions of the behaviors and their antecedents and consequences and hypothesized about functions motivating the incidents. These hypotheses were later summarized in themes based primarily on the functions of the problem behaviors. The authors note that more efficient assessment procedures have been recommended by other PBS researchers (O'Neill, Horner, Albin, Storey, Sprague, & Newton, 1997). As described in what follows, another core and definitional element of PBS is that the assessment also includes a careful analysis of family activity routines and of relevant aspects of their ecocultural niche.

Fettig et al. (2015) gave examples of the functions of three young children's problem behaviors as revealed through an FBA process. Jack, a 4-year-old boy with autism, refused to get out of the bathtub at the end of a bath. He had tantrums unless his father first also gave him a shower before getting out of the tub and drying off. The function of the problem behavior was determined to be escape from leaving a preferred activity, bathing. Emma, a 4-year-old girl, hid behind doors at meal time, screamed at her parents and siblings, and engaged in verbal battles with her siblings, thereby provoking the mother to try to redirect the girl and often yell at her. The assessment revealed that when the mother attended to the child throughout the mealtime, Emma remained in her seat and ate normally. The function of the behavior was to obtain parental attention. For the third child, Liam, a 6-year-old boy, the disrupted family routine was getting dressed and ready for school in the morning. He refused to get dressed, which caused time pressure and delayed successful accomplishment of the morning routine. The assessment suggested his problem behavior was motivated by escape from a task he did not like, getting out of bed and getting dressed. Based on the analysis and collaborative discussions, PBS interventions may recommend changes in the routine and/or ways to teach the child alternative ways of obtaining the same sought-after effects.

Assessment practices aim to thoroughly describe the context of problem behavior by identifying its antecedent conditions. These include setting events, those conditions that set the stage for problem behavior. For example, in a study by Lucyshyn et al. (2015) three setting events were identified for one of the children in the study: insufficient sleep, problem behavior at school prior to coming home, and illness. In some recent studies, researchers have also begun to identify motivating operations, which are antecedents that alter the reinforcing properties of conditions that immediately follow a problem behavior; that is, they intensify or weaken the reinforcement effectiveness of a consequence of the behavior (Call, Wacker, Ringdahl, & Boelter, 2005). Positive behavior support interventionists also try to identify the immediate triggering conditions of problem behavior. For example, Lucyshyn et al. (2015) demonstrated the way in which a parental directive such as a demand to put away a game can give rise within a few seconds to child problem behavior. Another triggering event was parent inattention to a child because of competing demands like talking on the telephone or concentrating on meal preparation triggered problem behavior motivated to gain attention for the child.

A third key feature of in-home PBS is that activity settings of daily routines in families are the primary unit of analysis for assessing the context of problem behavior as well as planning and conducting treatments. These routines are the common activities that make up family life. These are the patterned, repeated, and mundane ways in which families carry out basic aspects of their lives such as meal preparation, getting ready for school, watching TV, going to restaurants, answering the telephone, cleaning the house, treating a child's head cold, and so forth. Activity settings include tasks, the people involved in them, their cultural values, the meanings they give to the routines, and the patterned way in which they interact. Routines nested in activity settings make up the architecture of family life and are permeated with cultural, familial, and individual meanings (Gallimore, Goldenberg, & Weisner, 1993). In a middle-class family with two working parents, a dinner routine might involve frozen food that each family member microwaves individually and eats while seated in front of the television while watching a favorite TV show, whereas for a Chinese American immigrant family it might involve the whole family eating around the dining room table in silence while using chopsticks and each taking food from common serving bowls with cuisine prepared by the mother. For the first family, the values instantiated in the activity might be efficiency and shared enjoyment of entertainment, whereas for the second family values embedded and expressed in the mealtime routine might include family solidarity and gratitude for the meal.

Family activity routines are often modified in order to meet the needs of children with disabilities. Considerable problem-solving and creativity can go into making changes to routines for the family member with special needs, and often they work well for families (Maul & Singer, 2014). When children exhibit problem behaviors during these routines, the normal flow of events in a family can be disrupted and, to the extent that activities have to be modified in ways that are overtaxing and so demand a lot of extra time, energy, arousal of negative emotions, or attention, these disturbances of culturally constructed routines can become stressful. Inadvertent or deliberate modifications of routines to address challenging behavior can over time alter the basic pattern of family life and entrain distress. For example, a child who tantrums in many public settings may lead parents to decide to always have one parent stay at home with the child while the other parent takes siblings to community activities like eating out or going to movies. In families that value group solidarity and cohesion, this change may be perceived as detrimental and become a source of stress. Major changes in parents' and siblings' life trajectories can be the long-term molar outcome of smaller-scale distortions of desirable family routines, as in the case of a parent who gives up a career in order to care for a child with a severe disability because the child needs extra time and attention to manage problem behaviors in common activities.

A third characteristic of these studies is that they use multicomponent approaches combining several techniques as a coherent program. Lucyshyn et al. (2015) provide a detailed treatment plan for one of the children treated in their study. All had an extensive history of very serious problem behaviors, in most cases associated with autism. The plan, based on ecological assessment and FBA, presented strategies in four categories: setting events, preventive strategies, teaching strategies, and consequence strategies. Setting events identified in the assessment included too little sleep for the child the night before, sudden wake-up directives in the morning, parents' sole reliance on verbal directives to prompt routines without visual aids, absence of preferred items in routines, fatigue, return from home after an incident of problem behavior at school, insufficient noncontingent attention from the father, and illness. For each of these, a strategy was planned with parental input. For example, the interventionist coached parents to embed preferred items or stimuli into routines such as favorite breakfast foods in the morning and preferred homework topics for initiating homework. Visual schedules were provided to the boy to augment or replace verbal commands and give prior notification of verbal directives. Preventive strategies included providing advanced warnings before a transition away from a preferred activity, a statement of a positive contingency to motivate cooperation, prompting ahead of time to remind about an alternative replacement behavior ("Remember, ask me if you want a snack"). Teaching strategies included teaching skills for specific routines using systematic instruction methods including modeling, leading, testing, giving and fading prompts and rewards, and self-management checklists to teach skills such as table manners and homework competencies. Consequence procedures included contingent praise, positive attention, ignoring minor problem behavior, redirection, and withholding reinforcement or maintaining task demands when problem behavior occurred. These extensive plans required intensive and relatively long-term involvement from interventionists. Carr et al. also reported the need for extensive and protracted in-home work with parents in order to turn around long established and severe problem behaviors.

Postive behavior support interventions place a major emphasis on teaching replacement skills, that is, new ways of acting that are constructive and take the place of problem behavior. From its inception, PBS emphasized in particular instruction of communication skills designed to allow a person with problem behaviors to achieve the functional effect of a problem behavior through prosocial communication. In a classic study, Carr and Durand (1985) demonstrated that they could reduce problem behaviors in four children with DDs in a school setting. They first determined what motivated the tantrums, aggression, and self-injury exhibited by the children.

They tested two conditions based on direct observations of the contexts in which problem behaviors occurred—low levels of attention from the teacher and difficult tasks. After determining which of these conditions gave rise to problem behaviors, they identified skills that children could use to obtain the same outcomes—attention from the teacher and/or help with difficult schoolwork. They taught students to either say that they did not understand a required activity or to ask the teacher to comment on their work when they experienced lengths of time without attention from the teacher. Carr and Durand showed that these new skills only worked when matched to the right stimulus conditions. These communication skills were effective in replacing the problem behaviors when they were correctly matched such that children asked for teacher comments under conditions of low teacher attention and asked for help when faced with an overly difficult task. The researchers christened this kind of intervention functional communication training (FCT), which has become a common feature of many PBS treatment plans. A 2008 review of FCT research located 91 published studies in which over 200 individuals with DDs were taught to replace problem behaviors with communication skills (Tiger, Hanley, & Bruzek, 2008). Parents in home and community settings were the primary interventionists in some of these studies. Functional communication training is not a necessary component of PBS, but it is a common one. The teaching of replacement skills that may or may not be communicative is a basic component of PBS.

A fourth inclusion criteria and defining feature of home-based PBS intervention is that the scope of treatment goes well beyond reducing or eliminating problem behavior. It aims higher by evaluating the efficacy of a treatment by whether or not it improved the quality of life of the target individual and of the family. In part, these larger changes are achieved by making sure as part of the treatment that interventions generalize. Positive behavior support studies often aim to demonstrate functional impact of PBS practices on two or more family routines, which in combination result in radical improvements in the way family members experience a typical day. Buschbacher et al. (2004) coached parents on preventing problem behaviors and teaching new alternative behaviors in order to shape dinnertime, family television watching, and bedtime routines. In a classic study, Carr et al. (1999) conducted a longitudinal PBS intervention with three young people with severe disabilities across home, school, and community settings. Twenty-four activity settings in total for the three participants included a wide range of common tasks such as sweeping and mopping the floor, brushing teeth, riding an exercycle, and setting the table; these were all activities that occasioned serious and highly disruptive problem behaviors prior to treatment. They intervened in 16 different settings, including homes, supermarkets, buses, restaurants, churches, swimming pools, and school classes. By addressing the way activities are designed and coaching treatment providers to use more positive practices, these practices go beyond a sole focus on behavior to include features of the environment that can be changed in keeping with families' visions for how they want domestic life to be structured and the values expressed in it. The studies often include not only parents but also additional change agents including, in Carr et al., siblings, teachers, speech therapists, group home staff, job coaches, and bus drivers.

The goal of improving the quality of life of families and individuals with disabilities goes well beyond generalization. In their longitudinal studies, Lucyshyn et al. (Lucyshyn et al., 1997; Lucyshyn et al., 2007; Lucyshyn et al., 2015) noted many changes in families' lives in addition to problem behavior reduction. Carr et al. measured the extent to which participants were engaged in community activities as an outcome. Family quality of life measures are reported in some recent PBS studies as part of the evaluation. This emphasis grew out of clinical observations that earlier approaches to behavioral treatment were sometimes counted as successful when they succeeded in reducing problem behavior but when children remained in segregated environments and did not participate in normal community activities. While it is likely that families experience reducing or eliminating problem behavior as an improvement in their quality of life, these studies suggest that larger changes are feasible when families participate in planning, which encourages them to work toward family routines that not only are less stressful but also more closely approximate the ideals they hold for how family life should be enacted.

Finally, PBS interventions are defined in part by what they actively eschew—use of treatment methods that inflict pain or require prolonged restriction of access to common reinforcers. Postive behavior support originated in part out of moral revulsion at some practices that were prominent in the parent field of applied behavior analysis (ABA), including use of seclusionary time-out, restraints, electric shock, and some rarer but widely publicized exotic punishers such as helmets that administered white noise and water sprays to the face of individuals under treatment. Consequently, a defining feature of in-home PBS for families is that the treatments do not make use of aversive procedures either as routine treatment components or as emergency procedures although mild reprimands or very brief response cost procedures may be used.

When combined, the key features of in-home PBS establish an approach to family intervention that is quite distinctive. The defining features of in-home PBS can be seen in two seminal studies by Lucyshyn and his colleagues (1997). They used a multiple baseline design across four family routines. They evaluated the efficacy of an ecological approach to home-based PBS for parents of a child with multiple disabilities. The 14-year-old girl in this study had a diagnosis of severe mental retardation, functional blindness, and severe forefoot pronation. She had many problem behaviors, including extreme aggression toward family members (head-butting, kicking, etc.) and self-injurious behavior (eye poking). Her adaptive behavior scores on the Vineland Adaptive Behavior Scales (Sparrow, Balla, & Cicchetti, 1984) were in the severe deficit range. Her parents reported these frequent disruptive behaviors to be a chronic source of stress at home.

This multicomponent intervention combined functional analysis with an ethnographic assessment of the family to develop a behavior support plan that had a strong contextual fit (Lucyshyn et al., 1997). The researchers conducted an open-ended interview to gather information regarding family resources, goals, strengths, and sources of stress and support in order to determine valued family routines and to further individualize treatment (Albin et al., 1996). They also trained parents in conducting a functional analysis of their child's disruptive behaviors. Following this comprehensive assessment, an individualized PBS plan was developed to improve on behaviors in four environments or routines found to be important to the family: the dinner routine, a leisure routine, shopping at the grocery store, and eating together at a restaurant. The parents were provided with intensive coaching and guidance to carry out the support plan in one environment or routine at a time. This training included demonstrating the skills for the parents, direct coaching of parents to implement the intervention, teaching parents to monitor and evaluate their own performance, practicing these skills, discussing problem-solving, and eventually fading the support and training so that parents became self-sufficient in behavior management. The training sessions occurred one to three times per week and ranged in length from 20 to 75 minutes.

Lucyshyn and colleagues (1997) found that the child's total disruptive behaviors decreased significantly after the initial implementation of this ecological approach to PBS training for parents. Her self-injurious behavior and aggression decreased to near-zero levels in three of the four family routines, and significant decreases were noted in the fourth routine. Follow-up assessments 3 and 9 months later indicated disruptive behaviors remained at low levels. This study also reported significant collateral improvements in quality of life, such as increased child participation in community activities and a decrease in the mother's self-reported anxiety levels. While this case study may represent one family in particular, these findings had many implications for how home-based PBS training should be implemented.

RECENT CONTRIBUTIONS FROM IN-HOME POSITIVE BEHAVIOR SUPPORT RESEARCH

Recent PBS studies have addressed some of the deficiencies in the research literature on family support noted in our final chapter. There are a number of advances in respect to the design of treatments, the diversity of the participants in these studies, long-term maintenance of treatment gains, generalization of treatments effects, and the kind of problem behaviors addressed. Furthermore, recent work provides innovative explication of, and evidentiary support for, new theories regarding family processes and how to remediate undesirable, well-rooted, and complex patterns of negative behavior between family members and replace them with constructive family processes (Lucyshyn et al., 2015). Treatment designs represent considerable creativity in responding to the very real needs of families and their relatives with DDs. Compared with more traditional approaches from the original field of ABA from the 20th century, the extent to which these PBS treatments focus on prevention of problem behaviors and on instruction of skills to replace them is striking and illustrates substantial growth and development in this school of treatment practices. As noted, the treatment plans worked out jointly with family members in these studies include attention to antecedents of problem behavior and ways to replace them efficiently.

Single-subject design studies are particularly strong in establishing evidence for internal validity, an expression of the likelihood that an intervention results in a desired outcome. Because of the small numbers of participants in individual studies, SSDs have been less convincing in establishing evidence for external validity, generalization to representative populations across demographic characteristics, implementers, and locations. As noted in our final chapter, most of the research that purports to address family problems in fact focuses solely on mothers, most of whom have been White and from the middle class. Several PBS studies have begun to address this limitation. A study by Fox, Vaughn, Wyatte, and Dunlap (2002) with parents of young children included three Hispanics, six African Americans, two African immigrants, and one West Indian. Lucyshyn et al. (2015) included participants who were recent immigrants to Canada from China, Taiwan, Japan, and Iran. Two studies were conducted internationally: Erbas (2010) in Turkey and Blair et al. (2011) in South Korea. While these numbers are still very small, the trend is important and encouraging. In the same way, researchers have begun to include more family members in these studies. Cheremshynski, Lucyshyn, and Olson (2013) included one mother and one sibling; Lucyshyn et al. (2015), 10 mothers and fathers and 13 siblings; and Carr et al. (1999) included two mothers and two fathers.

When developing and implementing a home-based PBS program, it is important to consider the influence of a family's cultural values and beliefs. In a descriptive case study of a composite of Chinese American families, Wang, McCart, and Turnbull (2007) outlined several traditional Chinese values and perspectives that should be taken into consideration when designing a support plan. While the authors emphasized the variability in the cultural values of Chinese American families, they suggested the following values to be significant in developing culturally appropriate PBS for this population: promotion of the family as a unit, maintenance of harmony, high emphasis placed on education, negative perceptions regarding the cause of disability, and using punishment as discipline.

Research by Cheremshynski et al. (2013) combined experimental with qualitative analysis to explore the effects of a culturally informed home-based PBS plan. Participating in this study was a Japanese mother and her son. This family was from a middle-class, moderate-sized city. The 5-year-old boy had a diagnosis of autism and had no formal verbal communication, communicating instead by using picture symbols or gestures. He also had a history of disruptive behaviors including knocking items off tables and shelves, throwing objects, crying, and taking off his clothing. An SSD was used in this home-based PBS program (Cheremshynski et al., 2013). The authors used a cultural assessment tool based on one created by Chen, Downing, and Peckham-Hardin (2002) to create a PBS plan that was culturally informed and was based on values the family felt to be important. Semistructured interviews were conducted with the mother to gather more information about how the family's culture, values, and beliefs influenced their lifestyle.

Another qualitative component to Cheremshynski et al.'s (2012) study was having the interventionist working with the parent to keep an ongoing written journal of her thoughts, perceptions, and experiences related to working with a culturally and linguistically diverse family. This was used retrospectively in addition to the quantitative results to provide deeper insight about these experiences. Consistent with previous literature on PBS, an FBA was also conducted to develop a parent training intervention plan based on strategies for setting events, antecedent events, teaching new behaviors, and implementing consequences. From the cultural assessment, it was determined that the dinnertime routine was highly valued and previously unsuccessful, so this was chosen as the first environment for intervention.

Parent training occurred between one and three times per week and lasted from 15 to 30 minutes (Cheremshynski et al., 2013). There were seven sessions provided in total during a 5-week period. Similar to other studies, the training methods used included modeling, coaching, teaching self-monitoring and self-management, rehearsing the behavior, and problem-solving discussions. Also included in this intervention was a picture schedule of the dinnertime routine for the child and an implementation checklist to be used as self-management for the mother.

Child disruptive behaviors during the dinner routine were substantially reduced (Cheremshynski et al., 2013). When the intervention was briefly withdrawn, problem behavior increased, but after training was reintroduced, misbehaviors decreased again; this evidence suggested that the intervention was working as planned. The follow-up scores showed that disruptive behaviors remained at low levels. In terms of independent completion of dinner routine steps, the child completed 0% of steps at baseline and 100% at follow-up. This child was also able to stay in the dinnertime routine longer at follow-up than at baseline. The mother reported that the intervention resulted in a very close fit with what she had envisioned as ideal and that it quickly became natural to implement. Such results indicate the importance of considering cultural values when determining behavioral plans that fit the family context.

Evidence for longer-term maintenance of treatment effects has also been improving in this line of research. Carr et al. (1999) reported outcomes at 6 years after baseline, Lucyshyn and colleagues (2007) at 7 years, Feldman at an average of 107 weeks, and Lucyshyn et al. (2015) at between 11 months and 2 years. Carr et al. (1999) reported on the functional effects of multiple component PBS methods with three individuals with severe problem behavior over a period of 6 years. They found that regular monthly contacts with parents and group-home staff were needed to alert them to the emergence of new problem behaviors, as life conditions of families and the target individuals changed over time. It is very important for creation of effective service systems and adequate funding methods to develop this kind of understanding of what long-term maintenance of behavior change requires. In an impressive demonstration of long-term maintenance, Lucyshyn et al. (2007) published direct observation evidence showing that problem behavior reduction and generalization of appropriate behavior in the community maintained over a 7-year period after a PBS treatment for a child with autism and severe behavior problems. Parents were able to generalize treatment and maintain positive parenting skills embedded in family routines over a substantial period of time.

In an SSD study, Binnendyk and Lucyshyn (2009) aimed to lessen a child's food refusal by implementing a family-centered, multicomponent PBS intervention. Consistent with techniques of PBS, the researchers used functional assessments to determine what motivated and set the context of the problem behavior, developed a multicomponent support plan, and provided parent training as key components of the intervention. The family consisted of a 6-year-old boy with autism, his mother and father, two older male siblings (aged 9 and 11), and one younger male sibling (age 5) who was also diagnosed with autism. The parents expressed concerns that the 6-year-old had an extremely limited diet and would no longer eat many of the foods he used to. Prompting him to try food resulted in severe disruptive behaviors such as throwing or spitting food, self-injurious behavior (e.g., head banging), vomiting, screaming, hitting, or kicking. This study used an empirical case study design with five phases: baseline, intensive training with the therapist, parent training, generalization, and follow-up. The observation sessions of the child's snack routine were combined with the Behavioral Feeding Assessment Parent Interview (Budd, 1992) to determine specific areas of need for the feeding intervention. In addition to finding out what motivated the child's food refusal, Binnendyk and Lucyshyn learned which foods the child preferred and disliked to establish a hierarchy of acceptable foods and to determine what type of feeding intervention would be appropriate. Further, family ecology was assessed by discussing with parents what they perceived to be their family's strengths, goals, social support, and sources of stress. This information helped the researchers develop a PBS plan that was highly individualized to the needs of the family and child. For example, it was indicated by the mother that she did not possess the emotional strength or confidence to begin the intervention, so the support plan was modified and the child first received intensive training directly from the therapist in the home during the snack routine.

An escape-extinction procedure was implemented first by the therapist and then by the parent, who received in vivo coaching and feedback. Components of the PBS plan included modifying setting events (e.g., creating a set eating schedule), using antecedent strategies (e.g., pictures for visual prompts) and positive reinforcement statements (e.g., telling the child what rewards he will get for doing an appropriate behavior), and determining the right reward for the child (e.g., praise or a toy). The mother was also trained in ways to prevent the child from avoiding feeding (e.g., physically blocking him from leaving the mealtime area) as well as ways to de-escalate disruptive, aggressive, or self-injurious behaviors. Parent training sessions occurred once or twice a week (for a total of 15 sessions over 8 weeks) and on average lasted slightly less than an hour. Additionally, the therapist prompted the mother to instruct the father on implementing the mealtime PBS plan.

This comprehensive, PBS approach to handling food refusal was associated with significant gains in food consumption. The child ate no foods he disliked at baseline, ate 64% after intervention, and ate 56% at follow-up (Binnendyk & Lucyshyn, 2009). He completed more steps of his snack routine after intervention. He also spent more time at the dinner table. This study reported quality of life ratings for this family related to the areas of family interaction, parenting, health and safety, family resources, and supports for persons with disability. The data from these ratings suggest that the family's quality of life significantly improved, with the greatest improvements seen in the areas of family resources, support for persons with a disability, and health and safety.

Other innovations are notable in this collection of studies. L. K. Koegel et al. (1998) demonstrated the efficacy of PBS methods with sibling dyads. A serious problem that has been reported in some young families of children with autism is the onset of aggression by an older sibling directed at newborn or very young siblings whose entrance into the family alters established routines and can reduce parental attention to the older child. For example, Barry and Singer (2001) documented the changing nature of a brother's problem behavior at the arrival and subsequent development of a younger sibling. As the infant acquired mobility and new motor skills he would enter new environments within the home and interact with novel objects. These changing settings occasioned changing problem behaviors in the older brother. When the infant was confined to a baby carrier, the older brother would rub his nose on the baby's face and provoke scolding from their mother. When he was able to crawl, the older brother would entice the younger sibling to try to climb up a set of stairs that posed a hazard for the infant. Barry and Singer used instruction of positive replacement behaviors and self-management checklists to address each new problem as it emerged.

L. K. Koegel et al. (1998) addressed similar patterns of aggression in three families of siblings with autism and their younger brothers and sisters. A 5-year-old girl with autism engaged in hitting, yelling at, and pinching her infant sibling. In a second dyad a 4-year-old boy with a mixed developmental disorder with autism-like characteristics concerned his parents by hitting, pinching, rolling on top of, and grapping objects from his 7-month-old brother. In the third sibling dyad a 4-year-old boy with autism kicked, hit, pinched, squeezed, head butted, and poked his 6-month-old brother's head with his index finger. Needless to say, these interactions were highly stressful for the families. L. K. Koegel et al. (1998) cooperatively developed a multiple component treatment plan for each dyad based on an analysis of the conditions surrounding siblings' aggression and parent's routines and lifestyles. An assessment process identified the stimuli most commonly associated with the problem behaviors as well as replacement behaviors for the older siblings. Parents were taught to rearrange the environment to reduce setting events and triggering stimuli as well as how to teach replacement behaviors. For example, interviews and observations revealed that the older girl in the first dyad was most likely to become aggressive when her infant brother made a loud noise by kicking the tray on his high chair and by crying. Vocal noises and down times when children were left alone while the mother prepared meals also occasioned problem behaviors. The intervention demonstrates the way that physical as well as behavioral facets of activity settings for routines can be changed as part of a PBS intervention. The metal tray was replaced with a plastic one that was not noisy when kicked. The older sister was taught to give her infant sibling toys when he cried and to ask the mother to help him. Parents were also coached to increase interactions with the two children before and during mealtimes. Again a practical change in the meal preparation routine was part of the treatment. The interventionist recommended that the mother finish making meals before children were seated at the table so that they were not left alone right before meals. In the second dyad, one setting event that occasioned aggression was when the mother was occupied on the telephone and did not give attention to the children. The older boy was systematically taught to play independently for increasingly long intervals without parental attention so that he could tolerate his mother's phone routine. The interventions required only two or three sessions in which the interventionist prompted parents and a varying number of additional sessions to fade prompts so that parents implemented the practices independently. Problem behaviors in all three dyads were reduced to a zero level by the end of treatment. Follow-up observations of two dyads showed maintenance of the treatment effects at 6 months and 1 year for one dyad, and at 4 months post treatment for the second, with no follow-up reported for the third pair of siblings. A notable element of this study was that independent observers were asked to rate the children's affect from videos taken during baseline and later in the treatment phase. All children were rated as showing more signs of happiness after treatment. Parents' observed happiness levels also improved. They also documented an increase in the amount of time the mother in one of the families was able to engage in adult conversation during dinner time. This latter observation is an example of a quality of life change, which the parents valued as an untargeted emanative effect of the treatment.

In a related study, Duda, Clarke, Fox, and Dunlap (2008) used PBS procedures to reduce fighting between dyadic and triadic groupings of three siblings in the family of a child with autism. Reduction of sibling aggression may have important long-term effects for the sibling relationship. In a study of relationships in adulthood of nondisabled siblings and their brothers and sisters with IDs, Zeitlin (1986) found that those dyads that were mutually friendly and supportive in adulthood reported that they had been cooperative and played together as children, whereas dyads in which the siblings had little contact and were hostile in adulthood reported a long history of fighting during childhood. Although this retrospective study is suggestive but not definitive, it seems reasonable to believe that establishing positive sibling relationships early in life might contribute to longer-term supportive relationships. The issue is an important one for aging parents, who often need to rely on siblings to support adult children with DDs.

Blair et al. (2011), working in South Korea, showed that PBS could be effectively implemented in a combined home/school intervention in which teachers and parents were trained in the same PBS methods. This study makes a useful contribution to the PBS series, because it demonstrates that teachers and parents can be taught to implement multiple component treatments with fidelity and that treatment effects generalize across family and school settings. The study also included evidence of gains in untargeted appropriate behavior in classroom and playground settings with correlated reductions in problem behaviors. Direct observation data were collected during baseline, treatment, and follow-up phases on untargeted prosocial and problem behaviors, thereby developing convincing evidence of generalization effects as a function of the PBS practices.

Initial studies have begun to examine features of implementation, which account for strongest functional effects. Erbas (2010), a Turkish researcher, used an alternating treatment design across three children with DDs and their parents to show that when implementers added feedback to their consultation practices with parents, parents were better able to implement the PBS practices and children's problem behavior improved more when treatment fidelity was at its best. This kind of process research is valuable for clarifying the most impactful parent training practices. Understanding best practices for teaching parents to implement practices with fidelity are particularly important in multiple component behavioral treatments that require parents to learn several skills.

FUNCTIONAL COERCION AND POSITIVE FAMILY PROCESS THEORY

Lucyshyn et al. (2015) have contributed an important development in theory and theoretically derived intervention in the field of study on families of individuals with DDs. This paper is likely to be cited for many years as seminal in understanding the link between macro- and microsocial processes in families. Lucyshyn combined two key ideas in the behavioral study of family processes, functional analysis of the motivating causes of problem behavior, and family coercion theory based on the work of Gerald Patterson (1982) at the Oregon Social Learning Center. Patterson added a new finding in this literature concerning constructive family routines by describing them via microsocial sequential analysis and further by documenting the means by which coercive family processes can be replaced by positive parent–child interactions. Patterson focused on understanding and intervening in families of boys and adolescents with high rates of aggressive behavior, which predicted from an early age a host of negative life outcomes including imprisonment. Patterson carefully observed mothers interacting with highly aggressive young boys in home settings and found characteristic patterns in their social exchanges. This pattern of interaction was made up of escalating negatively toned and reciprocal social interactions in which mothers and sons each tried to terminate the other's interactive behavior by becoming increasingly demanding and aggressive. He called this pattern coercion and documented it using real-time sequential coding of key behaviors allowing him to characterize coercive processes in terms of probability equations and to show their ubiquitous presence in families with aggressive boys and troubled parent–child relationships. A typical coercive exchange in Patterson's studies began with a parental demand such as a request to pick up toys and put them away. In a second step in the prototypical coercive sequence, the child would resist by ignoring or refusing the demand. In response, the parent would then escalate the intensity of the demand and its negative affect by repeating the directive in a louder and/or angrier voice, which elicited a louder refusal by the child. In a typical next step in the reciprocal chain of behaviors the parent would threaten and/or yell, which would in turn bring out aggression from the child. In the next step the parent might become angry and punish the child. These interchanges often ends when the parent drops the demand and the child follows suit by calming down. Lucyshyn hypothesized that coercive interactions were likely to be motivated not only by terminating parental commands but also as a way for children to elicit attention or a desired item from parents. That is, coercive processes would vary as revealed by a functional analysis showing what motivated the child's problem behavior.

In the 2015 study, Lucyshyn and colleagues used real-time sequential coding to demonstrate a two-step and a four-step sequence of parent–child coercive interactions, which varied in their structure according to the child's motivation. This research team used conditional probability analysis to express the likelihood of predicted microsocial behaviors in a coercive exchange in terms of odds ratios. In families marked by frequent coercive exchanges motivated by a child's desire to escape from a parent's demand, the odds were comparatively high that a child would aggress, tantrum, or run away within four brief exchanges. Following a parent demand, the child would misbehave. The parent would withdraw the demand and the child would end or reduce the problem behavior. The researchers also showed that there were also predictable sequences in parent–child interactions when the child's problem behavior was motivated by obtaining parental attention or a desired item or activity. In this sequence, the parent at first was not attending to the child. In family routines, this lack of attention might occur while a mother is on the phone, looking at her e-mail, or engaged in the kitchen making dinner while children are in other rooms. In the step following parental ignoring, the child would typically enact a negative behavior. In the subsequent interval, the parent would respond by scolding the child. The intensity of the scolding would continue to increase if the child persisted in her problem behavior, which would eventually bring a more hostile response from the child. However, the child obtained the motivating attention from the parent, and so the stage was set for more of this kind of behavior in order to gain attention. When items or activities were the motivators, parental inattention to a child's efforts to obtain them led to negative behavior, which was in effect rewarded when the parent would provide the item or activity in order to terminate the child's negative actions. These exchanges are highly stressful for both parties and detract considerably from quality of life.

This team implemented multicomponent, assessment-driven PBS practices and showed that these coercive exchanges in families of children with autism and/or ID could be greatly reduced and replaced with constructive sequences in which parents made requests, the children complied, parents gave positive attention, and the child stayed engaged with the activity. The researchers called this, and related constructive patterns of dyadic exchange, positive family process. They delivered treatments to 12 families of children who were selected for the study partly because of a long-standing history of severe problem behavior. When coercive family processes were replaced by constructive family processes, the tone of home life changed; and researchers noted not only the extent of reduction of stress in the homes but also the development of new expressions of positive family cohesion and cooperation. This work would be an impressive contribution with any group of families, but it is all the more so given that the researchers deliberately selected study participants because of very serious problem behavior that was long-standing and had in some instances been resistant to prior treatment. The researchers evaluated PBS interventions with single-subject multiple baseline design studies across activity routines and across participants. Further they evaluated the change in parent–child dyadic interactions using statistical analyses of changes in dyadic interaction patterns at baseline and after treatment. Odds ratios were used to describe the probability that a targeted two-step or four-step behavioral sequence would lead to a designated negative or positive outcome. For example, in one family at baseline the odds ratio of parents terminating a demand after a child's aggressive behavior was 1.93, meaning that they were almost twice as likely to go through a sequence leading to a child's problem behavior and ending with parents dropping a demand than the likelihood they would go through a similar interactional sequence, not give up in face of the child's problem behaviors, and end the series of interactions with the child's compliance with the demand. After intervention, this odds ratio dropped to zero, meaning that the coercive sequence was no longer observed. In another family, the odds that a child would successfully obtain attention from a parent with aggressive or other negative behavior was 2.61 at baseline reducing after treatment to 0.8. Similar reductions in coercive processes were demonstrated in 9 of 10 families who received intensive in-home PBS treatments over a large number of weeks. In an indication of acquisition of positive family processes, the probability of parental requests leading to child compliance and parental praise were expressed in one family by an odds ratio of 0 at baseline and 2.70 on average after treatment.

One additional and very important aspect of the treatment design in this study is the delivery of adjunctive treatments to parents in addition to PBS parent training. Interventionists not only conducted ongoing assessments of the function of problem behavior, cooperatively designed multicomponent treatments, and coached parents to implement them, but they also observed interpersonal and intrapersonal problems that impeded uptake of the treatment practices and they intervened to address them. For example, for a parent who was often distracted and unable to respond contingently to her child, the researchers taught mindfulness. To parents who were fighting, they taught problem-solving and communication skills. For families with a history of isolation from the community, they encouraged community outings and participation in community life. A final strength of this report is the care with which information is provided about effective as well as less effective demonstrations of functional effects using SSD studies. Seven of 10 families demonstrated clear functional effects of PBS when evaluated with SSDs. By comparison, when evaluated with within-subject statistical comparisons, statistically significant improvements in coercive routines and gains in constructive routines were demonstrated using within-subjects statistical analysis of sequential data. When taken as a whole, the 2015 paper by Lucyshyn and colleagues is one of the most creative and potentially consequential for the field of family support of any of the studies reviewed in this book.

From our review of the literature, we are persuaded that in-home PBS is a sufficiently well delineated intervention that studies can be meaningfully grouped under its conceptual umbrella and that there are enough studies of sufficient quality to meet our standards for categorizing it as an established evidence-based practice. We are encouraged that this emergent school of practice offers considerable hope for more durable and socially valid interventions. It will be important in future work to demonstrate that severe problem behavior can be treated with less intensive applications of the treatment practices; or social policy and the funding it entrains will have to come to terms with the fact that some families and some individuals with severe problem behavior may simply require much longer term and more labor-intensive treatments than are now presently funded in many parts of the United States.

A notable feature of some of the in-home PBS studies reviewed here is that the researchers took pains to accept only participants with very severe and long-standing problem behaviors (Carr et al., 1999; Lucyshyn et al., 2015). Clinicians who work with individuals with DDs and their families are well aware that not all clients are as easily treated as others and that there is a small but socially important group of individuals whose problem behavior is often intractable in the face of more traditional behavioral treatments. These individuals can have devastating impacts on families and can be forced into lives as constrained as many prisoners in the penal justice system as a result of the limited and highly restrictive residential options available to them. From our own experience with this population, we believe that greater expenditures for treatment will be necessary and that these are well justified both for humanitarian and long-term economic benefits (Ganz, 2007). Costs of ineffective treatment over a lifetime not only are likely to be much higher than intensive treatment such as in home PBS but also involve a kind of social brutality that no humane society, particularly a wealthy one, should permit when effective treatments exist. Continued development of PBS as a school of treatment for this population is likely to pay large social dividends and help many individuals with DDs and their families provided there are sufficient investments in research and personnel development in this emergent field.

MODIFIED PROGRAMS

In the following discussion we review programs that were originally developed for a different population and then applied to parents of children with developmental disabilities. These represent a transfer of treatment methodology that usually required some important revisions to the original programs. This research strategy has been successful in several cases.

INCREDIBLE YEARS

The Incredible Years multicomponent intervention is a program created to address problem behaviors of young children at risk for oppositional and aggressive behavior. It has been adapted to also serve parents of young children with autism and developmental delay (McIntyre, 2008a, 2008b). We first describe the original program and subsequently McIntyre's adaptation of the model. The Incredible Years series uses a group training format to deliver instruction about behavior management and cognitive-behavioral techniques (e.g., team problem-solving, self-management, and self-talk) to parents of children with or at-risk for developing severe behavioral problems (Webster-Stratton & Taylor, 2001). In the Incredible Years BASIC program, trainers use videos and a parenting manual to demonstrate positive interactions with their child that are led by the child. For example, the program stresses "child-directed play," which encourages parents to engage with their children during play time and to allow the child to choose the toys and activities. The Incredible Years BASIC also teaches behavioral management skills, such as the ones discussed in chapter 3: differential reinforcement strategies (selectively and systematically rewarding positive behaviors), praise, direct commands, brief time-out, problem-solving, and natural consequences. Group discussion among parents about these instructional topics is encouraged during training sessions. The BASIC program takes place over 12 to 14 weeks with weekly 2 to 2 ½ hour sessions.

Whereas the focus of the BASIC program is on positive parenting strategies, the SCHOOL program emphasizes skills parents learned to support their child academically, including reading with their child, helping with homework, and building relationships with teachers. Consistent with other multicomponent treatments, the Incredible Years program also adopts a cognitive-behavioral approach to augment its behavioral and skills training. ADVANCED is a supplementary program in the series that teaches parent coping strategies and specifically teaches parents how to handle depression, how to access support, and how to communicate with other adults. The Incredible Years program efficacy has been tested in multiple RCT studies with generally positive results (Reid, Webster-Stratton, & Hammond, 2007; Webster-Stratton, Reid, & Hammond, 2001, 2004).

Although the Incredible Years program was originally developed for parents and teachers of children with behavioral and conducts disorders, it was adapted for the DD population. McIntyre's (2008b) small RCT study modified Webster-Stratton's Incredible Years parent training program (IYPT-DD) to suit toddlers and preschool age children with DDs. Twenty-one experimental families and 23 control families of children, ages 2 to 5, with developmental delay or disabilities were recruited for the intervention. Training took place weekly for 2½ hours per week over the course of 12 weeks at a preschool. The program used group discussion, videos of parent–child interactions, behavioral rehearsal, lectures, and weekly homework assignments to teach parents more positive parenting strategies (Webster-Stratton, 2001). McIntyre kept Webster-Stratton's main content areas of play, praise, rewards, limit setting, and handling challenging behaviors in this intervention, but based on feedback from preschool teachers and community members, the researcher incorporated elements from the Incredible Years toddler program to accommodate the developmental age of the participating children. While McIntyre mostly adapted the BASIC version of Incredible Years, this modified program has features that deviate from the traditional behavioral parent training approach. For instance, in the first session, the therapist asks parents to identify both blessings and challenges of having a child with developmental delays. In a later session, the therapist also discusses with parents strategies to form successful partnerships with professionals. During this session, information about how to access community supports and advocacy groups was handed out. (Specific programs that teach parents about navigating school and community resources and about parental legal rights are described in greater detail in chapter 6.)

McIntyre's Modifications

Since the emphasis of McIntyre's (2008b) intervention was to impact parenting behaviors to increase positive parent–child interactions, changes in parenting behaviors were assessed through observations of parent–child play activities. No significant differences were found in the amount of praise between the intervention and control groups, but inappropriate or negative parenting behaviors significantly decreased for the experimental group. Treatment group parents reported a greater reduction in child behavioral problems than did control group parents. Children in the treatment group also significantly decreased their internalizing behaviors. Overall, parents rated the intervention as somewhat to very useful, with parents who attended the training sessions with a spouse or with a support person more likely to find the intervention useful. Training attendance was also examined, and unsurprisingly, better attendance was found to correlate with better child behavioral outcomes.

Still, not every parent needs group training to develop better parenting skills. By the same token, some parents require more intensive assistance than a group training can provide. Therefore, Phaneuf and McIntyre (2011) created a multiple-tiered training with parents of children with DD to reduce child behavior problems. Their participants were eight mother–child pairs, with children, ages 2 to 4, who had autism spectrum disorder, speech/language delays, or global developmental delays. Furthermore, parents needed to demonstrate low levels of positive parenting to be eligible to participate. This means that the parents often failed to give direct and clear commands or they gave overly harsh consequences when their child misbehaved. The researchers were particularly interested in determining the appropriate level of support each participating parent needed. Phaneuf and McIntyre's three-tiered intervention was fashioned after a response-to-intervention model. Response-to-intervention is a method of monitoring and adjusting the amount of support given to the individual depending on how he or she performs. The parents were initially given basic, universal (tier 1) training. At this first tier, all parents were assigned to read materials related to praise, play, and behavior management or to listen to audiobook versions of these materials. Researchers pulled reading material from *The Incredible Years: A Troubleshooting Guide for Parents of Children 2–8 Years* (Webster-Stratton, 2006) and contacted parents intermittently to encourage reading. Then, they assessed the parents by observing how they responded to the intervention. If negative parenting strategies were not reduced and positive parenting strategies did not increase to meet a certain predetermined level/goal, then parents were given more intensive support (tier 2 training). At this tier, parents received group training based on McIntyre's (2008b) adapted Incredible Years Training program. If parents did not meet the researcher's goal, they then participated in individual sessions (tier 3). At the last tier, a therapist reviewed the parents' behaviors through video recordings of home interactions between parent and child, and then made home visits to demonstrate and practice with parents' positive interactional strategies. The therapist also provided praise and corrected parent skills until the observational data showed that parents met the goal or until three home video feedback sessions were completed.

In this single-subject changing conditions design study, data across the eight mothers were analyzed (Phaneuf & McIntyre, 2011). One parent responded to tier 1 intervention and so she was able to meet the goal with just the self-administered reading. Three mothers responded to the tier 2 intervention, and one mother withdrew from participation. Within tier 3, two mothers met the goal after one video feedback session, while one parent required two sessions. Results showed that, as a group, the rates of negative parenting decreased. At the 3-month follow-up, six parent–child pairs participated, and experimenters found that all six mothers still met the goal and either maintained or further reduced negative parenting levels. The researchers also wanted to evaluate child problem behaviors; observations and parent reports both indicated that problem behaviors significantly decreased from pre- to posttreatment. While more experimental trials of the Incredible Years, especially ones conducted by other research groups, are needed to validate the program's efficacy, the evidence here suggests that this intervention program could be very beneficial for the DD population.

PARENTS PLUS

Drawing from the video-modeling group training interventions of Webster-Stratton's Incredible Years, Sharry and Fitzpatrick's (1998) Parents Plus program helped Irish parents with their children's developmental and behavioral goals. Most Parents Plus interventions are purely behavioral parent training programs in nature, and thus, the structure of this program was described in detail in chapter 3. Parents Plus largely consisted of a group-based training to instruct parents in managing their children's problem behaviors and in assisting their children's play and communication skills. Many of the behavior management strategies were based on cognitive-behavioral principles (discussed in chapter 2) and social learning theory (Coughlin et al., 2009). Social learning theory explains that behavior can be learned through direct experience or by seeing how others behave (Bandura, 1971). In this program, parents spent time watching videos of actors and real parent–child pairs model strategies. The training also reflected a strengths-based philosophy, wherein therapists try to build on parents' strong suits in the areas of parenting skills that parents find most relevant to their own needs. Furthermore, the flexibility of the program allowed interventionists to address parental stress, parental self-care, and family listening strategies (Coughlin et al., 2009).

Coughlin and colleagues' (2009) study was the only study of the Parents Plus program that included parental stress management and self-care instruction. This study explored the treatment effects between children (ages 6 to 11) with developmental delay and children with severe behavioral problems, and hence, the treatment group consisted of these two subsample groups, compared with a treatment-as-usual control group. Coughlin et al. employed a sequential block design, in which 74 parents, recruited from children's mental health clinics and community settings, were assigned to the treatment or control group based on the date of their referral to treatment. In sequential block design, parent training was provided for a block of 12 to 15 parents in a group, and any newly recruited parents were placed on the waitlist control group until the parent training was made available. The interventionists offered nine group training sessions, which helped parents learn to provide positive attention, to conduct child-centered play, to establish routines, to encourage and praise appropriately, to use consequences appropriately, and to problem-solve with their child, among other topics. The final two group sessions specifically covered dealing with children's special needs, family problem-solving, and parent self-care. Although the foundation of the Parents Plus is behavioral training for parents, the program was flexible enough to accommodate parent self-care training and discussion of other topics that conveyed the program's multifaceted nature. Two individual parent trainings were provided. The individual sessions were meant to provide extra practice for families under the guidance of a professional. Again, the focus is on child-centered play and good routines, but the goals and needs of the family are incorporated into each session. For families who needed additional support in formulating a discipline system, trainers worked with those parents alone for additional one-to-one sessions. Weekly telephone support was also made available to parents.

The results of the intervention indicated that compared with the waitlist control group, the treatment group reported significant changes in total difficulties, in conduct problems, and in the impact of difficulties. Coughlin and colleagues (2009) also found that intervention parents achieved greater individual goal attainment, and these improvements were significantly larger than for the comparison group. Additionally, the Parents Plus group reported a significantly greater reduction in stress and a significantly greater increase in parenting confidence. Many of the Parents Plus intervention studies that did not incorporate cognitive-behavioral training failed to find significant changes in parent stress. The decrease in parental stress levels in Coughlin et al.'s study further demonstrates that stress should be explicitly targeted.

What Coughlin and colleagues (2009) found was that Parents Plus appeared to be equally helpful for both groups in certain areas but more helpful for families of children with behavioral problems than for families of children with delays in other areas of development. The program seemed to be equally effective for both groups of families in enhancing confidence in parenting and in helping parents overcome problems they defined at the beginning of the intervention. The program also lessened the impact of the children's difficulties, increased their children's positive social behavior, and reduced behavioral problems and parental distress for both parents of children DD and conduct disorders. However, compared with the DD group, PPCP reduced the total behavioral difficulties of the behavioral group children. Behavioral group parents also reported that the program helped reduce their children's problems with peers. What the results of this second analysis suggest is that, overall, there are similarities in the way parents of children with DD and parents of children with conduct problems respond to behavioral training and stress management treatment. Yet there are still differences that must be addressed with programs that target the particular needs of children with DD and their families.

SIGNPOSTS FOR BUILDING BETTER BEHAVIOR

A set of studies from Australia are important because they took a public health approach of making multicomponent family support interventions available on a much larger scale than previously reported in the DD literature. The strength of the Signposts for Building Better Behavior treatment is that it was specifically designed for parents of children with IDs. This family-centered intervention program offers parents training in managing child behavior, managing stress, and strengthening the family system (Hudson et al., 2003). This program was developed by A. Hudson and colleagues (2001) in Australia. The Signposts training curriculum contains eight information booklets. The first six booklets focuses on behavioral training: (1) *Introduction*; (2) *Measuring Your Child's Behavior*; (3) *Systematic Use of Everyday Interactions*; (4) *Replacing Difficult Behavior with Useful Behavior*; (5) *Planning for Better Behavior*; and (6) *Teaching Your Child New Skills* (Hudson et al., 2003). The last two Signpost booklets supplement the behavioral training curriculum with cognitive-behavioral support for parents: (1) *Dealing with Stress*; and (2) *Your Family as a Team* (Hudson et al., 2003). Videos were integrated into the curriculum, and therefore, the booklets intermittently directed parents to refer to certain video clips to enhance their understanding of material. The Signpost intervention was delivered either through the in-person individual mode, in-person group mode, telephone support to the individual, or an individual self-directed format (Hudson et al., 2003). In the group approach, a therapist ran six 2-hour sessions, covering the topics in the curriculum during sessions. For the telephone and self-directed approaches, parents received the behavioral-focused and supplementary booklets, the videos, and a workbook. While those in the self-directed mode did not get any other support, parents in the telephone-support mode received support from a therapist through 20-minute telephone calls to discuss progress and to go over problems encountered with learning and using the program.

Two intervention studies have been conducted with the Signposts program. Hudson et al. (2003) ran a quasi-experimental study examining the efficacy of the intervention on parent and child measures. The participants included 115 children who had ID and their mothers. A number of the children also had autism, epilepsy, vision impairment, hearing impairment, or cerebral palsy in addition to ID. Random assignment did not occur as planned because only the parents in the waitlist control group were randomly assigned into that condition. For the three intervention conditions (group support, telephone support, and self-directed mode), some parents were allowed to switch groups. The results of the study indicated positive outcomes for parents. Hudson's results indicated that the parents in the intervention conditions, on average, felt that they experienced less stress, that they were better able to handle being a parent, and that their needs were met after going through the intervention. Contrary to expectations, no differences in parent outcomes were found between the three intervention groups. This means that parents benefited no matter how they were presented with the behavioral management, stress management, and problem-solving skills. These changes were maintained at follow-up, 4 to 6 months after the end of the intervention. However, no differences were detected between the control and the intervention groups regarding changes in child behaviors.

Hudson and his colleagues Cameron and Matthews (2008) later implemented an 18-month large-scale intervention across the state of Victoria in Australia in another evaluation of Signposts. This study employed a matched group, repeated measures design with 1,790 families of children with ID ages 3 to 16. Unlike the previous study, this intervention incorporated all four intervention conditions, including individual support for parents. Contrary to previous findings, training format did appear to have an influence. Across the different intervention groups, large and medium effects were found for mothers participating in the individual support and telephone support modes. Medium and large effects were also found in child behavioral changes for mothers getting individual and telephone support. This wide-scale implementation of Signposts suggested the promise of the program, but as it was not an RCT study, outcomes cannot be entirely attributed to the intervention and must be interpreted with caution. Future Signposts evaluations would benefit from employing an RCT design to further establish its validity as a program.

STEPPING STONES TRIPLE P

The Stepping Stones Triple P (SSTP) (Sanders et al., 2004). is a multicomponent intervention, also developed in Australia, to help parents learn to manage their children's behavior and manage their own stress. The SSTP has undergone several incarnations. Similar to the Incredible Years and Parents Plus interventions, SSTP has roots in a program directed toward parents of children with behavioral rather than developmental needs. The SSTP is an adaptation of Sanders's (1999) Triple P—Positive Parenting Program. The original Triple P program was designed to "prevent severe behavioral, emotional, and developmental problems in children by enhancing the knowledge, skills, and confidence of parents" (Sanders, 1999, p. 72). Like Parents Plus, Triple P used positive parenting techniques based on social learning principles (Sanders, 1999). It was also structured in a multitiered model, akin to the response-to-intervention method that Phaneuf and McIntyre (2011) adopted for their Incredible Years study. Triple P gave support ranging from the lowest to highest intensity depending on parents' needs (Sanders, 1999). Results from randomized controlled trial studies in Australia have shown evidence of effectiveness for various populations, including for families of preschoolers at risk for developing conduct disorders (Sanders, Markie-Dadds, Tully, & Bor, 2000), as well as for families of preschool children with co-occurring behavioral and attentional/hyperactive needs (Bor, Sanders, & Markie-Dadds, 2002).

The Stepping Stones Triple P (SSTP) is a version of the Triple P program developed by Western Australia's Disability Services Commission and the University of Queensland to support parents of children with DD (Sanders et al., 2004). It is an important addition to the literature because the scale and scope are in line with the public health model. It initially kept the multitiered intervention system, revising the instructional topics to reflect issues more relevant to this population. Developers of the program incorporated strategies from the disability literature and feedback from parents of children with DD (Sanders et al., 2004). The first level of intervention was the "Universal Triple P." This level aimed at providing all parents with information about stimulating the development of their child, and it did so through an awareness campaign. The program sent out promotional flyers, posters, brochures, promoted through newspaper articles and radio announcements, and offered positive parenting literature to help families become more knowledgeable about developmental issues (e.g., play skills, communication skills) and about ways to address common behaviors (e.g., whining, problems with sharing). Parents seeking advice about a more specific behavioral difficulty (e.g., toilet training) could access the second level of intervention, the "Selected Triple P." At this level, an SSTP practitioner recommended solutions over two brief phone sessions or through an hour-long seminar. The third level, also called the "Primary Care Triple P," assisted parents who had difficulty managing discrete child behavior problems (e.g., tantrums, fights with siblings) or who required support in teaching their child self-help skills. During Primary Care Triple P intervention, practitioners gave advice and model parenting skills in four 20-minute phone or in-person sessions. The scope and scale of the program based on a public health model is an important contribution to the development of an applied research base for multicomponent interventions.

The standard Triple P parenting skills training was the fourth level of intervention. Typically, families of children with more severe behavioral problems (e.g., aggression) sought support at this level (Sanders et al., 2004). The standard Triple P program trained parents of children with disabilities in 25 core child management strategies (Plant & Sanders, 2007). Over the course of 10 training sessions, these skills were taught using modeling, role-play, feedback, and homework assignments. Several of the core strategies addressed children's development and self-help skills, such as activity schedules to help children with learning routines, tangible rewards and praise to reinforce good behavior, quality time with children to build positive relationships, incidental teaching to encourage children to initiate interactions and to communicate, and behavior charts to motivate students to reach behavioral goals (Plant & Sanders, 2007; Sanders et al., 2004). Other strategies helped parents handle inappropriate behaviors. These included setting rules, issuing clear and calm instructions, and conducting brief time-outs (Plant & Sanders, 2007; Sanders et al., 2004). Parents were taught a six-step planned activities routine so that parents were more likely to use these skills after the intervention ended (Plant & Sanders,

2007). Planned activities training (discussed in chapter 3) taught parents to be proactive in managing behavior by predicting and preparing in order to preempt their children's problem behaviors. Parents also learned to set goals and monitor their goal progress.

Parents who had children with very challenging behaviors and who experienced personal difficulties and stressors had access to the enhanced Triple P, the final tier in the multilevel SSTP program. This particular level ran from 11 to 16 sessions. In the enhanced program, parents not only received training on the core child management techniques but also learned stress coping strategies and partner- and family-support skills. The purpose of the program was to treat inappropriate child behaviors while helping parents deal with relationship conflicts, depression, and adjusting to disability in their children. Literature to supplement parent training was made available to families at every level of intervention.

Evaluations of SSTP have generally been limited to parent training in only the standard and enhanced levels of intervention. In one of several randomized, controlled trial SSTP studies with parents of children with DD (Plant & Sanders, 2007; Sofronoff et al., 2011), Roberts, Mazzucchelli, Studman, and Sanders (2006) examined the effectiveness of the standard and enhanced SSTP program with the families of 47 children ages 2 to 7 participating. The SSTP training taught parents in the treatment group the 25 cores strategies for promoting child development and managing child behaviors through the *SSTP Family Workbook*, videos, and consultations with therapists. The 10 sessions were delivered individually, with a combination of 2-hour clinic appointments and 40- to 60-minute home visits. During these sessions, therapists guided parents to select goals and rehearse strategies that achieved their objectives. The program encouraged parents to use these skills in different settings, especially after the end of the course; therapists helped parents plan for future challenges using the aforementioned planned activity training routine. Furthermore, 18 out of 27 treatment group families who wanted cognitive-behavioral support after the standard SSTP program were able to participate in the *Partner Support* module or a *Coping Skills* module of the enhanced SSTP curriculum. For instance, in the *Coping Skills* module, parents learned to deal with emotions by understanding how to recognize difficult emotions, like stress, anger, depression, that interfere with parenting. The therapist in the module then gave parents strategies, such reframing and rethinking their challenges, to enable them to overcome these unhelpful emotions. The modules also taught families to balance work and family life, to improve communication between partners, and to troubleshoot during conflicts.

Compared with the waitlist control group, treatment mothers in Roberts et al.'s (2006) study reported that child problem behaviors, on average, significantly decreased over the course of the intervention and even 6 months after. Curiously, there were no significant differences reported by fathers in the treatment group. While no effects were found for child noncompliance in the target setting (e.g., home setting), noncompliant behaviors for the intervention group did significantly drop in the generalization setting (e.g., community environments). There were also significant reductions in oppositional behavior, such as complaining and negative physical behavior, observed in intervention children that did not occur for control-group children. Parent discipline styles, measured by the Parenting Scale (Arnold, O'Leary, Wolff, & Acker, 1993), also differed across groups. Intervention fathers exhibited less negative parenting (i.e., being too lax or too verbose when disciplining) from pre- to postintervention and during follow-up 6 months later. Contrastingly, control-group fathers became more likely to engage in overly long reprimands with children over time. Intervention mothers were less likely to be overreactive during disciplining over time. The SSTP also appeared to lead to more parental positive social attention, such as praise, although not to giving specific instructions and other antecedents-based parenting behaviors. Additionally, parental stress did not seem to be affected by the intervention. A possible reason for this last finding is that not all treatment group parents attended the enhanced SSTP sessions devoted to stress management and coping skills training.

Roberts and colleagues (2006) noted that the enhanced modules of SSTP were not sufficiently tested for effectiveness, as not all parents participated in those modules. This research question was addressed by Plant and Sanders (2007) in a second RCT study of SSTP. The study assessed the difference between the standard Stepping Stones Triple P (SSTP-S) and the enhanced SSTP (SSTP-E), which featured the added components of teaching parents coping strategies beyond teaching parents behavioral management skills. Participants were parents of 74 preschool-age children with DD. Parents in the SSTP-S program received only the 10-week individual child-management training, whereas parents in the SSTP-E program received not only the 10-week individual training but also six more sessions that used a cognitive-behavioral approach to help parents cope with stress and strengthen their own social support. In particular, the adjunctive program discussed parents' reactions to having a child with DD and parental stress, as well as different coping strategies (e.g., relaxation, being aware of maladaptive thoughts) the parent could employ to mitigate the effects of depression, anger, anxiety, and stress. Sessions also taught parents to work together with professionals, to manage time better, and to bolster partner support or to strengthen the support from extended family and friends. Lastly, trainers discussed with parents the ways to problem-solve in order to promote maintenance post-intervention.

Measures on observed parent–child interactions and reported child behaviors, parental skills and competence, parental distress, and relationship satisfaction were taken. At immediate post-intervention, the treatment groups had better child outcomes than the waitlist control groups; however these results generally did not favor one treatment group over the other (Plant & Sanders, 2007). Compared with the waitlist control group, both the standard and enhanced SSTP-trained groups experienced significant decreases in observed negative child behavior and problem caregiving tasks. In comparison with the control, SSTP-S group reported less disruptive child behavior and the SSTP-E group reported fewer difficult child behaviors during caregiving. The enhanced SSTP group also outperformed the standard group in this latter measure. Although both treatment groups experienced significant improvements in parenting competence, contrary to expectations, only the standard treatment group saw significant gains in parenting skills when compared with the control. No differences among groups were found for negative parenting behaviors. Contrary to the researchers' predictions, neither intervention model significantly reduced mothers' distress. One year after the intervention, the same measures were taken. Results showed that there remained significant differences between the standard and enhanced SSTP groups in disruptive child behavior, with the enhanced treatment group having lower rates of difficult child behavior. Though again, no significant differences between treatment groups were found in parenting outcomes or in mothers' distress. Overall, getting treatment was better than receiving no treatment, but the 16-week behavioral- and CBT-based intervention did not produce considerably better parent outcomes over the standard behavioral training model. Plant and Sanders argued that parents in the enhanced treatment group may not have benefited from the additional support because they may not have needed the enhanced training in the first place. The major implication from this study is that interventions must be individualized for families. Implementing an initial assessment of families' needs prior to intervention may increase the efficiency of service delivery by allocating resources to parents who would gain the most from enhanced training.

Scholars continue to take steps to include a greater diversity of families and to deliver effective and cost-efficient training when designing SSTP interventions. An RCT study by Sofronoff et al. (2011) included 53 parents of children with a wide range of disabilities, including multiple disabilities, autism, ID, developmental delay, specific learning disability, acquired brain injury, cerebral palsy, vision impairment, and Maroteaux-Lamy syndrome. The intervention distilled the SSTP strategies into two 2-hour seminars. The first seminar topics focus on the positive aspects and challenges of having a child with a disability, as well as the core principles of positive parenting (e.g., ensure a safe, interesting environment, create a positive learning environment, use assertive discipline, be part of a community, take care of oneself as a parent, etc.). It teaches parenting strategies for managing developmental and behavioral issues. The second seminar covered strategies to teach children communication skills, problem-solving, play skills, independence. For each skill, a common procedure was taught: (1) identifying a target skill, (2) breaking the skill into smaller steps, (3) selecting reinforcers, (4) locating the appropriate setting for teaching, (5) using clear directions and physical guidance, and (6) monitoring and evaluating child progress. Parents were also made aware of common pitfalls and instructed on how to problem-solve to avoid those difficulties. Handouts of the strategies were provided at the end of each seminar. Post-intervention, a significant effect was found in the parental perceptions of the number of child problem behaviors, with the intervention group outperforming the control group. Intervention parents' reliance on dysfunctional parenting styles was significantly reduced. Parent conflict over child rearing decreased in the intervention group, but parent relationship quality, parental adjustment, and family functioning did not differ significantly when compared with the control group. The effects were maintained 3 months following intervention, which suggests that a shorter, group-based training may deliver similar results to the more intensive, enhanced, individual-based training delivered in past SSTP interventions.

Like other multicomponent programs, the development of the SSTP program has seen major changes. The initial multitiered program was a carryover feature from the original Triple P intervention model. While the standard SSTP training package found success in reducing child problem behaviors and reducing the use of ineffective parenting strategies, with the multitiered approach, researchers expected the more intensive training to deliver more promising results; this expectation has not been met, as results of the enhanced treatment with CBT-based components did not differ from those of the standard treatment (Plant & Sanders, 2007). In more recent RCT studies, the SSTP program has moved toward more cost-effective, shorter, group training sessions and has demonstrated similar effectiveness. Another growing trend evident in SSTP and other multicomponent programs is the continued adaptation of the program to include parents of children with more diverse challenges and needs. As these studies persistently showed promising results, researchers are interested in expanding the aims of the program to address the needs of different populations. The Stepping Stones Triple P Programs are supported by sufficient high-quality evidence to warrant a rating as established practices.

SUMMARY OF THE META-ANALYSIS RESULTS OF RANDOMIZED CONTROLLED TRIAL STUDIES AND CONCLUSION

In addition to a research synthesis of eight RCT or quasi-experimental design studies presented previously, we conducted a meta-analysis to generate effect sizes of all eight group comparison design studies. The procedures of running a meta-analysis were first introduced in chapter 1 and were also described in subsequent chapters (e.g., Chapters 2, 3, and 4). Table 5.3 presents the results of the meta-analysis with respect to dependent measures in each individual study and constructs of dependent measures. All the constructs of dependent measures were created conceptually and coded by this research team including all dependent measures at two tiers of constructs. Tier 1 constructs consist of Child Outcomes, Parent Outcomes, and Family System Outcomes. In Tier 2, the subconstruct of Child Outcomes comprises only one dependent measure on child's problem behaviors. The subconstructs of Parent Outcomes include parenting skills, parent adjustment, and reduced level of stress/distress. For the subconstruct of Family System Outcomes, it contains only one dependent measure on parent and child interaction. Table 5.4 lists the confidence intervals for each study's effect size.

The result of Q statistic test was statistically significant ($Q(41) = 76.445$, $p = .001$), suggesting that there is inequality of variances related to effect size calculation shared by all the studies included in the meta-analysis. Further examination needs to be taken to check the way that dependent measures are clustered to generate constructs and how average effect sizes of different dependent measure constructs can be calculated accordingly.

TABLE 5.3 RESULTS OF META-ANALYSIS OF MULTICOMPONENT INTERVENTIONS

				Intervention			Comparison				
Study	*Measure*	*Group*	*Outcome*	*N*	*Pre M (SD)*	*Post M (SD)*	*N*	*Pre M (SD)*	*Post M (SD)*	*F*	*d*
Coughlin et al. (2009)	Strengths and Difficulties Questionnaire (SDQ)—Total Difficulties	Child	Behavior	42	21.19 (6.15)	18.12 (6.23)	32	22.34 (7.33)	22.15 (8.30)	-	0.570
	Parental Stress Scale (PSS)	Parent	Stress/ Distress	42	47.76 (10.14)	43.07 (8.53)	32	44.51 (9.47)	44.20 (11.94)	-	0.110
	Parental confidence	Parent	Parenting Skills	42	4.14 (2.09)	6.48 (1.69)	32	4.15 (2.22)	5.10 (1.95)	-	0.770
	OVERALL										0.476
Durand et al. (2013)	Direct behavioral observation	Child	Behavior	17	-	-	18	-	-	0.380	0.208
	Questionnaire on Resources and Stress—Short Form (QRS-SF)—Pessimism	Parent	Stress/ Distress	17	-	-	18	-	-	0.130	0.122
	OVERALL										0.165
Hudson et al. (2003)	Parenting Sense of Competence (PSOC)—Efficacy	Parent	Parenting Skills	39	25.74 (0.00)	27.77 (0.00)	26	24.70 (0.00)	24.20 (0.00)	4.100	0.513
	Depression Anxiety and Stress Scale (DASS)—Stress	Parent	Stress/ Distress	39	11.29 (0.00)	9.78 (0.00)	26	13.30 (0.00)	15.10 (0.00)	5.750	0.607
	Parenting Hassles Scale (PHS)—Child Behavior	Child	Behavior	39	70.36 (0.00)	60.61 (0.00)	26	72.20 (0.00)	68.50 (0.00)	1.310	0.519
	Parenting Hassles Scale (PHS)—Parental Needs	Parent	Adjustment	39	41.11 (0.00)	36.84 (0.00)	26	42.60 (0.00)	42.30 (0.00)	4.210	0.290
	OVERALL										0.481

McIntyre (2008b)	Family Impact Questionnaire (FIQ)—Negative Impact	Parent	Adjustment	21	29.55 (13.40)	25.10 (11.67)	23	29.48 (11.48)	27.13 (11.83)	0.820	0.179
	Family Impact Questionnaire (FIQ)—Positive Impact	Parent	Adjustment	21	10.90 (4.74)	13.10 (4.43)	23	10.61 (4.74)	11.39 (4.56)	2.560	0.316
	Child Behavior Checklist (CBCL)—Total Problems	Child	Behavior	21	63.24 (9.58)	57.62 (9.03)	23	63.78 (12.70)	61.96 (12.25)	5.280	0.351
	Intervals inappropriate behavior (%)	Family	Interaction	21	52.91 (29.37)	11.98 (13.30)	23	47.06 (23.39)	46.19 (22.52)	19.520	2.142
	Child-directed praise	Family	Interaction	21	5.27 (3.33)	9.27 (8.02)	23	3.65 (3.03)	4.83 (5.46)	2.600	0.415
	OVERALL										0.568
Plant & Sanders (2007)	Family Observation Schedule (FOS-NCB)—% negative child behavior	Family	Interaction	50	28.27 (20.43)	17.51 (15.61)	24	27.11 (13.84)	28.77 (16.49)	-	0.781
	Developmental Behavior Checklist (DBC)—Disruptive	Child	Behavior	50	15.34 (7.77)	11.48 (6.71)	24	14.58 (8.49)	13.46 (8.89)	-	0.367
	Caregiving Problem Checklist (CPC)—Difficult Child Behavior	Child	Behavior	50	28.76 (7.40)	22.70 (5.73)	24	28.58 (8.25)	25.33 (8.18)	-	0.425
	Caregiving Problem Checklist (CPC)—Problematic care-giving tasks	Child	Behavior	50	9.58 (4.60)	5.44 (3.16)	24	8.63 (3.02)	8.92 (3.86)	-	1.301
	Parenting Scale (PS)—Total	Parent	Parenting Skills	50	2.96 (0.85)	2.55 (0.72)	24	2.87 (0.87)	2.96 (0.65)	-	0.720
	Parenting Sense of Competence (PSOC)—Total	Parent	Parenting Skills	50	57.12 (7.42)	67.00 (9.98)	24	57.13 (15.41)	58.46 (11.56)	-	0.814
	Family Observation Schedule (FOS-NCB)—% negative parent behavior	Parent	Parenting Skills	50	0.73 (1.60)	0.49 (1.18)	24	0.75 (1.72)	0.49 (1.01)	-	0.023
	Depression, Anxiety, and Stress Scale (DASS)	Parent	Stress/ Distress	50	27.16 (19.04)	19.54 (18.99)	24	31.96 (23.85)	28.33 (24.77)	-	0.190

(continued)

TABLE 5.1 (CONTINUED)

Study	Measure	Group	Outcome	Intervention			Comparison			F	d
				N	*Pre M (SD)*	*Post M (SD)*	*N*	*Pre M (SD)*	*Post M (SD)*		
	Abbreviated Dyadic Adjustment Scale (ADAS)	Parent	Adjustment	50	22.99 (4.95)	18.44 (10.51)	24	20.84 (7.27)	15.33 (12.42)	-	- 0.086
	OVERALL										0.484
Roberts et al. (2006)	Developmental Behavior Checklist—Total behavior problem score	Child	Behavior	17	67.47 (19.02)	49.65 (24.54)	15	64.13 (26.52)	67.20 (27.36)	-	0.807
	Depression, Anxiety and Stress Scale (DASS)	Parent	Stress/ Distress	14	14.07 (10.32)	9.14 (8.39)	15	10.27 (7.36)	9.93 (8.45)	-	0.545
	Family Observation Schedule—Noncompliance (target)	Child	Behavior	17	0.15 (0.21)	0.12 (0.24)	15	0.21 (0.15)	0.19 (0.22)	-	0.043
	Family Observation Schedule—Noncompliance (generalized)	Child	Behavior	17	0.18 (0.15)	0.03 (0.04)	15	0.12 (0.13)	0.14 (0.15)	-	1.595
	Family Observation Schedule—Oppositional behavior (target)	Child	Behavior	17	0.29 (0.32)	0.03 (0.08)	15	0.14 (0.12)	0.17 (0.22)	-	1.799
	Family Observation Schedule—Oppositional behavior (generalized)	Child	Behavior	17	0.16 (0.14)	0.03 (0.04)	15	0.15 (0.17)	0.09 (0.11)	-	0.868
	Family Observation Schedule—Appropriate behavior (target)	Child	Behavior	17	0.63 (0.21)	0.85 (0.24)	15	0.68 (0.16)	0.72 (0.29)	-	0.680

	Family Observation Schedule—Appropriate behavior (generalized)	Child	Behavior	17	0.71 (0.17)	0.85 (0.24)	15	0.73 (0.21)	0.72 (0.29)	-	0.567
	Parenting Scale—Laxness	Parent	Parent Skills	14	2.96 (0.93)	2.42 (0.81)	15	3.03 (0.65)	2.92 (0.76)	-	0.545
	Parenting Scale—Overreactivity	Parent	Parent Skills	14	3.59 (0.77)	2.79 (0.82)	15	3.37 (0.79)	3.33 (1.01)	-	0.823
	Parenting Scale—Verbosity	Parent	Parent Skills	14	3.24 (0.78)	2.80 (0.67)	15	3.21 (0.79)	3.27 (0.97)	-	0.596
	OVERALL										0.768
Singer et al. (1989)	Beck Depression Inventory (BDI)	Parent	Stress/ Distress	28	9.62 (6.80)	5.57 (5.59)	21	7.93 (7.98)	11.13 (11.75)	-	0.828
	State-Trait Anxiety Inventory-Trait Scale (STAI)	Parent	Stress/ Distress	28	40.75 (10.86)	35.07 (9.18)	21	41.13 (11.01)	41.37 (12.16)	-	0.561
	OVERALL										0.692
Sofronoff et al. (2011)	Eyberg Child Behavior Inventory (ECBI)	Child	Behavior	26	-	-	27	-	-	5.990	0.672
	Parenting Scale (PS)	Parent	Parenting Skills	26	2.97 (0.71)	2.47 (0.60)	27	2.88 (0.66)	2.86 (0.66)	-	0.760
	Parenting Sense of Competence Scale (PSOC)	Parent	Parenting Skills	26	-	-	27	-	-	3.123	0.486
	Parent Problem Checklist (PPC)	Parent	Adjustment	26	4.73 (3.91)	2.95 (2.66)	27	4.50 (2.72)	4.33 (3.55)	4.452	0.512
	Relationship Quality Index	Parent	Adjustment	26	34.59 (9.56)	35.04 (8.45)	27	34.50 (8.27)	33.38 (7.83)	0.683	0.193
	Parental adjustment and family adjustment	Parent	Adjustment	26	-	-	27	-	-	0.638	0.219

(continued)

TABLE 5.1 (CONTINUED)

Study	*Measure*	*Group*	*Outcome*	*Intervention* *N*	*Intervention* *Pre M (SD)*	*Intervention* *Post M (SD)*	*Comparison* *N*	*Comparison* *Pre M (SD)*	*Comparison* *Post M (SD)*	*F*	*d*
	OVERALL										0.469
All Studies											
		Child									0.662
		Parent									0.434
		Family									1.082
			Behavior								0.662
			Adjustment								0.258
			Parenting Skills								0.591
			Stress/ Distress								0.396
			Interaction								1.082
	OVERALL MULTICOMPONENTS										0.553

TABLE 5.4 EFFECT SIZES AND CONFIDENCE INTERVALS OF MULTICOMPONENT STUDIES

Study	*Measures*	*d*	*95% CI*
Coughlin et al. (2008)	B + D + E	0.476	[0.205, 0.746]
Durand et al. (2012)	B + E	0.165	[-0.304, 0.635]
Hudson et al. (2003)	A + B + D + E	0.481	[0.229, 0.733]
McIntyre (2008)	A + B + C	0.568	[0.292, 0.844]
Plant & Sanders (2007)	A + B + C + D + E	0.484	[0.318, 0.65]
Roberts et al. (2008)	B + D + E	0.768	[0.545, 0.991]
Singer et al. (1989)	E	0.692	[0.280, 1.104]
Sofronoff et al. (2011)	A + B + D	0.469	[0.245, 0.692]
Overall		0.553	[0.431, 0.674]

d and 95% CI

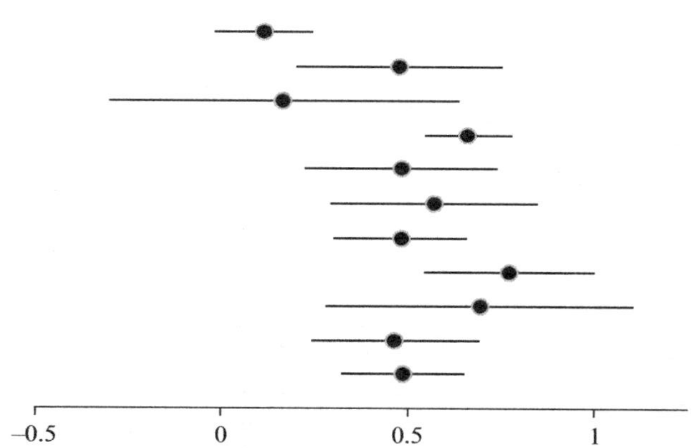

Note. A = Adjustment; B = Behavior; C = Interaction; D = Parenting Skills; E = Stress/Distress.

Unweighted effect sizes of all dependent measures and constructs of dependent measures are reported in Table 5.4, ranging from a small negative effect of -0.086, to the lowest positive effect size of 0.024 (close to no effect), and then to the largest positive effect size of 2.142. Also shown in Table 5.4, the overall effect size of the multicomponent programs is 0.553, suggesting a sizable effect of treatment for all multicomponent programs. As shown in Table 5.4, the average effect sizes of the constructs of Child Outcomes, Parent Outcomes, and Family System Outcomes are 0.662, 0.434, and 1.082, respectively. So the multicomponent programs seem to have a treatment effect on the child outcome (d = 0. 662) and on the construct of parent outcomes (d = 0.434). A smaller number of comparisons (n = 3) suggests they may also impact positively the family system (d = 1.082). In particular, for the construct of Parent Outcomes, effect sizes range from a treatment effect of a multicomponent program on parent's reduced level of stress/distress (d = 0.396), parent psychological adjustment (d = 0.258), and parenting skills (d = 0.591). Overall the effect sizes are impressive, given the ongoing long-term challenges that family caregivers encounter.

In conclusion, taken as a group, the work of the researchers presented in this chapter represents considerable innovation, an injection of new ideas in this area as well transfer of methods from related work with other groups of children. We find it heartening to see the continued vitality in this line of work. It bodes well for improving the quality of life in help-seeking families. Two of the interventions reviewed here meet the criteria as established evidence-based practices: in-home PBS, and the SSTP program. All of the other programs reviewed we categorize as promising, and in most cases these programs simply await further replication to be rated as established practices.

6

ADVOCACY AND SELF-HELP PROGRAMS AS EVIDENCE-BASED PRACTICES FOR FAMILIES OF CHILDREN WITH DEVELOPMENTAL DISABILITIES

Yeana W. Lam, Mian Wang, George H. S. Singer, and Jiyeon Kim

Family involvement in schooling activities typically contributes to more successful outcomes for students with developmental needs and disabilities (Anderson, Meyer, & Somers, 2006; Hill et al., 2004; Simon, 2001). Parent involvement is also a hallmark in special education due to the mandates of special education law, specifically the Individuals with Disabilities Education Act (IDEA, 2004), which requires parents of children with disabilities to participate in setting and evaluating educational and transition goals (Anderson et al., 2006). Congress envisioned parents as central stakeholders in the planning and execution of special education services. They are given more authority and legal rights than what is normally available to parents of typically developing children. It is assumed in the law that parents will be advocates for their children and will participate as full members of interdisciplinary individualized education program (IEP) teams. Subsequent court rulings have established the IEP as having the legal status of a contract between parents and schools regarding the amount and kind of services that will be provided to a child as well as specific educational goals and placement in specific educational settings. Despite the fact that participation is legally supported and expected in special education, collaboration does not always occur. In fact, one primary source of parent–school conflict is school's de facto exclusion of families from the educational process, a conflict that some parents characterize as "us versus them" (Mueller, Singer, & Draper, 2008). The mechanisms of exclusion are complex, but they result in IEP meetings in which parents, if present, passively ratify plans that have been developed in advance by the professional members of the IEP team. The IDEA establishes a sequence of due process measures available to parents in the event they disagree with special education decisions. Although the percentage of parents who enter into disputes with schools is a very small, the threat of legal action has had a powerful influence in school systems (Mueller & Carranza, 2011).

Along similar lines, the IDEA also requires that adolescents with disabilities also be involved in meetings concerning their IEPs and their transition to adult life. Yet only about half of all students with IEPs attend their meetings (Trach & Shelden, 2000), even though it has been found that students who participate meaningfully in their IEPs tend to develop better self-advocacy and communication skills (Mason, McGahee-Kovac, Johnson, & Stillerman, 2002). Moreover, survey results of adults with developmental disabilities have indicated that a greater sense of self-sufficiency is associated with better employment status, with independent living, and with financial independence (Wehmeyer & Palmer, 2003; Wehmeyer & Schwartz, 1997). Such findings have encouraged researchers to explore ways to help students exercise more personal control in school, home, and community settings. Their mandated inclusion in transition planning in IEP meetings from age 14 on is one outgrowth of these efforts.

Therefore, a number of intervention programs have been developed to mitigate family–school conflicts and to promote family and student inclusion in decision-making processes. These interventions include home–school collaboration programs, parent advocacy trainings, parent-to-parent programs, family-involved student self-determination trainings, and IEP interventions. Empirical studies done on these programs are listed in Table 6.1. This chapter examines these interventions more closely and discusses related issues and concerns.

HOME–SCHOOL COLLABORATION

Although home–school collaboration is lauded as a necessary component to student success, there exist serious structural and psychological barriers to initiating home–school partnerships in general and special education. For schools, lack of funding and training, pressure from national and state accountability measures, stereotypes about families, and wariness of conflict can hinder their willingness to engage with parents (Brantlinger, 1991; Christenson, 2004; Minke & Anderson, 2005; Muscott, Mann, & LeBrun, 2008). Likewise, parents encounter their own set of barriers that limit collaboration with schools: lack of role models; insufficient knowledge, resources, time, and

TABLE 6.1 RESEARCH SYNTHESIS OF ADVOCACY AND SELF-HELP INTERVENTIONS

Author(s)	*Design*	*Participants*	*Intervention*	*Results*
Baker & Brightman (1984)	Quasi-experimental design	15 parents of children with intellectual disabilities (e.g., Down syndrome, other intellectual disability, autism, and cerebral palsy of average age 5.7), randomly assigned to *Parents as Teachers* or *Parents as Advocates*	The Parents as Advocates course taught parents IDEA rights and procedures and how to participate in their children's IEP meeting. The Parents as Teachers course trained parents on behavioral principles and teaching methods.	Parents with advocacy training significantly improved on the IDEA knowledge questionnaire and on the simulated advocacy activity. Parents with behavioral training significantly improved on behavioral knowledge measures and on IDEA knowledge.
Balcazar, Keys, Bertram, & Rizzo (1996)	Pre- and posttest (treatment group only)	21 parents of children with developmental disabilities and three adults with disabilities	Partners in Policymaking (see Zirpoli, Hancox, Wieck, & Skarnulis, 1994)	Participants made significant gains in number of advocacy actions performed (phone calls, meetings, letters and mass mailings, media reports). Active advocates at baseline performed the majority of the advocacy actions during follow-up and reported the most outcomes from advocacy (school inclusion, legislative changes, community education activities, appointments to decision-making boards, etc.).
Blair, Lee, Cho, & Dunlap (2011)	Single-subject design	Three children (ages 4.5 to 5.5 with autism and intellectual disability or autism and cerebral palsy) in South Korea, their mothers, and their teachers	Mothers and teachers received individualized positive behavior support (PBS). Team members received training in collaborative teaming, and in developing, implementing, monitoring, and evaluating a behavior support plan.	Children's problem behaviors significantly decreased, appropriate behaviors increased, and results generalized to other settings. Positive mother–child and teacher–child interactions increased, and negative interactions decreased. Results maintained at 3-week follow-up. Social validity was found to be high across participants.

(*continued*)

TABLE 6.1 (CONTINUED)

Author(s)	*Design*	*Participants*	*Intervention*	*Results*
Brinckerhoff & Vincent (1986)	Randomized controlled trial	14 parents of children (aged 2–5 years) with IEPs, school/community liaisons	School/community liaisons were trained individually to prepare parents for the IEP process. Liaisons met with the six experimental families prior to the IEP to discuss family routines, family functioning, and quality of home, development and adaptive skills of child, as well as IEP procedures and roles of stakeholders.	Treatment parents were found to contribute more frequently, to make more decisions, generate more goals alone and jointly with school staff, compared with the control group. School staff in the experimental group made fewer decisions, compared with the control group.
Buelow, Johnson, Perkins, Austin, & Dunn (2013)	Randomized controlled trial	31 primary caregivers of children between ages 7 and 16 who have epilepsy and mild intellectual disability or serious learning problem	The Creating Avenues for Parent Partnership (CAPP) program was a 1-day program educating parents on effective communication skills with professionals, on caregiver and student rights, and on developing partnerships with school personnel and healthcare professionals. Four booster sessions provided opportunities to reinforce concepts and real-life practice.	Caregivers rated the intervention useful but not very easy to implement. No significant differences were found in family empowerment, in family needs, or on the emotional and time aspects of the family quality of life measure. A significant difference was found in the activities aspect of family quality of life but was in favor of the control group.
Chadwick, Momcilovic, Rossiter, Stumbles, & Taylor (2001)	Randomized controlled trial	62 families of children (ages 4–11) with cerebral palsy, Down syndrome, autism, or epilepsy	Parents receiving training in behavioral analysis and behavioral techniques were assigned to participate in the group intervention, individual-based intervention, or control. Teachers also received 2-day training on behavior management, functional analysis, and the need for mutual support.	Results indicated parents found the intervention useful and that there were short-term reductions for the individual training group in children's problem behaviors, but no significant differences among groups were found at the 6-month follow-up. No significant differences were found in parental stress among the three groups.

Goldstein & Turnbull (1982)	Randomized controlled trial	45 parents of elementary-age children with learning disabilities	One treatment group of parents were sent questions about child's educational goals and potentials and the IEP process prior to the IEP meeting. Another treatment group had a school counselor serve as a parent advocate at the meeting, directing questions to parents and encouraging parental input.	Parents in the second treatment group, who had a parent advocate at the meeting, verbally contributed more to the IEP conference, compared with the control group parents. No significant differences were observed between the first treatment group and the control group. No differences were found in parents' ratings of satisfaction and level of participation in meeting.
Hagner et al. (2012)	Randomized controlled trial	47 youths (aged 16–19 with ASD)	The transition planning intervention consisted of a group training for families that discussed transition planning, problem-solving, services, financing, and taking action. Students and parents also participated in person-centered planning, in which facilitators helped families develop a transition plan based on students' history, strengths, support network, vision, and goals.	Compared with the control group, the intervention group saw increased student expectations and parent expectations for the future, gains in self-determination, and vocational decision-making.
Hoffman & Field (1995)	Quasi-experimental design	77 high school students with disabilities (14.3% with intellectual disabilities)	The Steps to Self-Determination curriculum instructs students to engage in the cognitive, affective, and behavioral components of self-determination. Families are invited to participate in the orientation to support students in becoming self-determined.	Intervention group significantly improved, compared with the control group, in the knowledge of skills presented in the curriculum. Measures of student behavior also demonstrated increases in self-determination.
Kim & Park (2012)	Quasi-experimental design	24 middle school students (with intellectual disabilities or autism) in South Korea, their teachers, and their parents.	The family-involved self-determined learning model of instruction (SDLMI) guides students to self-direct their own learning with a set of 12 questions. Parents monitor and facilitate discussion about children's learning at home.	Intervention students were found to have significantly increased their academic engagement compared with peers in the control group in the behavior checklist and direct observations of behavior. Intervention students also experienced significantly greater goal attainment. Participants generally found the intervention favorable.

(continued)

TABLE 6.1 (CONTINUED)

Author(s)	*Design*	*Participants*	*Intervention*	*Results*
Miner & Bates (1997)	Quasi-experimental design	22 high school students (aged 14–21 with intellectual disabilities) and their families	Person-centered planning activities were used to prepare families and students for IEP/transition meeting. Activities incorporated active family and student participation to identify supports at home, school, and community; acknowledge student preferences and strengths; and develop a vision based on student's desires.	Treatment families participated in transitional IEP meetings significantly more than control families did. No significant differences were found in the frequency of postschool topics discussed. There were also no differences in parent satisfaction immediately after the IEP meeting but satisfaction was higher at the 6-month follow-up survey.
Pierce & Schreibman (1994)	Single-subject design	3 boys (ages 6–9 with autism)	Intervention consisted of training participants to use self-management techniques via picture prompts to learn to perform functional skills (e.g., getting dressed, setting the table, making the bed, etc.) independently.	Observational data indicated that on-task behaviors increased and inappropriate behaviors decreased post-treatment. At the generalization and the 2-month follow-up, two of three participants were able to perform the task without pictorial prompts.
Powers, Turner, Ellison, et al. (2001)	Randomized controlled trial	20 adolescents with disabilities (8 with mild intellectual disabilities)	The TAKE CHARGE for the Future intervention included an individualized coaching session with students regarding self-determination; workshops for students, families, and community mentors; community activities with mentor; and telephone and home visit support for families.	Intervention students experienced significant improvements on psychosocial adjustment, empowerment, and number of accomplishments. No significant differences were found in disability-related self-efficacy between the intervention and control groups. A majority (97%) of short-term goals were attained in the intervention group.
Powers, Turner, Westwood, et al. (2001)	Randomized controlled trial	43 students (aged 14–17 with learning, emotional, orthopedic, or other health disabilities) that did not currently participate in transition IEP meetings; families also participated	TAKE CHARGE for the Future was implemented with the additional component of professional development for transition staff.	Intervention students experienced significant gains in educational planning involvement, transition awareness, and empowerment; they engaged in higher levels of initiation and participation in transition meetings. Parents' educational planning and transitional awareness increases were also significant. Educators' educational planning involvement also significantly increased.

Ruble, Dalrymple, & McGrew (2010)	Randomized controlled trial	35 special education teachers, randomly selected child (aged 3–8) with autism from each class, and the child's parents or caregivers	The Collaborative Model for Promoting Competence and Success (COMPASS) is a behavioral consultation program that helps teachers and parents develop IEP goals, teach skills, and evaluate IEP goal attainment addressing social skills, communication, and independence.	Intervention student–teacher dyads made greater gains in IEP goal attainment. The IEPs of the intervention dyads were also of higher quality. Intervention teachers were satisfied with COMPASS. Teachers and parents reported that intervention was implemented with fidelity.
Sheridan, Eagle, Cowan, & Mickelson (2001)	Single subject design	52 students (grades K-9) and their parents and teachers. Participants were identified with having disabilities (14% with intellectual disabilities) or at risk for academic failure.	Behavior consultants implemented conjoint behavioral consultation (CBC) through four problem-solving trainings/interviews with parents to identify children's problem behaviors, to analyze the problem, to treat the behaviors through implementation of a behavior plan, and to evaluate the treatment.	Large average effect size was found in observations of target behaviors at home and school. Larger effect size was present for older clients with less severe symptoms and with younger clients with severe symptoms. High ratings of effectiveness and acceptability were also found. Consultants collectively met at least 80% of objectives for their cases.
Singer et al. (1999)	Randomized controlled trial	128 parents of children with disabilities	The Parent to Parent program matches trained veteran parent volunteers with parents who need one-to-one emotional and informational support.	Intervention parents were found to be significantly more accepting of disability. Treatment parents with low parenting efficacy pretreatment made significant gains in parenting efficacy over the course of intervention. Qualitative results suggested effects of intervention might depend on perceived sameness of experience between paired parents, social comparison of parents' situations, ready availability of support, and mutuality of support.

(*continued*)

TABLE 6.1 (CONTINUED)

Author(s)	*Design*	*Participants*	*Intervention*	*Results*
Stormshak, Fosco, & Dishion (2010)	Randomized controlled trial	377 families in three public middle schools	The school-based, multilevel intervention Family Check-Up (FCU) delivered family-centered services through the family resource center (universal level), FCU program (at-risk level), and individual family consultation (high-risk level). Family resource center provided information and brief consultations. FCU consisted of a home visit and interview, assessments, and feedback session. Family management curriculum was implemented in the individual consultation level.	FCU implementation was associated with gains in self-regulation from grade 6 to 7. Grade 7 self-regulation was related to reduction in depression throughout middle school, and grade 8 self-regulation was associated with increased school engagement.
Wehmeyer, Palmer, Shogren, Williams-Diehm, & Soukup (2013)	Randomized controlled trial	371 high school students with intellectual disabilities or learning disabilities	Teachers implemented the self-determined learning model of instruction together with a choice of ChoiceMaker curriculum, Self-Advocacy Strategy, Whose Future Is It Anyway?, or NEXT S.T.E.P. curriculum in this longitudinal study. Of these programs, NEXT S.T.E.P. was described to have a family involvement component.	Intervention students significantly increased their capacity and opportunity for self-determination (AIR Self-Determination Scale). Only students with intellectual disabilities in the intervention group increased their scores on the ARC's Self-Determination Scale, which evaluates the characteristics of self-determination the students have.
Zirpoli et al. (1994)	Within-group, posttest only	35 participants, including 30 parents of children with disabilities (whose mean age was 6.5) and five adults with disabilities	The Partners in Policymaking program taught empowerment and self-advocacy in the area of developmental disabilities in a series of 2-day training sessions. Each participant completed a major advocacy project by the end of the training.	Participants rated program positively: at 6-month follow-up, the majority of participants reported they had contacted government officials about their needs. The majority had self-advocated or educated others about disabilities. They also reported an increase in confidence, knowledge, and access to the system.

childcare; feelings of inadequacy; and linguistic and cultural differences (Brantlinger, 1991; Christenson, 2004). Family characteristics may play a role in how involved parents are in their children's schooling experiences. For families of children with developmental disabilities, family resources (especially knowledge of information), expectations for schooling, attitudes about participation, and perceptions about school characteristics (e.g., whether parents think teachers seek their input) are significant predictors of involvement in activities at school (Coots, 1998).

Even if a collaborative relationship between the family and school is established, additional obstacles can emerge. One of these challenges is the differences in levels of trust among parents and teachers. Parents of both typical children and children with disabilities tend to have significantly higher levels of trust in teachers than teachers have for parents (Adams & Christenson, 1998). Professionals are viewed as possessing expertise, and this expert knowledge is usually favored over parents' subjective knowledge of their children (Kalyanpur, Harry, & Skrtic, 2000). Another obstacle is the discrepant expectations for student learning that teachers and parents bring into the relationship. Beebe-Frankenberger, Lane, Bocian, Gresham, and MacMillan (2005) examined teacher and parent ratings of social skills in adolescent students previously identified as at risk for academic or behavioral concerns. Teachers universally valued cooperation skills in students with problem behaviors because cooperation in class maximizes expedience in instruction. Conversely, parents' ratings indicated that social skills that demonstrate responsibility, self-control, and assertion—rather than cooperation—were most critical to home success. Appropriate behavior may be more difficult to reinforce when expectations are different across settings, and it may be difficult for parents and teachers to align their hopes and goals for students in some educational domains. There must be congruence in messages (Reschly & Christenson, 2009); that is, the expectations of the student and the interactions between adult and student should be consistent across school and home environments. This requires a level of coordination that goes well beyond annual IEP participation.

A number of recommended practices to professionals have been proposed to overcome these barriers that prevent parents and teachers from entering a collaborative relationship. Reschly and Christenson (2009) argued that practitioners and researchers must orient themselves to look at the quality of the relationship. Building mutual trust and respect is critical for shifting home–school relationships from one of merely "parental involvement" to an active model of family–school collaboration or partnership (Minke & Anderson, 2005). Schools must create opportunities for parents and teachers to build rapport and trust, such as holding regular informal events that encourage interaction (Adams & Christenson, 1998). Hoover-Dempsey et al. (2005) suggest that a crucial variable in establishing trust between parents and school personnel is simply the number of school invitations to events providing opportunities for interactions with family members. Both the invitations and the events should be designed in ways that enhance parental knowledge, sense of empowerment, and motivation to continued engagement with the school.

Related to interventions, Dunst, Trivette, and Hamby (2007) expressed that family-focused services should exhibit relational help-giving (practices that give positive beliefs about family strengths and capabilities) while providing knowledge and skills training. Relational help-giving is characterized by respect for families, empathic listening, and clear communication. Participatory help-giving practices center on providing meaningful mechanisms for parents to contribute to planning and design of supports as well as to have a say in the governance of the services that provide them. This latter form of help-giving has been less common and more difficult to achieve than the former (Dunst et al., 2007). Effective family-centered practices, both relational and participatory, were found to strongly relate to outcomes such as ratings of parent satisfaction with program services and of parent self-efficacy. It is likely that these psychological variables may also be linked to more distal outcomes (e.g., child behavior, parenting behavior, and personal/family well-being; Dunst et al., 2007). Some necessary types of participatory support that schools can offer are to help parents feel more empowered to advocate for their children and to help parents be an integral part of the decision-making process for their children's education (Minke & Anderson, 2005). As reviewed below, there is some research guidance about how to accomplish these aims.

Scholars' recommendations in developing and sustaining healthy home–school interactions convey optimal practices. Practitioners and researchers have created interventions that include family members and school staff with the purpose of improving behavioral outcomes for students with developmental disabilities. Home and school collaborations interventions fall under three distinct types of interventions: parent and teacher trainings, individualized behavioral support or consultation, and multitiered behavioral support.

PARENT–TEACHER JOINT TRAININGS

In parent and teacher training programs, researchers instruct teachers and parents to know basic behavioral principles, to collect data, to formulate hypotheses about the behavior functions, to collaborate with other team members to generate a behavior plan, and to implement these plans as a team across settings. One such study by Chadwick et al. (2001), introduced in chapter 3, evaluated intervention methods designed to familiarize parents and teachers with the principles and methods of teaching appropriate behaviors and reducing inappropriate behaviors, and this study's design included a control. This study showed modest short-term success; the authors indicated that future programs should be longer in duration. Results of children's behavior ratings showed that there was a significant difference in the reduction in the severity of problem behaviors between the baseline and immediate postintervention assessments, with the individually based intervention group showing greater improvement than the group intervention and the control. Yet these differences were no longer significant at the 6-month follow-up. Children's problem behaviors occurred significantly less frequently with families in the individually based training group immediately after intervention, but this reduction again was not significant when examining the baseline-to-follow-up time points. There is a need for research on maintenance of parent-teacher coordinated behavioral practices.

BEHAVIORAL CONSULTATION

Another model of behavioral intervention featuring home–school collaboration component is individualized behavioral support or consultation. Like the coordinated parent–teacher training programs, training is provided to both parents and teachers in this model, but support for data collection, analyses of behavioral functions, instruction of specific behavioral strategies, development of a behavioral plan, and continuous monitoring and evaluation of intervention progress are tailored to the family. In Blair et al.'s (2011) study, the researchers examined whether individualized positive behavior support (PBS, discussed in chapter 5) through family–school collaboration increased appropriate behavior and decreased problem behaviors across classroom and home settings for preschool-age children with developmental disabilities in South Korea. Additionally, they investigated whether these results maintained after the culmination of the intervention, generalized to other nontargeted classroom and home routines, and increased mothers' and teachers' positive interactions with children while decreasing negative interactions. Three children participated in Blair and colleagues' (2011) multiple baseline, single-subject design study. The school staff, parents, and research team of each child met to plan the process of working as a team, to discuss strengths and interests of the child, and to establish shared goals for intervention. Team members then participated in a 10-hour training to learn skills in the areas of collaborative teaming, conducting a functional behavioral assessment, identifying and confirming strategies, implementing support strategies at home and in the classroom, and monitoring and evaluating outcomes. Furthermore, the training focused on staff and family collaboration in the process of individualized behavior support and their roles and responsibilities. Each child's team then developed a behavior support plan, with specific strategies selected by the researcher to fit the teachers' and families' abilities, resources, and needs (e.g., increasing peer, sibling, and adult involvement in play, increasing the number of novel activity materials). After the teachers and mothers participated in an additional 2- to 3-hour training consisting of modeling systemic teaching and response procedures, the teachers and mothers jointly developed plans of action and implemented the behavior support plans based on the child's preference and interests. Home–school communication was ongoing throughout implementation.

Team members participated in weekly or biweekly meetings during the intervention phase to review progress and to receive technical assistance in implementing the behavior support plan across home and school. Teachers and mothers engaged in brief discussions during drop-off and pick-up times around the implementation of the plan and their child's progress. Daily school–home notes with checklists indicated occurrence or nonoccurrence of child's target behaviors in each setting. Results showed that the problem behaviors significantly reduced during intervention and appropriate behaviors increased with a stable pattern of high levels over time (Blair et al., 2011). These patterns were also maintained during follow-up. Collateral effects from intervention were also present in nontargeted activities, namely at the community playgroup. Furthermore, interactions between the target children and the participating adults, especially the mothers, improved significantly as well. The authors credited the positive results to family–school collaboration in this individualized PBS investigation.

This study is an important contribution to the literature. It highlights the importance of creating and maintaining teamwork between school personnel and parents, in this case mothers. The study was conducted in Korea and should be replicated in the United States to test its replicability in a different cultural setting.

Similar to individualized PBS, conjoint behavioral consultation (CBC) is a form of therapeutic service in which parents, teachers, and other support staff work together to address the academic, social, or behavior problems of a student. As part of a larger 5-year study, Sheridan et al. (2001) investigated the effects of a CBC intervention on parents and teachers of 52 students with different disabilities or at-risk for academic failure, whose grade levels ranged from kindergarten through ninth grade. Data were collected as single-subject experimental cases in Sheridan et al.'s (2001) study on CBC interventions. Substantial positive behavioral changes were indicated by visual inspection of the data. The program appeared to be more effective for younger students or for those with fewer problem behaviors. Parents and teachers also reported high levels of satisfaction with the consultant and consultation experience. Replication with more children with severe problem behavior is called for.

MULTITIERED BEHAVIORAL SUPPORT

The final model of behavioral interventions described in the home–school collaboration research is multitiered approaches, which embed varying levels of behavioral supports within an academically and behaviorally diverse schoolwide setting. The first tier of intervention typically involved basic, universal supports available to all students, families, and professionals; the second tier related to more targeted supports administered in small-group or individual settings; the third and last tier included intensive supports and intervention that involve more comprehensive individualized planning and intervention (Eber, Sugai, Smith, & Scott, 2002).

Reinke, Splett, Robeson, and Offutt (2009) targeted student behavior in the schoolwide setting using the Family Check-Up (FCU). The FCU model is a family support system conducted in school settings to support and sustain healthy academic and social behaviors (Reinke et al., 2009). The FCU is an example of a second-tier intervention that uses motivational interviewing and feedback to help parents identify risk factors and promote the use of specific helpful resources. Evaluations of their program have shown that families assigned to the experimental condition tended to have children who were less involved with deviant peer groups, less likely to display antisocial behavior, and less likely to engage in substance use than those in the control group. Stormshak et al. (2010) specifically used the FCU as a parent training model in the school setting to test the hypothesis that FCU would directly support development of youths' self-regulation, which in turn would promote improved psychological functioning (i.e., reduced levels of depression) and school engagement. A 4-year longitudinal study was conducted across three public middle schools in an urban area with 377 adolescents and their families, with 277 families randomly assigned to the intervention condition and 100 families randomly assigned to the control condition. Of the families in the intervention condition, 46% received consultation from a parent consultant and 38% received the full FCU intervention. Results indicated that participation in FCU was associated with increases in self-regulation from sixth to seventh grade. That is, a relatively brief, family-centered school-based approach to intervention led to a positive effect on self-regulation. Seventh-grade self-regulation was negatively associated with youths' depressive symptoms throughout middle school, with a small to medium effect size. Eighth-grade self-regulation was associated with a medium effect size increase in school engagement by ninth grade. This study is an important contribution because it provides a feasible tiered model of service delivery housed in a public school. Replications are necessary to bolster the case that the FCU is the proximal cause of changes in middle school students' self-regulation.

Overall, there is evidence from these studies that behavioral intervention programs involving family–school partnerships are associated with positive behavioral changes in students with developmental disabilities. Many of these studies have demonstrated that a critical feature of the program is the attention to the priorities and goals of the family. However, as not all of these studies were randomized controlled trials or single case studies, there is a need for future work in home–school collaboration to incorporate high-quality experimental design.

PARENT ADVOCACY TRAINING

Rather than wait for schools to extend home–school collaboration opportunities, families can proactively enhance their participation in their children's education by becoming advocates for their children (Trainor, 2008). Barriers such as the bureaucratic nature of the school system and its emphasis on efficiency (e.g., electronic IEP writing programs, tightly scheduled meetings) often adversely affect family–school interactions and prevent schools from meeting students and families' individualized needs (Bacon & Causton-Theoharis, 2012). While school and service personnel need to help correct this imbalance by shifting their perspective about engaging families and employing more cooperative practices (Bezdek, Summers, & Turnbull, 2010; Christenson, 2004), school and service staff also need to answer to the needs of the organizations they represent (Trainor, 2008). This conflict of interest on the part of school personnel means that parents themselves must, at times, take initiative and advocate on behalf of their children to obtain information or resources.

Parent Advocacy

We define advocacy broadly as a type of parent participation that intends to ensure "that the educational rights of youth with disabilities are met" (Trainor, 2008, p. 36). Closely related to the term "advocacy" is the construct *empowerment*. Empowerment has been described as the process of individuals or groups attaining mastery over matters that they perceive to be important (Zimmerman, 1995). In the context of the relationship between families and service delivery, empowerment means "parent's active agency and sense of control over themselves, their child, and their family" (Nachshen, 2005, p. 67).

Not all parents possess the social capital, including intrapersonal skills and knowledge (i.e., the ability to self-motivate, self-manage, adapt, and problem-solve) to advocate successfully on their own (Trainor, 2008), and so a number of parent advocacy training models have been created in both the special education and mental health fields to increase family involvement. Research in this area has yet to establish a consistent programmatic profile. Many of the training programs target parent empowerment but vary greatly in the content, in the delivery of the content, in the intended outcome of the training, and in the actual related effects of the training. Likewise, the methodologies used to evaluate the interventions have also been diverse, with very few controlled, randomized experimental studies.

Developed by Baker and colleagues, the Parents as Advocates curriculum within the *Steps to Independence* program taught parental rights and advocacy skills to parents of young children with ID as part of a larger parenting program (Baker & Brightman, 1984). This 14-hour program is delivered to parents in a group setting over the course of seven weekly sessions, using lectures, small group problem-solving discussions, videos, role-play with peer feedback, handouts, and homework assignments (e.g., finding their special education coordinator). The emphasis of the program is on parents' understanding of their IDEA rights and procedures and preparing for their children's IEP. In a randomized study of this program, parents were assigned to either the advocacy or the behavioral training program (Baker & Brightman, 1984). The seven parents in the advocacy education group were assessed using a questionnaire on their knowledge of special education law; they were also assessed using direct observation of their response to hypothetical advocacy situations. On average, this group of parents significantly improved on both measures after the completion of the course, compared with the results from parents randomly assigned to the behavior training program.

While advocacy interventions may enhance parent knowledge, it may not always result in intrapersonal and behavioral empowerment outcomes. Buelow et al. (2013), in a recent study, focused on the pilot intervention program Creating Avenues for Parent Partnership (CAPP) in Canada. Participants in a previous qualitative study on the intervention program found the 1-day training acceptable (Buelow, 2007), and so, a larger-scale, randomized controlled trial study, with a waitlist comparison group, was implemented that followed this model (Buelow et al., 2013). The 1-day training lasted 6 hours and was provided to 31 parents of children identified with having both epilepsy and intellectual disabilities or significant learning problems. During the training, participants were exposed to informational presentations, discussion, problem identification, and problem-solving on the topics of gathering information on their children's disabilities and building partnerships with health providers and school personnel. Additionally, three 2-hour booster sessions were administered monthly after the initial training. Homework was assigned for parents to implement the action plans developed during the 1-day workshop and the first two booster sessions. Progress on these action plans was then discussed, with feedback and encouragement provided, during the subsequent sessions. The trainers also discussed parents' and students' rights, information about the school system, and effective ways to communicate with school staff and healthcare professionals.

Buelow et al.'s (2013) study found the CAPP intervention to be acceptable and feasible for parents; however, it also found that the intervention only marginally improved parents' sense of empowerment, as measured on the Family Empowerment Scale (FES), and parents' concern for child's emotional limitations, as measured by a family quality of life scale (Child Health Questionnaire—Family Scale [CHQ-FS]). No significant changes were found for families' perception of their needs. The effect sizes were generally small (ranging between 0.00 and 0.20). In fact, for the activities limitations subscale of the family quality of life measure, which produced the largest effect size (-0.20), the waitlist control group actually performed significantly better than the intervention group. Buelow and colleagues cited the small sample size and the lack of consideration of treatment fidelity as issues that may have affected the results.

Unlike many other parent education programs that focus on advocacy knowledge affecting individual families' interactions with educators or health professionals, Partners in Policymaking aimed to train adults and family members to actively advocate in larger social and political domains. This federally funded program based in Minnesota provided adults with developmental disabilities and families of children with developmental disabilities with information regarding local, state, and federal issues regarding disability, advocacy organizations and advocacy skills, employment, nonaversive behavior management skills, severe physical disabilities, and educational issues (e.g., IEPs, family participation, availability of services; Zirpoli et al., 1994). This training consisted of eight 2-day sessions that included presentations given by experts on developmental disability topics, local and state legislators, and staff members of congressional representatives and senators. Participants were also given homework assignments that required the trainees to contact policy makers, to attend community meetings, to make presentations, and to complete an internship or organize a meeting with public officials. Although preintervention measures were not taken, and therefore the change in the participants' empowerment was not assessed, postintervention survey results indicated that a majority of participants (57%) rated the program as "excellent" in improving their self-advocacy skills. Participants also responded positively to items about accessing services and being an effective advocate.

To further assess the effectiveness of Partners in Policymaking, Balcazar et al. (1996) implemented the intervention in Illinois with pre- and postintervention measures. Balcazar and colleagues were interested in examining the differential effectiveness of this program on advocacy actions of those that were classified as beginner, involved, and activist advocates. The researchers hypothesized that individuals at different developmental stages of advocacy—based on the frequency of advocacy actions (e.g., phone calls, office visits, letters, media reports, school presentations, fundraising, membership in advocacy group, etc.) performed—will influence the impact of the program. These advocacy actions could be intended to effect change on the personal, local, state, or national level. Participants in this training included individuals with disabilities, but a majority (21 of 24 trainees) were parents of children with developmental disabilities. Results from the 9-month training revealed that all groups, regardless of the advocacy developmental stage, made significant increases in levels of advocacy actions. Those in the activist group still performed the greatest number of advocacy actions at the end of training (activists reported 63% of all advocacy actions). The authors presumed that members of the activist group were likely already connected to local and state networks and were likely more knowledgeable about taking action. Nonetheless, those in the beginner and the involved groups also made significant gains in number of advocacy actions, suggesting that the program was beneficial to all groups.

With regard to the content of the training, these four programs taught parents specific knowledge about the child's disability or condition, the school or service system, parental rights within those systems, and the available resources within those systems and the community. These programs also addressed advocacy skills, such as identifying and solving problems and communicating and partnering with school staff, providers, or community members. Procedural knowledge about participating in IEP meetings was stressed in one of the parent education programs. In addition, self-efficacy and assertiveness skills were taught and reinforced in some programs.

The associated effects of training sometimes did not reflect the components of empowerment outcomes that were specifically targeted in the interventions. For example, the Parents as Advocates training taught systems and procedural knowledge (Baker & Brightman, 1984), and their results noted a rise in participant knowledge. However, for Buelow and colleagues' (2013) evaluation of the CAPP training, support in knowledge of skills, confidence, and advocacy behavior was provided, and yet there was no change in overall family empowerment after training. One major factor that may have impacted the effectiveness of that program was the length of training. Parent advocacy trainings involving short-term courses may have less of an influence than emotional and informational support provided over a longer period of time. A closer examination of the measures used in this study may also shed light on the weak effects. For example, several items on the Family Empowerment Scale relate to public forms of advocacy including political actions; these may not have been targeted by some of these programs.

One practical implication of these studies is the importance of focusing on parents' needs in the implementation and the content of the curriculum. Advocacy training programs must be sensitive to the needs of the particular parents they serve. Cunconan-Lahr and Brotherson (1996) surveyed and interviewed participants of an advocacy program and found the major barriers to advocacy were time and cost, as well as the taxing emotions that become involved in the advocacy process (e.g., embarrassment and reactions to stigma and fear from educational and service systems). There are also obstacles that affect specific families.

Most studies and evaluations on parent advocacy programs fail to consider the needs and experiences of culturally, linguistically, and socially diverse groups. Interventions have found success in delivering parent–professional trainings in the home language of the participants (Whitbread, Bruder, Fleming, & Park, 2007). Beyond that, training developers must also realize that parent advocacy and participation manifest differently depending on the cultural capital (i.e., material resources and knowledge) and social capital (i.e., social networks and connections) that the parents possess (Trainor, 2008). In advocacy situations, low-income families have been found to rely on their intuitive knowledge, which is more often dismissed by professionals when compared with their higher-income peers who have more sophisticated knowledge about special education laws (Trainor, 2008). Parents from racial-ethnic minority groups are less likely to employ a stance of expertise on disability-related topics, a more successful advocacy approach (Trainor, 2008). There is a clear need for support and advocacy programs to impart self-efficacy skills, as well as knowledge on disabilities, special education legislation, and the educational and service systems to racial and ethnic minority families. Without such research and development, parent advocacy will remain the privilege of White middle- and upper-class parents. At this early stage of development, parent advocacy programs must be considered unproven and await further development.

PARENT TO PARENT PEER SUPPORT

The special contribution of peer support programs is the capacity to provide resonant, experiential empathy (Corcoran, 1981; Meissner, 2010). Parents when they voluntarily assist one another can be a trusted source of information, encouragement, and a relief from social stigma. In previous work, we have defined peer support in the following way:

> Peer support is freely given assistance from individuals who share a difficulty or identity that is important to their well being. It is particularly valuable to individuals who experience social stigma and problems which others find difficult to understand. (Singer, Hornby, Park, Wang, & Xu, 2012)

Parents and siblings whose families experience relatively rare problems, particularly if they commonly are socially devalued, may be able to establish resonant empathy with others through peer support programs (Davison, Pennebaker, & Dickerson, 2000). Social support is usually discussed as *informal* when it comes from family and friends or *formal* from people in helping professions; informal social support is among the most crucial resources that families draw on to cope with stressors (McCubbin et al., 1980; Trivette & Dunst, 1992). Supportive social networks are associated with higher parental well-being and more positive parent–child interactions (Dunst et al., 2007) between mothers and their young children with developmental disabilities. In some studies of mothers of children with developmental disabilities, the most powerful predictor of depression and anxiety was perceived lack of social support (Boyd, 2002). In studies in which parents have been asked to rank social support by how helpful it is, they attribute their informal support network, usually other family members and friends as the most helpful (Santelli, Turnbull, Sergeant, Lerner & Marquis, 1996). In two-parent families informal support from spouses has proven to be a powerful moderator of child-related stress in families of children with intellectual disability and developmental disability (Bristol, Gallagher, & Schopler, 1988; Konstantareas & Homatidis, 1989).

Some parents of children with disabilities can experience a particular kind of loneliness from feeling that their family is substantially different from most families and that their experiences are difficult for most people to understand. A survey study of over 2,800 parents of individuals with intellectual disability asked parents to rate items on a list of 32 kinds of services and supports by rating them on a 3-point scale as "not a problem, some problem, or a major problem." When asked how much of a problem it was "having someone to talk to that understands what I deal with," over half reported it was problematic, with 36% who said they had some problem and 25% who rated it as a major problem. They also reported problems from within the family. When asked about "getting cooperation and assistance from other family members," over half rated it as problematic, 34% reporting it was *some problem*, and 24% said it was *a major problem*. Given the need and its importance, it is not surprising that parents of children with disabilities connect with one another and provide mutual support (Santelli, Turnbull, Marquis, & Lerner, 1995).

One form of informal support that has been popular among parents of children with disabilities in the United States is informal social support from peers obtained through parent support groups and Parent to Parent (P2P) volunteer programs emphasizing one-to-one links between a helping parent and a parent seeking help. Peer support offers social provisions that are qualitatively different from those available from professionals and family members. Parent to Parent programs have arisen from the grassroots beginning in 1980 in a program in Omaha, Nebraska. By 2014, there were P2P programs in most states in the United States and in several nations around the globe. The core function of P2P is to match a help-seeking parent with an experienced parent who has volunteered to be on call to serve as a resource to others. The experienced parents receive several hours of training with a focus on family adaptation and listening skills. Over the past decade, a national umbrella organization, P2PUSA, has been established through volunteer efforts of grassroots leaders from state and local organizations. It maintains a directory of state programs, offers technical assistance to new and emergent programs, and brings grassroots leaders together for national meetings. It maintains a website that provides a map with contact information for programs in every region of the country (see www.P2PUSA.org).

Typically, in P2P group interventions, groups of 8 to 12 parents meet once a week for 6 to 8 weeks. The meetings are structured and run by professionals who discussed coping skills and stress management.

Parent to Parent programs maintain a list of parents who want to serve as volunteers to provide one-to-one emotional and informational support to parents who contact the program asking for assistance with a problem. Volunteers are trained to cover a broad spectrum of concerns including parents' feelings of isolation, requests for information about community resources, help with navigating complex or recalcitrant bureaucracies, and troubles with spouses or siblings of children with disabilities. One-to-one contacts can occur as few as a one-time-only phone call to many and frequent contacts over a long period of time. When new relationships are established, they may evolve into long-term mentoring or friendships.

Parent to Parent programs have been described in considerable detail in books and journal articles (Santelli et al., 1995; Santelli, Turnbull, Marquis, & Lerner, 1997; Santelli et al., 1996). In a randomized controlled study of P2P programs in six states in the United States (Singer et al., 1999), parents were randomly assigned to either a treatment group ($n = 56$) or a waiting list control group ($n = 72$). The average ages of the children with disabilities were 6.9 years in the treatment group and 7.7 in the control group. In the treatment group, 5.5% were African American, 3.5% Latino, and 91% Anglo-Caucasian. Parents in the treatment group called participating P2P programs in their area. Once they chose to enroll in the study, they received a packet of measures in the mail and again 2 months after contacting a helping parent. The outcomes measured were cognitive adaptation, parenting efficacy, empowerment, and progress toward solving a current problem. The measure used to determine whether P2P promoted positive cognitive adaptation was the Source of Strength and Family Closeness scale of the Kansas Inventory of Parent's Perceptions (KIPP; Behr, Murphy, & Summers, 1992). The 7-item scale measured positive attitudes about the child with a disability and impact on the family. For example, two items about parental attitudes asked parents the extent of their agreement with the statement, "I am more accepting of things" and "I am grateful for each day." Two items about family attitudes and adjustment stated: "My family has become closer because of a child with a disability" and "We are more in charge of ourselves as a family." The measure of empowerment was the Family Empowerment Scale (Koren, DeChillo, & Friesen, 1992). It consists of three scales, the first measures a sense of empowerment in caring for one's family, the second tests empowerment vis-à-vis the service system, and the third measures empowerment as expressed through community and political participation. The Parent Coping Efficacy Scale (Blanchard, Powers, Ginsberg, Marquis, & Singer, 1996) was used to assess whether or not being matched with another parent influenced the sense of coping efficacy as a parent. The measure was made by the researchers on this multisite study. The 24-item measure has two scales, one measuring efficacy in dealing with family needs and the other, efficacy in caring for the family. The scales ask parents about how capable they have felt in the past week at several parenting tasks. For example, one item asked, "Over the past week how capable have you felt in dealing with your child's day care or childcare needs?" The Family Scale asked about the parent's sense of competence at caring for the family as a whole. The final measure asked parents to rate the extent to which they had made progress in dealing with the problem that first brought them to contact P2P.

After being matched with an experienced parent for 2 months, there were significant positive effects on the KIPP subscale with an effect size *d* of 0.25. For parents who entered the study with a low sense of parenting efficacy, significant differences were found using the PCES. There were no significant differences pre and post between the two groups on the measure of empowerment. When the treatment and control groups were compared on an indicator of progress addressing a problem, the treatment group was significantly higher than the control group with an effect size of $d = 0.56$. Furthermore, Singer et al. (1999) found that over 80% of the participants in peer support programs rated them as helpful and reported making progress with the initial problem, which motivated them to contact the P2P program, compared with little or no such progress in the waiting list control group.

Qualitative interviews have also been used to learn why parents believed P2P was effective or ineffective (Ainbinder et al., 1998). Four reasons for its success with parents who rated it as very helpful were: (1) perceived sameness of experience, (2) comparable situations for learning relevant skills and gathering useful information, (3) the ready availability of support, and (4) the mutuality of support. Parents were quite elegant in explaining their positive experiences. For example, the mother of a child with intellectual disability who has behavior problems found that her matched parent was not judgmental and seemed to understand her experiences. She stated,

> There's a compassion there and there's still an outpouring of love instead of a label and just annoyance that she (the daughter) is disrupting them in some manner, and it doesn't feel like their eyes (strangers) are boring in on you.... And then once you pass through it (a difficult flare up of problem behavior), they're there to put their arms around you and just (say) "that was a rough one." (p. 103)

The sense that the helping parent had been through similar experiences of social judgment and the discomfort of dealing with problem behavior in a public setting made her expressions of compassion more believable to the parent who called P2P for help.

There are some problems with the rigor of this study, most particularly in its choice of measures, which had less psychometric data supporting their utility than the measures used in most of the studies in chapter 2. The authors explained that the study was conducted as participatory action research (PAR), in which P2P leaders determined the outcome measures. A replication study is needed, one in which more standard measures are used. Given some weakness in its rigor and the need for replication, we judge the practice of P2P to be promising.

FAMILY-INVOLVED STUDENT SELF-DETERMINATION PROGRAMS

As children with disabilities develop into adults, roles and responsibilities often start to shift from the parent to the individual. The individual with disability begins to make increasingly more important decisions that affect the life course. The role of advocating for support and services also often shifts from parent to the individual during these transitional times. Increasingly, self-determination has been perceived as a long-term objective for people with developmental disabilities (Developmental Disabilities Assistance and Bill of Rights Act, 2000), and has also been examined as a possible predictor for better outcomes for people with developmental disabilities (Wehmeyer & Schwartz, 1997).

The construct of self-determination has been defined as a "dispositional characteristic" rooted in the belief that the individual must "act as the primary causal agent in one's life" in order to "maintain or improve one's quality of life" (Wehmeyer, 2005, p. 117). That is, individuals are self-determined when they act according to their own will. One definitional model proposed by Wehmeyer (1997, 1999) and colleagues (Wehmeyer, Sands, Doll, & Palmer, 1997) conceptualizes self-determined behaviors as comprising the characteristics of autonomous, self-regulated, psychologically empowered, and self-realizing behaviors. Behavioral autonomy may not require total independence or absolute control in all areas of daily functioning (Wehmeyer, 1997), but it does signify that the behavior is performed without "undue external influence or interference" from others (Wehmeyer et al., 1997, p. 307). According to Wehmeyer (1997, 1999) and his colleagues (Wehmeyer et al., 1997), these four characteristics are associated with a number of component skills and attributes, such as choice making, decision-making, problem-solving, goal-setting and attainment, self-efficacy, and self-advocacy. Depending on contextual variables, these self-determination characteristics may be expressed differently.

Another important theme in self-determination definitions is the pervasive influence of the environment (Trainor, 2002). All settings within an individual's life may have some impact on one's self-determination, but one critical environmental factor to consider is the child's family. Although self-determination stresses autonomous behavior, interdependence is increasingly recognized as a positive outcome for individuals with disabilities, and that some influence from family members is natural and acceptable (Wehmeyer, 1997), especially if it motivates further growth in individuals making decisions in their own lives. Research has discussed the influence of family characteristics on the development of self-determination (Brotherson, Cook, Erwin, & Weigel, 2008), though not all studies have found that family demographics (e.g., socioeconomic status or racial-ethnic group) relate to self-determination capacity or opportunities (Carter, Owens, Trainor, Sun, & Swedeen, 2009). The home context may also matter because family members can serve as role models for students in the application of self-determination skills (Field & Hoffman, 2002).

The literature has consistently linked self-determination skills with improved academic and life outcomes for individuals with disabilities (Field & Hoffman, 2002; Wehmeyer & Palmer, 2003; Wehmeyer & Schwartz, 1998). Consequently, strategies and interventions have been developed to guide professionals to better promote self-determination in youths with developmental disabilities. Scholars encourage families to use specific techniques to support engagement, autonomy, and choice making in young children with cognitive and physical disabilities. The instruction of daily living skills and self-management skills at home will help students become more self-sufficient, and experimental research has been done to investigate the effectiveness of this approach. Pierce and Schreibman (1994) found that children with autism can be taught to use pictures to learn to independently manage functional behaviors (e.g., setting the table, making lunch, doing laundry, getting dressed) in home settings. A greater number of interventions have been developed to teach self-determination skills in the school setting with older children. A few such programs include the family and community as critical components. Powers, Turner, Ellison, and colleagues (2001) promoted a multiple component model, TAKE CHARGE for the Future to enhance student involvement in planning their own transition into adulthood. The intervention included activities in the student's school, at home, and in the community. In a randomized controlled trial field test of this intervention, 20 adolescents with physical disabilities and chronic health conditions between the ages of 12 and 18 participated. Of the participants, eight were also identified as having intellectual disabilities. Participants were randomly assigned to the intervention or the waitlist comparison group.

The field test of Powers, Turner, Ellison, and colleagues' (2001) program consisted of four intervention components implemented over 5 months. In the first component, an individual, 50-minute, weekly coaching session was delivered to students assigned to the intervention group. At these sessions, coaches helped students develop short-term, activity-based goals, come up with solutions to attain goals, and prepare for actual goal achievement. The second component of the program involved community activities that mentors share with the youths, such as applying for vocational rehabilitation services, visiting the mentor's college or workplace, or doing recreational activities. Mentors were adults with disabilities from the community, who represented role models for the youths and were matched to individual students based on gender, interests, and similarities in disability. These workshops provided an opportunity for students, parents, and mentors to discuss topics related to high school, supports and services in college, employment, personal finances, and independent living. The third element was monthly community-based workshops for the students, parents, and mentors. The fourth component was telephone and home visit support for parents. Parents not only received a TAKE CHARGE for the Future guide but also received information about their children's progress and ideas about strategies through phone communication with the intervention coaches. The parent support coordinator of the program also made phone calls and home visits to provide emotional support and community resource information. Significant differences in the improvement of outcomes overtime were found between the treatment and the waitlist control group in Powers, Turner, Ellison, and colleagues' (2001) study. Students in the TAKE CHARGE for the Future intervention group made significant gains in measures of adolescent empowerment, personal adjustment, and level of personal accomplishment. However, no significant differences between groups were found for student self-efficacy. Still, the effects of this intervention showed immense positive gains in many of the characteristics and components elements of self-determination.

In another randomized, controlled trial study evaluating TAKE CHARGE for the Future, Powers, Turner, Westwood, et al. (2001) solicited the participation of four high schools across four US states. Forty-three adolescents, age 14 to 17, were recruited from these sites and were randomly assigned to the intervention or the waitlist control group. The students represented a wide range of disabilities (i.e., learning disability, orthopedic disability, multiple disabilities, emotional disability, and health impairment). A fifth component added to the model was an in-service education for the transition school staff. Intervention results of the Powers, Turner, Westwood, and colleagues (2001) project were once again positive. Youth involvement in transition planning was measured by a researcher-developed scale and direct observations of student participation in transition meetings. Awareness of transition planning requirements and resources was assessed in parents and students. Lastly, a family empowerment measure evaluated how much students accessed services and advocated on behalf of others. There were significant differences between the intervention and control groups over the time period of the study in student educational planning, student empowerment, parent educational planning, parent transition awareness, and educator educational planning. The results also indicated that treatment effect sizes were all least moderate (all < 0.40). During transition planning meetings, the intervention group demonstrated more engaged and responsive behavior than students, parents, and staff in the control group. While these results pertained to students without developmental disabilities in this second study, that the results were positive for students with histories of behavioral problems is encouraging.

The work of Powers and her colleagues is exemplary in that the intervention is thoroughly developed and explained in a published guide, it has been tested in the context of public school programs, and it is supported by two high-quality randomized control trials. The outcome measures used in these studies include direct observation of the kinds of behavior that self-determination programs are designed to promote and as such are highly encouraging that these skills can be taught and students motivated to implement them. To meet standards as an established intervention it needs to be replicated by an independent group and compared to another intervention. Consequently, we rate it as promising and strongly recommend that practitioners and researcher interested in this domain should value it highly.

Hoffman and Field's (1995) self-determination curriculum also included a family component. In their curriculum, *Steps to Self-Determination*, one of the important points in its design is family or friend participation and support (Hoffman & Field, 1995). For example, students are asked to invite a family member or another important adult to a workshop at the beginning of the curriculum. At the workshop, students and the adult engage in activities focusing on the "know yourself" and "value yourself" components, such as considering how the relationship between the adult and the student may change as the student becomes more self-determined (Field & Hoffman, 2002). Another way family involvement has been structured is through worksheets that parents could complete with the student, in which the responses from the worksheets are used in a later classroom activity. The *Steps to Self-Determination* curriculum was field-tested in a controlled study on a sample of students with diverse disabilities, including intellectual disabilities (Hoffman & Field, 1995). On the researcher-developed test of self-determination knowledge, the experimental group score significantly increased compared with the control group score, with an effect size of 1.02. On the Self-Determination Observation Checklist (SDOC), which is an observation checklist counting the frequency of behaviors associated with self-determination, the treatment group again showed a significant increase in desired behaviors. Involving the family not only supports students in becoming more aware of their own strengths, needs, and preferences, but also supports positive relationship-building skills, such as accessing resources and negotiating with others, which are important as students become more independent. The curriculum showed tremendous promise; however, there are limited empirical studies that demonstrate the program's effectiveness since this initial field test.

In another study, Wehmeyer et al. (2013) conducted a randomized, control-group, longitudinal study using a menu of interventions to evaluate their efficacy on overall self-determination skills, with some of the interventions expecting parent participation. In this 5-year longitudinal study, 50 high schools were randomly assigned to either a control group or to the treatment group. In the treatment group, teachers at the school were able to select from a list of intervention options (i.e., *ChoiceMaker Curriculum, Self-Advocacy Strategy, Steps to Self-Determination, Whose Future Is It Anyway?* and *NEXT S.T.E.P. Curriculum*) a program that they think is most suitable for their classroom and best serves their students. Additionally, all teachers were trained to implement an additional intervention model, the self-determined learning model of instruction (SDLMI). The SDLMI is a teaching model consisting of three phases that, with some support from parents, guide students to set their own learning goal, take action in completing that goal, adjust their goal, or plan their action (Wehmeyer, Palmer, Agran, Mithaug, & Martin, 2000). A quasi-experimental study of South Korean students with autism showed that the SDLMI is associated with gains in language attainment and in more self-regulated learning behaviors (Kim & Park, 2012).

The 371 students in Wehmeyer et al.'s (2013) study had either intellectual disability (28%) or learning disability (72%). Student participants were assessed on two self-determination measures: the ARC's Self-Determination Scale (SDS; Wehmeyer & Kelchner, 1995), which examines the different components of self-determination, and the AIR Self-Determination Scale (AIR-S; Wolman, Campeau, Dubois, Mithaug, &

Stolarski, 1994), which measures capacity and opportunity for self-determination. Results showed that the intervention group experienced significantly more positive increases in capacity and opportunity for self-determination over the duration of their program. Interestingly, the only intervention group that experienced significantly greater increases in self-determination (SDS scores) over time was students with intellectual disabilities. The rate of growth in self-determination scores was similar between intervention and control groups for students with a learning disability. The authors proposed that self-determination interventions do significantly help short-term changes in skills, attitudes, and opportunities for self-determination (AIR-S scores). While some of the interventions made available for selection do include a parental involvement component (i.e., *Steps to Self-Determination, NEXT S.T.E.P. Curriculum,* and SDLMI), the control group was also administered a training pertaining to parent involvement, which may negate any potential effects of parental involvement in the experimental group. It is unclear whether the combination of parent involvement with the self-determination curricula made an impact on self-determination. Further research into the effects of different components (e.g., parent-involvement vs. non-parent-involvement) may be helpful in answering this question.

Youth at all age ranges with various developmental disabilities have been found to benefit from programs that support self-determination component skills. Still, no studies conducted follow-up measures to assess whether the gains from the intervention were short-term or more permanent. Scholars could only speculate that the effects would persist (Wehmeyer et al., 2013), but future studies could examine whether improvements in self-determination would maintain. Moreover, one of the main purposes of self-determination is to enable students and their significant others to voice their background, point-of-view, interests, dreams, and goals. Since new technology is increasingly used as a prominent mode of communication, it would be helpful for students to access these tools to develop and exercise their self-determination skills. Skouge and colleagues (2007) encouraged the use of new technologies for youths with developmental disabilities to look critically at his or her environment, supports, and needs, to establish future plans based on this examination, and to communicate his or her story to the family, school personnel, community members, and friends at transition meetings. However, limited studies have examined the impact of technology on students' self-determination. Future interventions must consider incorporating new media to promote self-determination in youths with developmental disabilities.

When taken as a whole, the literature on promoting self-determination skills in adolescents with disabilities is encouraging. Although the practices differ in specifics, they share a sufficient family of practices that we believe they warrant an overall evaluation as a group. Interventions reported here have been supported by adequate RCT studies and we thus rate self-determination programs that include parent involvement as established practices.

INDIVIDUALIZED EDUCATION PROGRAM INTERVENTIONS TO INCREASE PARENT PARTICIPATION

The bulk of the literature on self-determination interventions focuses on helping students develop more agency in the IEP process. Family engagement is required in the IEP process for students with developmental disabilities, yet parents sometimes judge the act of guiding planning activities to attain goals to be exclusively the role of teachers and the school (Zhang, Wehmeyer, & Chen, 2005). Still more barriers to parent involvement in the IEP process have been acknowledged and summarized by scholars. Mitchell, Morton, and Hornby's (2010) review pinpointed common obstacles discussed in the IEP literature: (1) the scheduling of IEP meetings at inconvenient times for parents, (2) the transportation and childcare needs of parents, (3) the poor seating arrangement and lack of privacy in IEP meeting settings, (4) teachers' use of technical language that alienates parents, and (5) the lack of cultural sensitivity of school staff. These barriers may perhaps explain why 20% to 27% of parents have been found to be dissatisfied with their IEP experiences (Fish, 2008; Garriott, Wandry, & Snyder, 2001).

Scholars and innovative school personnel have also presented strategies to counteract these obstacles to effective parent participation, most of which are similar to approaches that encourage overall family–school collaboration. For instance, schools can maintain good working relationships with parents, develop IEP manuals for parents, communicate to parents prior to the meeting about student progress, hold pre-IEP meetings to discuss their thoughts about their child's needs, arrange for childcare and transportation for the IEP meeting, provide language interpreters, and employ nontechnical language (Mitchell et al., 2010). Families have also advocated for teachers and school staff to adhere more closely to IEP protocol and have suggested more parent education on special education law as ways to improve IEP meetings (Fish, 2008).

There is an immense need for interventions to promote parental and student control in the IEP meetings; however, only a handful of programs have been developed to encourage parents' contribution to meetings. A recent study evaluated the effectiveness of a specific IEP development program targeting families of children with autism. The Collaborative Model for Promoting Competence and Success (COMPASS) approach focuses on promoting collaboration between school personnel and parents when generating interventions (Ruble et al., 2010). As this approach has been specifically developed for the population of children with autism, it emphasizes acquisition of functional skills (i.e., social skills, communication, and independence) and accompanying environmental supports to prevent problem behaviors. COMPASS is implemented within the context of the child's existing IEP development, implementation, and evaluation process. For Ruble et al.'s (2010) controlled, randomized group study, 35 special education teachers, a randomly selected child (ages 3 to 8) with autism from each class, the target student's parents or caregivers, and special education directors participated. First, parents completed consultation assessment forms that identified teachers' and parents' concerns. Then, parents, teachers, and consultants gathered in an initial consultation to discuss general background information about COMPASS. Team members then translated the concerns from the assessment forms into IEP goals that fit the functional skill domains COMPASS targets. Following the development of objectives in the three targeted skill areas, consultants worked with teachers to develop teaching plans for those objectives. Consultants also made visits to classrooms to observe, coach, and evaluate teachers' instruction of these IEP objectives, with summaries of these visits made available to teachers and parents. Parents and teachers reported on intervention fidelity and satisfaction during the last stage of consultation. The results from the study indicated that COMPASS intervention teachers had significantly higher goal attainment progress than did nonintervention teachers ($d = 1.0$). The authors also found that ratings of teachers' adherence to coaching recommendations positively correlated with goal attainment progress ($r = .589$). IEPs were also of higher quality ($d = 0.81$), and teacher satisfaction with intervention was high. A major component of this program was joint parent–teacher planning, including meetings to work together on assessment and goal development.

The few interventions that seek to improve parent involvement at IEP meetings include a randomized controlled trial study by Goldstein and Turnbull (1982), which tested two intervention strategies. In one treatment group, 15 parents of elementary-age children with disabilities were provided questions before the IEP conference about their child's educational goals, academic potential, and the development of an IEP. The second treatment group consisted of 15 parents, whose IEP meetings were joined by a school counselor acting in the role of parent advocate. These counselors asked parents and other IEP committee members questions, verbally reinforced parental responses, and summarized the discussion at the end of the conference. Lastly, another group of 15 parents served as the control group, which received treatment as usual. The outcomes of the study suggested that parents were significantly more likely to offer input and make comments with the presence of a parent advocate at the meeting, compared with the control group. Goldstein and Turnbull's investigation highlighted that changing the way school professionals treated parents at IEP conferences could elicit more parental involvement.

Similarly, Brinckerhoff and Vincent's (1986) study demonstrated that a short training of parents of children with disabilities and school/community liaisons can considerably change IEP meeting interactions. School and community liaisons were trained individually by researchers to teach six families in the experimental group to document daily family routines as a way to provide more information to IEP teams about family activities, family functioning, and quality of home interactions. Moreover, liaisons were trained to teach treatment parents to informally assess the development and adaptive skills of their children. Before students' IEP meetings, liaisons met with treatment parents to complete these two tasks. As further preparation, liaisons discussed the purpose of the IEP meeting, the procedures of an IEP, the role of various IEP team members, and the role the prior activities had in the IEP meeting. Parents who were randomly assigned to the control group did not receive this training. Compared with this control group, treatment parents were observed to contribute more to IEP meetings, to make more decisions, and to generate more goals, while school IEP team members made fewer decisions. In addition, joint decisions made by parents and school staff increased in frequency for the experimental group in comparison with the control group.

Person-centered planning is another example of transition-planning process that seeks to maximize student and family participation and input during IEP and transition planning meetings. Miner and Bates (1997) examined the relationship between the implementation of person-centered planning and parents' contribution to transitions and IEP meetings, satisfaction with meeting process, and outcomes. In this study, 22 high school students with intellectual disabilities and their families were randomly assigned to either the person-centered planning intervention or to a control group condition. Students and families acknowledged individuals in the student's life that could be a source of support of the student, identified community settings in which these supports or opportunities for independence may take place, recognized things that work or fail to work for the individual, and enumerated the strengths of the student. A vision of the student's future, his or her goals, and a plan to attain these goals were then drafted with the input of the participants. Three outcome measures were assessed in Miner and Bates's (1997) project, including direct observation of the frequency and content of parent input, satisfaction with the meeting immediately post-meeting, and satisfaction with meeting outcomes 2 months after the intervention. Intervention families were found to speak more often than control families, yet there were no statistical differences between the two groups in terms of percentage of time postschool issues were discussed and in terms of postmeeting satisfaction. This suggests that one person-centered planning meeting may not immediately increase future-oriented discussions. However, parent satisfaction was significantly higher in the intervention group compared with the control group 2 months post-intervention. A larger study on the effects of person-centered planning was conducted by Hagner and colleagues (2012). This randomized controlled trial intervention examined how person-centered planning may influence the self-determination of students with autism, based on *Specific Planning Encourages Creative Solutions* curriculum (SPECS). Those students and families who received person-centered planning training scored significantly higher in the student expectations for the future and parent expectations for the future over time. Their scores on the standardized Arc Self-Determination Scale and the standardized Vocational Decision-Making Interview-Revised also showed that treatment group students significantly improved on overall self-determination skills and on decision career decision-making ability. This study further suggested the potential of a person-centered planning intervention with family engagement.

A criticism of person-centered planning, which can be equally levied toward IEP interventions in general, has been discussed in the literature. Kim and Turnbull (2004) observed, "Typically, person-centered planning approaches have focused almost exclusively on promoting the quality of life of the individual with the disability, only indirectly addressing the family's quality of life as a priority outcome" (p. 55). Too often, IEP interventions only target students' and school staff's behaviors, overlooking the possibility of promoting a dynamic exchange and joint collaboration among parents, students, and other IEP team members. They also seem to ignore the possibility that school services can directly enhance the quality of home life by teaching students skills that are helpful at home and in the community and by promoting community participation in ways that are valued in families' cultural and social class niches. Paralleling the points raised by Burke (2013) regarding parent advocacy training, scholars are calling for more holistic considerations of the effect of intervention. Kim and Turnbull proposed that a person–family interdependent model be developed as a new approach to enhancing the quality of life for both the individual and the family. Their orientation is based on the premise that families—while being a resource for the individual—have needs, values, and preferences that should be considered as well. For IEPs, and especially transition IEPs, to truly support students in reaching their goals, Kim and Turnbull call for more comprehensive policies and programs that address families' social and emotional needs, as well as financial limitations.

SUMMARY AND CONCLUSIONS

In this chapter, we discussed the importance of enabling parents of individuals with developmental disabilities to advocate for their families and to access the support they need. We also described various parent advocacy and self-help programs that have been developed over the past few decades. Among these programs are interventions that seek to promote productive and harmonious partnerships between families and the school. Though, as many parents of children with disabilities can attest to, even with the advent of home–school collaboration programs, harmonious partnerships do not always take place. Therefore, parents must also be ready to inhabit the role of advocates; interventions have been created to help parents navigate the school and service systems. Peer parent programs have also become more common, offering a method of informal support to families. Still, parents of children with disabilities will one day become parents of adults with disabilities. Self-determination interventions reflect a growing movement to transfer the role of primary decision-maker and advocate from parent to the individual. The IEP meeting can be a great site for that transfer, and so programs that enhance child and family participation in the IEP process will ultimately empower families.

When examining the 16 studies of these parent advocacy and self-help programs, we find that the level of evidence for their efficacy varies depending on the type of program. For programs that promote family-involved self-determination, the three randomized trial studies, (Powers, Turner, Ellison, et al., 2001; Powers, Turner, Westwood, et al., 2001; Wehmeyer et al., 2013), two quasi-experimental studies (Hoffman & Field, 1995; Kim & Park, 2012), and one single-subject design study (Pierce & Schreibman, 1994) suggest that these programs are established practices. The IEP intervention with family involvement, with three randomized trial studies

(Brinckerhoff & Vincent, 1986; Ruble et al., 2010) and one quasi-experimental design study (Miner & Bates, 1997), also qualifies as an established practice. Similarly, home–school collaboration interventions present strong evidence as an established practice, with two randomized controlled trial studies (Chadwick et al., 2001; Stormshak et al., 2010), one single-subject design study (Blair et al., 2011), and one synthesis of single-subject studies (Sheridan et al., 2001). The one randomized controlled trial P2P study (Singer et al., 1999) demonstrates the promise of the peer support model; this intervention type would benefit from replication to be judged as established. Finally, as its one randomized trial (Buelow et al., 2013) showed little to no effect, parent advocacy training's evidence stems from one single-subject study (Baker & Brightman, 1984), and is therefore still yet to be a proven practice. This latter model deserves further investigation and demonstration of its efficacy.

7

BARRIERS AND FACILITATORS FOR IMPLEMENTATION OF EVIDENCE-BASED PRACTICES

GOING TO SCALE

George H. S. Singer and Mian Wang

Studies of implementation suggest a model in which there are predictable stages of development from early discovery of a practice through its use as standard practice on a broad scale. It is an idealized model useful for organizing complex observations and findings, but not an exact road map. The model is as follows: At first, applied research undergoes a period of discovery and development in which new practices are defined and revised through small-scale studies in controlled settings. Once the practice has emerged as a definite set of processes, it can be field-tested under semicontrolled circumstances. At this early stage, the goal is to establish the efficacy of a new practice. Efficacy in this context is a term for "successful working" under controlled or partly controlled conditions. These first two steps are usually undertaken by university-based researchers with grant funds that are used to study and support a new practice. Research studies from university-based researchers can resemble hothouse plants. They are often grown under carefully controlled circumstances and are tended to in detail and with great care. Initial research is usually supported with grant funds, which may or may not reflect available funding in the community where the new practices are ultimately to be used. The level of care with which interventions are developed and evaluated in academia is difficult to replicate later in applied settings, so that there may be a decline in fidelity or adherence to the practices as originally designed. Much of the published academic research is conducted by advanced graduate students who are highly motivated and energetic. Again, the level of dedication they bring to implementing research in the early stages of determining efficacy is difficult to replicate later under community conditions.

The "hothouse" environment in universities gives way to augmented field sites in the next stage of development. The original researchers try out the new practice in model sites, such as model schools or local social services staffed by recent university graduates from the institution originating the new practices. The host organization might receive additional resources from the researchers via grants. In a next step, the practice may be studied under more typical conditions. This process often takes several years or longer until its claims for efficacy are supported with adequate evidence.

If the new practice continues to do what it was designed to do and the developers continue to garner resources to keep the development process going, it may then begin to be taken up by others under less-supported and often very different conditions. Ideally, controlled evaluation research is conducted too at this stage, when the people who implement the program are the "real-world" practitioners who practice it in the classrooms, homes, clinics, or community settings where it is meant to be helpful. In the best of circumstances, large randomized trials are conducted. For example, schools or school districts may be randomly assigned to two groups, one which continues with business as usual, the other which implements the new practice with technical assistance from the developers.

Sometimes developers at this stage are able to spin off a separate small organization dedicated to disseminating a practice by training and supporting practitioners and the organizations where they work. When there is sufficient evidence that the practice works as planned in many varied conditions, it may be claimed to be effective. "Effective" in this usage means that research verifies that a practice works successfully in "the real world" on a large scale. The standards for evidence to support a claim of effectiveness have yet to be developed or are not yet agreed on in education, psychology, and medicine. Social scientists at present are still learning to accept and use new guidelines for establishing effectiveness.

One de facto way that has emerged to determine whether a new practice is effective is via synthesis of the evaluation research. Meta-analyses have become common tools for defending or rejecting claims for effectiveness at this point in development and dissemination of interventions. This kind of literature review, meta-analysis, combines the findings from many studies in order to characterize the average strength of the intervention and to determine whether variables that moderate effectiveness can be identified.

In the final stage, effective practices become standard practices in a profession and service system. If the new practice continues to hold promise as a way to successfully address an important social problem, it may be funded to be implemented in several sites over time, on a large scale and in many places, ideally helping many people. This stage requires that practices be sustainable and be taken up and taught as part of professional training in the relevant field. Of the practices we have reviewed, behavioral parent training (BPT) and cognitive-behavioral therapy (CBT) have become standard practice. Unlike BPT, interventions based on CBT are standard practices for treating many different mental health problems. However, they are not widely available as standard practice by social service agencies for parents of children with disabilities. In some states the service system has not been designed to provide assistance to families. We hope that the evidence presented in this book might help to encourage DD services to make group CBT programs available to parents. Behavioral parent training and its relative, positive behavior support (PBS), are used widely in DD services, early childhood special education and early intervention, and special education programs. The BPT programs are usually implemented by behavior analysts, who increasingly are required to have higher education training at a master's degree level, undergo an extended supervised internship, and to pass an examination before attaining a certification as a board certified behavior analyst. Additionally, special educators in the United States are taught to implement PBS and to teach others to use behavioral methods. They also are required to meet standards set by the state departments of education and the federal law, the IDEA. For both behavior analysts and special educators, knowledge of behavioral practices is required.

Not all practices follow a trajectory through the stages we have described in order to become validated and taken up on a large scale. Some are first created and practiced outside of the formal research/service system. Parent to Parent (P2P) programs have gone to scale and have become available in most states in the United States. They have proven to be sustainable and have established standard practices for training and maintaining quality. We rated P2P as a promising practice that is supported by evidence from one randomized trial. Before P2P can be claimed to be an established intervention, P2P programs will require at least one more randomized trial comparing P2P with another effective practice. Parent to Parent was created outside of the system of universities and the domain of funded research. It has been a grassroots program developed at first informally, often on a very small scale, and it has gradually grown into a valuable resource available to thousands of families. It has been specifically focused on serving families of children with disabilities based on self-help principles.

In this book, we set out to see what practices can be said to have efficacy in supporting families of children from early childhood through adulthood who experience intellectual disability (ID) or autism. We followed a set of standards that have been agreed on by Division 12 of the American Psychiatric Association and the Council for Exceptional Children for experimental group comparison research and single-subject design (SSD) research. We have presented evidence for supporting a claim that a number of practices can be considered as having efficacy at least for White Anglo mothers in the short term. Although they meet standards for efficacy and show up as reasonably strong in meta-analyses, these practices are not yet widely available for families of children with disabilities in many parts of the country. The availability of family support services varies according to state policies and the funding for the DD system. In urban areas, parents can usually find behavior analysts who accept insurance or private payments for teaching parents skills for interacting positively with their children. These parent training programs are not, however, routinely available through early intervention and public school special education programs and availability is often limited to upper-middle- and upper-class families.

LIMITATIONS IN THE EFFICACY RESEARCH

Practices that are efficacious do not always become effective. Sometimes the problems that impede implementation grow out of gaps in the original knowledge base about new practices. An initial problem with going to scale is posed by limitations in the knowledge base around family support interventions. Some of these limitations include a relatively small number of randomized controlled trials (RCT) with small numbers of subjects for most practices, the paucity of detailed treatment manuals to guide replications, the lack of evidence about long-term or even middle-term outcomes, and limitations in the representativeness of the participants in evaluation studies compared with contemporary demographics of the US population. Of particular concern is the relatively small number of participants in the studies we have reviewed who live near or below the poverty line or who come from nonmajority ethnic groups. One assured conclusion from our review of these studies is that systematic replication research with larger and more diverse samples in RCT and SSD studies is vital to continuing development and acceptance of the evidence-based practice (EBP) movement in DDs. While researchers have come a long way in learning how to assist families, the United States is at an early stage of creating a service system which provides EBPs as standard practice.

THE NEED FOR RESEARCH ON FAMILIES LIVING IN POVERTY

Researchers have been better at identifying the conditions that increase suffering in homes than in the more recent effort to understand the contributors to salutatory outcomes. From four decades of research we know that those conditions that reduce the quality of life for all families increase stress in families of children with disabilities. Poverty is perhaps the largest of these negative conditions. Fujiura and Yamaki (2000) found that 26% of children with disabilities lived in poverty compared with 16% of children without disabilities. Rates of disability are elevated in low-income families for a variety of reasons. These include limited access to healthcare and adequate nutrition, dangerous housing in unsafe neighborhoods, racism, threats to adequate mother–child interactions in the development of language, higher exposure to environmental toxins, and elevated birth rates in the low-income population of teenage single mothers, to name a few of the pressures in the ecological niche many such families occupy.

In the United States, poverty is associated with elevated vulnerability for families of children with and without disabilities (Park, Turnbull, & Turnbull, 2002). The social safety net for US families has been weakened so that low-income and impoverished families bear the brunt of both large-scale and local destructive forces and events. These ecological forces include the erosion of the job market for decently paid low-skill employment: economic recessions, war, extreme weather events and other natural disasters, reductions in support programs (e.g., long-term unemployment insurance and food stamps), dangerous neighborhoods, and low achieving schools. These have impacts that amplify stress in caregiving families.

Given the impact of poverty and low income on families, an important missing facet of the research reviewed in this book is demonstrations of effective programs for these families. There are a few exceptions, such as the Triple P Parenting program, the problem-solving program evaluated by Berry, Elliott, Grant, Edwards, and Fine (2012), Project CLUES (2012), and Phillips (1999) sibling support intervention, but overall, little is known about the efficacy of these treatments for low-income families. Similarly, the evidence base of studies with participants who come from linguistic and ethnic minorities in the United States is very limited. As a result, one barrier to large-scale implementation of EBPs is limited evidence for generalization to the full range of families in need of support. Researchers who have worked with low-income families of children with disabilities have stressed the importance of multiple component intervention packages capable of addressing interfamily problems that interfere with BPT (Lutzker & Campbell, 1994). These include elevated depressive symptoms and other mental health problems in mothers, marital discord in two-parent families, substance abuse disorders, and behavior problems of nondisabled adolescent siblings. In order for parents to engage in parent training and implement positive parenting methods, they may need support to counter some of these contextual problems. Treatments for these problems have been conceptualized as adjunctive treatments needed to support BPT. However, in some families these treatments may well be primary, whereas parenting skills are of less concern.

Early intervention programs have been addressing complex needs in multiply stressed families for many years. Those home-visiting programs and center-based programs that have been effective for young children and their families ought to be evaluated experimentally when modified and extended to families of older children. Successful supports for families over longer periods of time may require extending family-centered care from early childhood to junior and senior high school in public school systems (Dunst, 2002).

LACK OF REPRESENTATIVE EVIDENCE

With a few exceptions, the research that we have reviewed does not represent the makeup of the contemporary United States. A majority of the studies did not report any data on the ethnicity of the participants; out of 98 studies, only 31 reported on race and/or ethnicity. The demographic makeup of the United States has changed remarkably over the past 30 years. The two-parent families who were most often represented in earlier research make up a substantially smaller proportion of families in the contemporary United States. The diversity of family forms that has proliferated is gradually being met with acceptance. Children with disabilities are now growing up in single-parent mother-led households and single-parent father-led households. They live with same-sex parents, in recombined families, and in millions of documented and undocumented immigrant families.

In 2010 over a third of all households with children were headed by single mothers with roughly half of this group cohabiting with a partiner but unmarried (Cherlin, 2010). Most of them were employed or looking for work while raising children. Simultaneously a growing percentage of families were responsible for providing care to elderly family members. A dual caregiving role is becoming commonplace as the baby boomer generation ages and parents of children with disabilities are called on to provide support for both children with disabilities and aging parents. As we have pointed out elsewhere, if the United States hopes to adequately address the needs of its elderly and its citizens with disabilities, it will need to embrace public policies that are more supportive of family caregiving for family member with disabilities regardless of the nature of their cause (Singer, Biegel, & Ethridge, 2010).

The change in the ethnic makeup of the US population has shifted to such an extent that White Anglo citizens are expected to become a minority by the middle of the 21st century. In California as of 2014, there was no longer a single majority ethnic group served by the public schools, and over 100 different languages were spoken there. The percentage of citizens who were Latinos in 2010 was 16.9%, Asian 3.6%, and African American, 12.1%. Nationally, 60.5 million people reported speaking a language other than English at home.

Culture has a pervasive effect on all aspects of family life. Families define who is a member differently across cultures and who is responsible for child rearing. Definitions and beliefs about disability are also diverse. For example, traditionally Mexican and Central American immigrants did not have a word for mild ID, which was thought of as a condition experienced by only those with the most severe disabilities. Ideas about authority figures, relationships with professionals, and the overlap of home and school life are subject to great variation. Whether or not people find it appropriate to share their problems with a group or with anyone outside of the family also varies. Whether help seeking and help receiving are viewed as a normal part of social life or as humiliating and a source of shame is another cultural construct. Given its profound impact on human thought, emotion, and behavior, it is somewhat surprising to find that studies of how to provide support to diverse families are rare in the literature we have reviewed. At this point, the experience and craft knowledge of many practitioners has far outrun the knowledge gathered in the research literature. This limitation in formal knowledge can make dissemination and implementation of EBPs difficult at best with a large percentage of families in the United States.

PROBLEMS IN RECRUITING AND RETAINING SUBJECTS IN EFFICACY STUDIES

Another threat to generalization of effective treatments is evidence of low levels of response to recruitment and a failure of many participants to complete some of the programs. Durand et al. reported that of 54 families who entered his study, 35 completed the eight session treatments, a drop-out rate of roughly one out of three parents (35% noncompleters, 65% completed the treatments). Durand specifically recruited pessimistic parents who would be more likely to drop out, so this level of attrition may be elevated. Nonetheless, these completion levels are comparable to those in other parent psychoeducational programs for parents of troubled children without disabilities (Roberts, Mazzucchelli, Studman, & Sanders, 2006). Singer, Goldberg-Hamblin, Peckham-Hardin, Barry, and Santarelli (2002) aggregated several studies that presented data on attrition. They calculated that fewer than half of the parents who have been contacted initially to participate in studies actually enroll, see the program through, and learn enough to implement practices accurately. If correct, this means that to be effective on a larger scale these problems in foundational research will need to be overcome.

LACK OF KNOWLEDGE ABOUT LONG-TERM EFFECTS

A further limitation in the evidence supporting the treatments reviewed is the relatively short-term duration of the evaluations. Only a handful of studies conducted follow-up assessments beyond 3 to 6 months post treatment. Kirkham (1993) and Lucyshyn, Albin, Horner, Mann, and Wadsworth (2007) were exceptions; they assessed at follow-ups of 2 years and 7 years respectively. In the United States 65%–85% of adult children with ID live at home well into middle age (Fujiura & Yamaki, 2000) and family members often remain committed to supporting adults with disabilities lifelong. Interventions with 3-month follow-ups represent a very limited period of time in comparison with the duration of caregiving over the lifespan. One encouraging example of a longer-term view of efficacy is a study by Lucyshyn et al. (2007), which reported on results of a 7-year follow-up in a case study of a child with multiple disabilities who at baseline had severe problem behaviors and whose behavior was not problematic 7 years after the initial intervention with a bundle of PBS interventions.

LIFESPAN SUPPORT

Family support over the lifespan will require services that families can call on for help as conditions in the family change over time. Family life consists of developmental processes through the life cycle. These changes continue to establish the antecedents and consequences of both adaptive and maladaptive behavior for individuals with a DD. For example, Barry and Singer (2001) documented a transactional process in which a boy with autism responded to the birth and subsequent development of a younger brother by matching problem behaviors to new steps in the infant's development. Approximately every 4 months, the infant's behavior would become more complex and independent and would afford new opportunities for the older brother to get attention by developing a new problem behavior. Each new problem also presented the opportunity for the older brother to learn new helpful ways of getting along with the baby. When the newborn brother was largely immobile, his mother sometimes put him in a portable car seat, in which he was strapped down for safety. His older brother would touch his nose to the infant's face and make loud sounds. His mother was worried this close contact, nose to nose, would give the infant a cold. She would raise her voice and scold the older brother who then increased his attempts to rub faces together. Months later, when the infant was able to stand with support in a seat on a long rope hanging from a ceiling beam, the older brother would shake the baby up and down rapidly, making him cry. Again his mother's scolding reinforced the problem behavior. Once the baby could crawl, his brother would entice him to climb stairs, which could lead to a dangerous fall. As the topography of the infant's behavior developed, his brother's problem behavior evolved in response. Barry and Singer used a self-management procedure to teach the boy with autism how to behave as a helpful older brother, coaching him to replace each new problem behavior as it appeared with appropriate and helpful interactions. The older brother kept data on his own prosocial behaviors. For this sequence it was necessary for the interventionists to return to work with the older brother on six occasions over a 26-month period. The intervention required brief instruction with the child and discussion with his mother. Over time, his mother stopped talking about putting him in foster care. In this example, the developmental dynamics were shaped by the infant's developing repertoire. Family life is ever changing though often structured by a core of routines. These culturally established patterns evolve and necessitate new family adaptations, and sometimes new forms of support or renewal of older ones.

Changing conditions can set the stage for both new problems and new opportunities to create and establish effective accommodations. In our clinical experience we have seen the need to provide brief discussions or in-home coaching when family dynamics changed over time. Research is needed that would study this kind of follow-along treatment over several years. Ideally, the original intervention would teach parents such adaptive and powerful skills that they would manage their own adaptation over time. Lucyshyn's case study demonstrated that this goal could be attained in one family for a decade. Based on clinical experience, we believe that for some families occasional coaching is necessary to help parents or other families adapt to new stages of the family lifecycle. For interventions to go to scale and to be sustained over time, research and demonstrations are needed to demonstrate long-term efficacy and effectiveness.

WE KNOW ABOUT MOTHERS, NOT FAMILIES

A stark fact about the evidence base is that most research has been centered on mothers. A small number studied supports for fathers, and fewer for siblings. We were unable to find any controlled studies of practices to support grandparents. When all of the studies we reviewed were tallied, the number of studies that include fathers were 51 out of 137 (37.22%). We were only able to identify two evaluations of supports for siblings. Family systems theory, an almost universally accepted framework in the general family literature, holds what impacts on one family member affects the other members in the family system. In the research on family support this model has yet to be validated. Little is known about how to support and strengthen the caregiving capacity of family members other than mothers. *None of the studies we judged to be eligible for review attempted to support whole families.* Researchers who have evaluated family support programs for families of individuals with severe mental illness have had more experience with whole-family interventions (McFarlane, Link, Dushay, Marchal, & Crilly, 1995). This neighboring literature may be a resource for those working with families with members who experience DDs.

LIMITATIONS IN COMMUNITY-BASED SYSTEMS OF CARE

Evidence-based practices have been and will continue to be developed and validated. In this domain, they represent a major milestone in a long-term effort to base human services on science. While this part of the research-to-practice enterprise is underway and has made considerable progress, the next stage in moving research to practice is sorely underdeveloped. Evidence-based practices require a vehicle for delivering, sustaining, and improving on them. Most of the research establishing EBPs has been conducted by university-based researchers and their doctoral students. Research-performing universities have well-worked-out systems of practice, tradition, and support to maintain a lively movement around creating and evaluating EBPs. They may be, however, a poor vehicle for translating experimental treatments into standard practices. That is, universities are rarely the sites for going from development and evaluation of interventions to delivering them with fidelity on a large scale. There have been some notable exceptions, which ought to be studied to learn what kinds of leadership, organization, funding, and evaluation is required to bring and sustain practices on a large scale.

Fixsen, Naoom, Blase, and Friedman (2005) have developed a framework for identifying common elements of implementation projects in medicine, education, and mental health systems. They point out the need for *host entities* with the capacity to learn and sustain EBPs under everyday conditions of scarce resources and competing needs. The goal of effective implementation efforts is to embed EBPs in organizations with the missions, resources, and community supports to adopt them with fidelity and to sustain their delivery over the long term. In education, the host organizations are clearly established, the public schools. In medicine, these organizational units may range in size from individual physician's practices to state and national public health programs. For some practices it may be necessary to establish new schools as in the charter school movement or to create new medical service entities such as regional health maintenance organizations.

In regard to family support programs, once children with disabilities outgrow early childhood, there is no widely established host organization for housing, providing, improving and sustaining evidence-based family supports. All states have some community-based service system for adults with DDs, although they differ widely in the scope of services they provide. Some states like New Hampshire, Massachusetts, and California have had 30 or more years of experience in establishing and maintaining community-based service systems. Others have more recently entered this arena and have lesser commitments. In some states, regional service centers contract with private providers to deliver services. Of the EBPs that we consider established, BPT is associated with the longest history of sustainable host organizations. These are usually but not always private nonprofit or for-profit professional services designed to deliver in-home behavioral treatments. They are usually staffed by at least one behavioral treatment expert with graduate-level training and paraprofessionals. Some states have been offering behavioral services since early in the history of the deinstitutionalization movement. A fundamental practice of applied behavior analysis is collecting and using treatment data based on direct observation to evaluate treatments while they are being delivered. This approach to ongoing assessment is one that other agencies and systems ought to consider, because this kind of data allows for informed decision-making during interventions. It is a key to making any particular individual application of an EBP truly evidence-based during individualized intervention.

There is presently no widespread comparable system for providing the CBT stress management treatments we have reviewed. There is such variation in service entities that the processes involved in going to scale and making EBPs standard practice will need to be extremely flexible and sufficiently robust to withstand varying levels of treatment fidelity. In some states, one of the first barriers to implementation that must be overcome to make EBPs widely available and standard practice is the need to find organizational homes for their practitioners.

Advocacy and self-help programs may be positioned to host EBPs, but presently they usually rely on private fundraising, so that may result in entities such as state-level P2P programs leading a hand-to-mouth existence. Because of federal legislation, all states have DD councils charged with assessing and addressing shortcomings in community systems. The US Department of Education has funded parent information centers, which have housed advocates in every state. An even larger system of support for advocacy and self-help consists of national organizations devoted, in part, to supporting parents in advocacy efforts. Parent to Parent programs have a presence in many parts of the country, and many disability-specific advocacy and self-help organizations have active websites where family members can acquire information, referral, and assistance with obtaining needed help.

The very fact that advocacy is so necessary attests to the limitations in the system of care. Ideally, over time there might be less need for parents to take on the role of fighting for their children's rights and for adequate family support.

PERSONNEL SHORTAGES

Another barrier to implementation is a shortage of trained personnel to provide family support. Most states currently have shortages in personnel for early intervention and special education programs. These affect every level of the personnel development system; the higher education system in the United States lacks sufficient numbers of young professors to staff special education and early intervention programs (Smith & Salzberg, 1994).

In the mental health service system, it has been recognized for many years that there are not enough trained psychologists and allied mental health professionals to meet the need for treatment. It is estimated that 40% to 50% of cases of serious mental illness go untreated partly because of the limited availability of trained personnel and because funds have not been available to millions of citizens through public or private insurance to pay for mental health treatments (Kessler et al., 2001). Stigma and the belief that services will not be helpful also contribute to this problem. At the time of writing this book, two major public policy changes offer considerable hope that over time these resource restrictions may be overcome or at least reduced. Federal law now requires insurance companies to provide parity for treatment costs with medical coverage in mental health coverage. Further, the Affordable Care Act may make such insurance available to many, although by all means not all, US citizens. Treatment for the 11 million noncitizens in the country is still problematic, a problem largely untouched by recent reforms.

WHAT WE NEED TO KNOW

Here are some research questions that need to be asked in order to establish the effectiveness of most of the practices we have reviewed. The following are important unanswered questions about BPT, PBS, CBT, stress management, and multiple program models:

Does this practice have efficacy for fathers, grandparents, and siblings?
What impacts does this practice have on the whole family?
Does this practice have efficacy for families living in the lowest quartile of the income distribution in the United States?
Does this practice have efficacy when implemented with ethnically diverse populations?
Does this practice work as well for adolescents and adults as for younger individuals with ID or DD?
How long in time do EBPs continue to be implemented and effective?

Are long-term booster sessions needed, and if so, how often should they be offered, when, and by whom?
How do these practices need to be revised as the children grow older or family conditions change?
A small group of individuals with ID or autism exhibit extreme problem behavior, which can lead to bodily harm for the interventionist, parent, and the individuals themselves. What services are necessary to address this problem?
Is there a way to attract, enroll, retain, and successfully train more families in programs that are evidence based?

In addition, the following questions should be asked about P2P programs, advocacy programs, and home/school models:

Are these programs effective when implemented with large numbers of families in widely different geographical and cultural settings?
Can manuals, video demonstrations, and live online coaching be offered on a large scale and is it efficacious? Is it effective?
What family variables predict dropping out or terminating treatment early?
What can be done about these?
What organizational/personnel variables predict failure to deliver the treatment program?
What can be done about these?
How much does it cost to implement these programs with fidelity of implementation?
Using cost-benefit analysis, how much money will be saved over the lifespan?
What changes in public policy needed to assure widespread availability of EPBs at scale?
What ethical questions arise when these practices are implemented widely?

We do not mean to imply that established and promising interventions should not be implemented until these questions are answered. We believe that a practitioner or parent can trust that there is sufficient confidence in the evidence to use the established practices with the understanding that they have not yet been fully validated. It is only fair to note that the questions above have rarely if ever been answered for any interventions in education and applied psychology.

In summary, we have identified shortcomings at two levels in the research evaluating some of the key interventions that meet the criteria for established or promising practices. That said, there is nothing inherent in these limitations that cannot be overcome by even a few well-designed, large RCT studies. Regrettably, a barrier to this kind of research is the reluctance of funding agencies to put money into replication studies and a devaluing of replication research in the competitive world of academic research, where a premium is put on innovation rather than replication. We believe that these attitudes are likely to change as it become more evident that they are impeding the dissemination and uptake of intervention practices on a large scale.

FACILITATORS

The influence of social and medical research on the helping professions predates the current expansive trend toward identifying and disseminating EBPs. Graduate schools educating helping professionals have long drawn on research in training their students although the quality and quantity of the research and the weight given to empiricism has varied greatly. Four long-standing trends have accelerated the adoption of EBPs and increased their importance. First, consumers as well as funders, including government and insurance agencies, have insisted on more accountability and have increasingly required empirical support for the potential benefits of practices as a warrant to expend public funds on particular interventions. In addition, the quality of practice and intervention research has gradually improved over the past half-century, so that its validity and trustworthiness has overcome some of the common skepticism about the relevance of research-to-professional practice. As part of this developing trust, the growing acceptance of meta-analysis since its inception in the early 1970s has provided practitioners with a succinct way to identify practices and quantify the effectiveness of specific interventions. It has also allowed researchers to come to conclusions about a group of studies other than the formerly common finding that studies were inconclusive and more research was needed. Finally, many of the helping professions have had to cope with practice fads that have often been unscientific but nonetheless have gathered large followings. The field of DDs has been marked by the promotion of unvalidated and sometimes frankly preposterous treatments ranging from fad diets to dolphin therapy. Unfortunately, fads based on unscientific beliefs have often offered false promises while consuming limited resources for better substantiated practices (Jacobson, Foxx, & Mulick, 2005).

As a counter to such fads, development and evaluation of interventions that meet standards for established treatments are important steps in the evolution of family support services and have the potential to help improve the quality of support services and ultimately the quality of life of many families. It is necessary to determine which interventions have sufficient evidence of high enough quality supporting claims of efficacy that are made about them. In this context, efforts to develop and validate science-based interventions represent an important effort to see that stakeholders can be reasonably assured scarce resources will be allocated for, at the least, potentially beneficial and effective programs.

In addition to changes in the research world, there are several applied trends and resources that can contribute to the gradual widespread dissemination and adoption of EBP's. In all states there is at least a rudimentary community infrastructure of services required by federal law including early intervention, special education, and vocational rehabilitation programs. Early intervention is already designed to be family centered and is one logical platform for offering EBPs. Further, all states have a DD service system, often designed on a regional basis. These range from minimal services to large centers for supporting access to generic community life and specialized programs specifically addressing the needs of adults with DD. Most regional centers have been primarily responsible for meeting the needs of adults, however there are now several states that have decades of experience of using these systems for small-scale family support programs. These regional centers in many states make natural host organizations for delivering EBPs to families. Family support programs in the United States range greatly in the amount of funds states dedicate for them. An encouraging trend has been slow growth in funding. In 1990 only 3% of DD funding was allocated for supporting families; by 2009 the allocation had grown to 8% (Braddock et al., 2011).

An encouraging trend in state DD services is a rethinking of service system designs. The disability rights movement has had a substantial impact on the extent to which people with disabilities and their families are empowered to design and manage their own support plans. The trend has been away from top-down planning for individuals as well as away from bureaucratically managed allocation of resources to families. In their place are newer ways of serving families by providing them with maximum choice in how they plan for and use public resources. At the core of these newer approaches are ways of planning that are meant to make family support and individual assistance plans much more responsive to the needs of consumers and to the expressed preferences of family members with disabilities. Person-centered planning and family-centered planning may contribute to the processes of going to scale with EBPs. These planning practices at best are flexible, individualized, and designed to elicit family members' own perceptions of the kinds of support, if any the family desires. The EBPs we have designated as established or promising were usually developed to meet the expressed problems of families, and so they may be in greater demand as families become more enabled to identify their needs for assistance.

MOVING TO A POSITIVE PSYCHOLOGY OF FAMILY SUPPORT

Support practices are more likely to be in demand and to ultimately be effective if they are designed with a realistic understanding of the breadth of experience families have as they live with and love their family members with ID or autism. When the dominant view among professionals was that a child with DD was an inevitable disaster for a family, there was a mismatch between the variety and range of parents' experiences and the ways that they appreciated their roles. To reiterate a point from chapter 1, we again quote Glidden and Schoolcraft: "Providing supports for families to help them make accommodations to their children is a very different enterprise from helping them deal only with their pain and tragedy" (Glidden & Schoolcraft, 2003, p. 251).

Efforts to place practices on a firm scientific foundation lag behind the rate of change in what are believed to be best practices in the professions concerned about people with DD and their families. It can take many years for enough high-quality evidence to accrue to establish a treatment as having efficacy. During these years, new values or treatment philosophies sometimes change the context dramatically. For example, over the three decades needed to establish CBT as helpful, the positive psychology movement has arisen, and it ought to influence our beliefs about the goals of family support. By moving away from a sole emphasis on the problems families face, the goals may be shifting from reduction in mental health problems in parents to promotion of a better quality of life for the whole family. As Glidden and Schoolcraft (2003) have stated elegantly, the universal assumption of family tragedy has given way to a much more nuanced and complex understanding of children's impacts on families. Recent research on family responses to raising a child with autism or ID report evidence of positive adaptation in families as well as strain in other families related to long-term caregiving stress. Over the long course of caregiving, it is likely that a majority of families find ways to adapt positively as well as living through intermittent times when stress and its negative impacts intensify before returning to more manageable levels. There is sufficient evidence that many, perhaps most, families are resilient over the long term and that many find benefit in parenting a child with DDs (Hastings & Taunt, 2002). Positive adaptation does not mean that families do not need support; even the most positive of families may endure times of crisis in which they feel overwhelmed. Furthermore, it may well be that part of why families recently have been seen as more adaptive and as attaining considerable psychological growth is that the service system and the network of parent self-help groups is sufficient to bolster positive adaptation.

Now that we acknowledge the wide range of families' experiences, the goals of family support systems ought to change from a sole emphasis on amelioration of suffering to prevention of stress and distress and promotion of positive adaptation. One implication of adopting these three goals is that service providers (special educators, social workers, pediatricians, etc.) should no longer expect elevated distress in families as a given and should no longer view parenting children with disabilities as a family tragedy. To the contrary, they should be educated in such a way that they understand the full range of family responses and appreciate that positive well-being for the whole family can be an attainable outcome over time.

POSITIVE INTERVENTION PRACTICES

An example of this shift in emphasis is Durand, Hieneman, Clarke, Wang, and Rinaldi's (2013) positive family intervention (PFI). Several of the components of their positive parenting treatment have long been recognized as effective parenting techniques in BPT, and the positive attitude treatment based on Seligman's (2002) work appears to be the same as traditional CBT. However the emphasis and language of support has shifted. Parents not only learn to challenge their pessimistic mindset, as in traditional CBT, but also work toward replacing it with a sense of efficacy and the growth of appreciation for their roles. These are not illusions, many family members do find true benefits in time. Similarly in their stress management and multiple component treatment studies, Singer et al. (Singer, Irvin, & Hawkins, 1988; Singer, Irvin, Irvine, & Hawkins, 1989) led discussions in the classes for parents. These focused on parents' successes during the week as a central topic of discussion. Empathy between members of the groups for the difficulties they shared and support for everyday successes, bolstered positive outcomes.

POSITIVE BEHAVIOR SUPPORT

A similar shift toward promotion and prevention is embedded in positive behavior support (PBS). When PBS practitioners carry out parent training they focus on designing and implementing the kinds of *family routines* that family members want to attain (Lucyshyn & Albin, 1993). For example, a father might wish to establish a time after dinner when he tosses a football back and forth with his son. At baseline the interviews and observations might reveal that the father rarely enjoys this kind of activity because his son often tantrums after dinner. The treatment goal as described would be not only to make tantrums a thing of the past but to work with the father and son until a new routine is established, one that is enjoyable to the father and his child. The building of several routines, designed the way the family chooses, can make a major change in their perceptions of the quality of their family life. A more traditional treatment, for example, might teach the parents to ignore their child with no scolding or raising their voices while he tantrums. Reduction or elimination of predictable, frequent tantrums would certainly be welcome as a goal. However, the therapist and the family might not go the next step as expected in PBS, one consisting of learning about how the family would like their common routines to be reconstructed and then helping them to establish new routines. We believe that this shift in the emphasis in support programs is likely to make them more attractive to families and to contribute to adoption of more positively oriented family activity routines.

GENERALIZING EFFECTIVE TREATMENTS TO OTHER FAMILY MEMBERS

The low representation of fathers in the research we reviewed is a problem that needs to be addressed. It is likely that interventions will be more stable and sustainable if parents in two-parent families can coach one another. In the BPT study by Adubato, Adams, and Budd (1981) (see chapter 3), the researchers first taught mothers positive parenting skills and then encouraged them to teach their husbands. The fathers learned the skills, and the children who originally had problem behaviors were better behaved after fathers began to use the skills. Given the percentage of children living in single-parent homes, a concerted effort is needed to find effective ways to support single parents and grandparents.

In addition, almost nothing has been published as empirical evidence about divorce and reconstituted family formation.

TREATING KEY FAMILY PROBLEMS

Currently one of the most promising lines of work for helping whole families centers on addressing coercive processes in families (Lucyshyn et al., 2015). "Coercion" is a process in which parents and children fall into patterns inadvertently increasing child problem behavior and ineffectual parenting over time. Commonly, parents give directives, children misbehave to get away from the demand, parents withdraw it, and children stop misbehaving. These processes can become habitual and spread throughout the family system in time. These processes can become habitual, can begin in early childhood as parents and children learn to respond to one another and they can intensify over time. Lucyshyn and colleagues have studied these processes in families of children with DD who have very severe problem behaviors. Through intensive PBS, families were able to learn new ways of interacting, which over time generated a positive momentum in which benign habits for living together developed and became adaptive. New practices for supporting families indicate considerable vitality in the development stages of the EBP process.

NEW MEDIA FOR DISSEMINATION AND TECHNICAL ASSISTANCE

Barretto, Wacker, Harding, Lee, and Berg (2006) used a telehealth system to provide BPT to parents living far away. Even less expensive systems have become widely available. Heitzman-Powell, Buzhardt, Rusinko, and Miller (2013) used telemedicine to conduct functional behavioral assessments of children at a distance in rural Iowa. Nefdt, Koegel, Singer, and Gerber (2010) demonstrated the efficacy of an interactive Web-based program for teaching pivotal response training to parents at a distance. A randomized comparison study using video tapes of parent–child interactions as outcomes showed that parents could take up and correctly implement these methods. It has long been known that a key to implementation is to provide direct coaching to people learning new skills. Joyce and Showers (2002) reviewed the literature on in-service training for schoolteachers. Her conclusions are now widely quoted. She reported that only a small percentage of teachers learned new teaching methods and applied them in their classrooms if the in-service training consisted only of lectures and reading about new practices. When modeling and role-playing are added, a somewhat larger percentage of teachers take up the skills and use them correctly. In order to train most teachers so they actually can implement the new practices, direct instruction and feedback based on in vivo observations and coaching are required. Direct instruction with in vivo coaching appears to be a sine qua non for large percentages of practitioners to take up a new practice. The research indicates that coaching is best done during the times the learners (teachers in this case) use the new skills.

PARENT-PROFESSIONAL PARTNERSHIPS

Ideas about professionalism and helping relationships in this field have undergone a thorough critique and establishment of new ways to conceptualize the crucial relationship between family members and the many professionals they encounter over the lifespan. The Beach Center on Family and Disability has contributed greatly to this effort by defining partnerships and studying what they look like in practice. Based on this research, they have offered several practical guidelines for these relationships. Stronger alliances between professionals and P2P programs could increase the rate and breadth of dissemination of EBPs for families. The P2P movement has proven to be a resilient one. As discussed in chapter 6, we rated one-to-one, parent-to-parent programs as promising based on one RCT. Parent to Parent USA is an national umbrella organization for these programs in over half the states in the country. It has established quality standards for local P2P programs and offers technical assistance to local- and state-level programs. In this model, program coordinators identify experienced parents who are positively adapting to parenting a child (or adult child) with a disability and who want to volunteer to assist other parents. The P2P organizations offer training for volunteers. These help-giving parents often possess valuable funds of knowledge about the resources available in local communities. Above all, they know what it is like to live day by day with a son or daughter with ID or autism and find benefit in parenting. These volunteers can serve as partners with professionals in delivering a range of programs. For example, Family Voices of Minnesota and the pediatrics department of a major hospital teamed up to provide clinics for families whose children have chronic illness and/or DDs (Woods & Singer). An evaluation of this program found that the addition of family support workers to the clinics enhanced physician's knowledge of their patients and their communities. Further, parents who participated in a parent-to-parent match were more actively involved in doctor–patient interviews. They asked more questions and more frequently offered useful information about their children's health. The clinics served low-income rural communities of native Americans and diverse low-income city neighborhoods, communities of predominantly African American and Latino families. The coordinators of the P2P programs were from these ethnic/racial groups and from poverty-impacted neighborhoods. By allying themselves with the P2P programs, physicians and nurses were able to gain access to knowledge about communities and cultures that was otherwise out of reach.

THE NEED FOR EVIDENCE-BASED SOCIAL CHANGE

We have pointed out the need for further research to determine what modifications will be needed to make interventions efficacious with diverse families and with whole families including siblings, fathers, and grandparents. The participants in the research will need to become more representative of the US population in the 21st century. The programs will have to be taken up and sustained by common community services and organizations.

While the size of the challenge can appear daunting, it is important to remember that only a few decades ago very few of the programs we have evaluated as evidence based existed. Public schools were not required to serve all children, discrimination on the basis of disability was not illegal, early intervention was not offered in many parts of the country, and large institutions were the main recipient of federal funds for people with DD. In 1970 very little was known about how to treat children with autism; the condition was considered intractable and the children uneducable. Parent organizations that first formed in the 1950s had not yet begun to influence national policy. There was no infrastructure on which to build supports for families, whereas presently several state and private entities have the capacity to expand services, invent and evaluate new interventions, and make communities more fully inclusive to citizens with DDs and their families. Based on these historical trends there is reason for hope that EBPs will go to scale.

Evidence-based practices are only the beginning—the ultimate goal needs to be evidence-based social change. The knowledge and skills that we have reviewed as established or promising represent a considerable achievement by parents, researchers, policy makers, and practitioners over the past four decades. Programs that have been developed and disseminated from the research universities in the United States need to become standard practice as part of a community-based system of care. That is, they need to "go to scale." Even this stage will not be sufficient to adequately support family home caregiving in a way that ensures a positive quality of life for families and their loved ones with disabilities. At the time of the writing of this book, over one in five children in the United States is living in poverty. Many parents, often single mothers, are struggling with unemployment or underpaid jobs, dangerous neighborhoods, and inadequate public schools. Over 11 million undocumented immigrants in the United States live in fear of being caught, arrested, and deported. They work without the normal protections of employment laws and access to the remaining social safety net. As presently constructed, the United States offers people living in poverty little realistic hope for social mobility despite a national myth to the contrary. While the problems of poverty in the United States go well beyond the purview of this book, they are intertwined with the challenges faced by a disproportionate number of families of children with disabilities.

RESOURCE ALLOCATION

In order to go to scale so that EBPs are widely available, there will need to be some public policy changes that, in turn, should be evaluated for their efficacy and effectiveness. Currently, less than 8% of the DD public budget goes to supporting families. Roughly five times as much of these funds are still given to support the small number of people remaining in large institutions, despite evidence that they are better off living in the community. There needs to be a funding stream dedicated to supporting family caregiving and providing community organizations with the information and training needed to make generic organizations fully inclusive and capable of supporting families. Medicaid needs to be restructured so that the waiver program is replaced by a dedicated funding stream for community programs including family support and dissemination of EBPs. Medical insurance similarly needs to be reformed to meet the long-term needs for mental and physical healthcare for caregivers who can benefit from the kinds of psychosocial programs reviewed in this book.

Furthermore, the budget for research on family support will need to be bolstered, particularly if the United States is to acquire the knowledge needed to meet the needs of the burgeoning population of citizens with autism through the lifespan. Service systems are only as good as the practitioners who work for them. There is a shortage of people who can carry out EBPs, and there is a large and growing shortage of professors in the fields of special education and early intervention. They constitute the infrastructure for educating the professionals required for going to scale. Funds will need to be channeled to make higher education affordable for future practitioners, researchers, and educators.

TOWARD NATIONAL FAMILY AND DISABILITY POLICIES

We have argued in previous work for more attention to the possibility of identifying and meeting the common needs of caregivers regardless of the kind of disability a family member experiences (Singer, Biegel, & Ethridge, 2010).

Presently, there is very little exchange of ideas and programs across the disciplines and service systems that are focused on caregiving for people with serious mental illness, the frail elderly, people with dementia, people with traumatic brain injury, individuals with serious chronic illnesses, and individuals with DDs. A good starting place would be frequent exchange of ideas between the disciplines, which currently exist in "silos." For example, one of the shortcomings we have pointed out in the research is the lack of interventions for the whole family. In the field of support for families of people with schizophrenia, interventions for working with several whole families together have been developed and evaluated (Lucksted, McFarlane, Downing, & Dixon, 2012). Research on caregivers for the elderly has included several evaluations of the efficacy of programs, which appear to be almost identical to some of the CBT and multiple component interventions in this book. Currently there are no scholarly journals dedicated to research on caregiving, and university programs for direct service practitioners rarely include experience and instruction about caregiver stress. These are difficulties that we believe could be readily overcome if they were to rise to the level of the public agenda for higher education.

Finally, this review of research leaves us hopeful despite much that needs to change. In a segment of society that was considered hopeless for centuries, considerable progress has been made. The possible life trajectories of people with severe disabilities and their families have multiplied and improved. Tens of thousands of people with disabilities and their families have benefited already from EBPs. Parent advocacy has meaningful influence in the political system, and people with disabilities have been successful in placing their concerns on the public agenda. There is good reason to believe that these trends will continue so that research will be translated into assistance that improves family quality of life in the United States and other nations.

REFERENCES

Abidin, R. R. (1990). *Parenting Stress Index (short form)*. Odessa, FL: Pediatric Psychology Press.

Adams, K. A., & Christenson, S. L. (1998). Differences in parent and teacher trust levels: Implications for creating collaborative family-school relationships. *Special Services in the Schools, 14*(1/2), 1–22. doi:10.1016/S0022-4405(00)00048-0

Adubato, S. A., Adams, M. K., & Budd, K. S. (1981). Teaching a Parent to Train a Spouse in Child Management Techniques. *Journal of Applied Behavior Analysis, 14*, 193–205. doi:10.1901/jaba.1981.14-193

Ainbinder, J. G., Blanchard, L. W., Singer, G. H. S., Sullivan, M. E., Powers, L. K., Marquis, J. G., & Santelli, B. (1998). A Qualitative Study of Parent to Parent Support for Parents of Children With Special Needs. *Journal of Pediatric Psychology, 23*, 99–109. doi:10.1093/jpepsy/23.2.99

Albin, R. W., Lucyshyn, J. M., Horner, R. H., & Flannery, K. B. (1996). Contextual fit for behavior support plans: A model for "goodness of fit." In L. Kern Koegel, R. L. Koegel, & G. Dunlap (Eds.), *Positive behavioral support: Including people with difficult behavior in the community* (pp. 81–98). Baltimore, MD: Paul H. Brookes.

Aldred, C., Green, J., & Adams, C. (2004). A new social communication intervention for children with autism: pilot randomised controlled treatment study suggesting effectiveness. *Journal of Child Psychology and Psychiatry, 45*, 1420–1430. doi:10.1111/j.1469-7610.2004.00338.x

Aldred, C., Phillips, R., Pollard, C., & Adams, C. (2001). Multidisciplinary social communication intervention for children with autism and pervasive developmental disorder: The Child's Talk project. *Educational and Child Psychology, 18*(2), 76–87.

Allen, K. D., Kuhn, B. R., DeHaai, K. A., & Wallace, D. P. (2013). Evaluation of a behavioral treatment package to reduce sleep problems in children with Angelman Syndrome. *Research in Developmental Disabilities, 34*, 676–686.

Altman, B. M., Cooper, P. F., & Cunningham, P. J. (1999). The case of disability in the family: Impact on health care utilization and expenditures for nondisabled members. *Milbank Quarterly, 77*, 39–75. doi:10.1111/1468-0009.00124

Amendah, D., Grosse, S. D., Peacock, G., & Mandell, D. S. (2011). The economic costs of autism: A review. In D. Amaral, D. Geschwind,& G. Dawson (Eds.), *Autism spectrum disorders.* (pp. 1347–1360). New York, NY: Oxford University Press.

American Psychiatric Association & DSM-5 Task Force. (2013). *Diagnostic and statistical manual of mental disorders: DSM-5.* Washington, DC: American Psychiatric Association.

Anastopoulos, A. D., Shelton, T. L., DuPaul, G. J., & Guevremont, D. C. (1993). Parent training for attention-deficit hyperactivity disorder: Its impact on parent functioning. *Journal of Abnormal Child Psychology, 21,* 581–596. doi:10.1007/BF00916320

Anderson, C. M., & McMillan, K. (2001). Parental use of escape extinction and differential reinforcement to treat food selectivity. *Journal of Applied Behavior Analysis, 34,* 511–515.

Anderson, J. A., Meyer, L. D., & Somers, J. W. (2006). The impact of system-of-care participation on school functioning: Exploring caregiver and teacher perspectives. *Preventing School Failure: Alternative Education for Children and Youth, 50,* 13–20. doi:10.3200/PSFL.50.3.13-20

Anderson, L., Larson, S. A., & Wuorio, A. (2011). *2010 FINDS National Survey Technical Report Part 1: Family Caregiver Survey.* Minneapolis, MN: University of Minnesota, Research and Training Center on Community Living.

Antonovsky, A. (1987). *Unraveling the mystery of health: How people manage stress and stay well.* San Francisco, CA: Jossey-Bass.

Arno, P. S., Levine, C., & Memmott, M. M. (1999). The economic value of informal caregiving. *Health Affairs, 18,* 182–188. doi:10.1377/hlthaff.18.2.182

Arnold, D. S., O'Leary, S. G., Wolff, L. S., & Acker, M. M. (1993). The Parenting Scale: A measure of dysfunctional parenting in discipline situations. *Psychological Assessment, 5,* 137. doi: http://dx.doi.org/10.1037/1040-3590.5.2.137

Aurand, J. C., Sisson, L. A., Aach, S. R., & Van Hasselt, V. B. (1989). Use of reinforcement plus interruption to reduce self-stimulation in a child with multiple handicaps. *Journal of the Multihandicapped Person, 2,* 51–61.

Autism Society of California (2012). Autism in California 2012 survey. Retrieved from http://www.scdd.ca.gov/res/docs/pdf/Whats_New/ASC_Survey_April_2012.pdf

Bacon, J. K., & Causton-Theoharis, J. (2012). "It should be teamwork": A critical investigation of school practices and parent advocacy in special education. *International Journal of Inclusive Education.* Advance online publication. doi:10.1080/13603116.2012.708060

Baer, D. M., Wolf, M. M., & Risley, T. R. (1968). Some current dimensions of applied behavior analysis. *Journal of Applied Behavior Analysis, 1,* 91–97.

Bagner, D. M., & Eyberg, S. M. (2007). Parent–child interaction therapy for disruptive behavior in children with mental retardation: A randomized controlled trial. *Journal of Clinical Child and Adolescent Psychology, 36,* 418–429. doi:10.1080/15374410701448448

Bailey, D. B., Golden, R. N., Roberts, J., & Ford, A. (2007). Maternal depression and developmental disability: Research critique. *Mental Retardation and Developmental Disabilities Research Reviews, 13,* 321–329. doi:10.1002/mrdd.20172

Baio, J. (2012). Prevalence of autism spectrum disorders: Autism and developmental disabilities monitoring network, 14 sites, United States, 2008. *Morbidity and Mortality Weekly Report. Surveillance Summaries, 61*(3), 1–19. Centers for Disease Control and Prevention. Retrieved from http://files.eric.ed.gov/fulltext/ED530639.pdf

Baker, B. L. (1996). *Parent training.* Retrieved from http://psycnet.apa.org/books/10203/022.pdf

Baker, B. L., & Brightman, R. P. (1984). Training parents of retarded children: Program-specific outcomes. *Journal of Behavior Therapy and Experimental Psychiatry, 15,* 255–260. doi:10.1016/0005-7916(84)90034-X

Baker, B. L., Brightman, A., & Blacher, J. (1997). *Steps to independence: Teaching everyday skills to children with special needs.* Baltimore, MD: Brookes.

Baker, B. L., Brightman, A., Heifetz, L. J., & Murphy, D. M. (1976). *Steps to independence.* Champaign, IL: Research Press.

Baker, B. L., Heifetz, L. J., & Murphy, D. M. (1980). Behavioral training for parents of mentally retarded children: One-year follow-up. *American Journal of Mental Deficiency, 85*(1), 31–38. Retrieved from http://psycnet.apa.org/psycinfo/1980-28450-001

Balcazar, F. E., Keys, C. B., Bertram, J. F., & Rizzo, T. (1996). Advocate development in the field of developmental disabilities: A data-based conceptual model. *Mental Retardation, 34,* 341–351. Retrieved from http://mn.gov/web/prod/static/mnddc/live/pipm/pdf/Advocacy_Development-Retardation-Journal.pdf

Bambara, L. M., Mitchell-Kvacky, A. A., & Iacobelli, S. (1994). Positive behavioral support for students with severe disabilities: An emerging multicomponent approach for addressing challenging behaviors. *School Psychology Review, 23,* 263–278.

Bandura, A. (1971). *Social learning theory.* New York, NY: General Learning Press.

Barretto, A., Wacker, D. P., Harding, J., Lee, J., & Berg, W. K. (2006). Using telemedicine to conduct behavioral assessments. *Journal of Applied Behavior Analysis, 39,* 333–340. http://doi.org/10.1901/jaba.2006.173-04

Barry, L. M., & Singer, G. H. S. (2001). A family in crisis replacing the aggressive behavior of a child with autism toward an infant sibling. *Journal of Positive Behavior Interventions, 3,* 28–38. doi:10.1177/109830070100300105

Barsch, R. H. (1961). Explanations offered by parents and siblings of brain-damaged children. *Exceptional Children, 27,* 286–291.

Bastien, C. H., Vallières, A., & Morin, C. M. (2001). Validation of the Insomnia Severity Index as an outcome measure for insomnia research. *Sleep Medicine, 2,* 297–307. http://doi.org/10.1016/S1389-9457(00)00065-4

Baxter, C. (1989). Investigating stigma as stress in social interactions of parents. *Journal of Intellectual Disability Research, 33,* 455–466. doi:10.1111/j.1365-2788.1989.tb01501.x

Bayat, M. (2007). Evidence of resilience in families of children with autism. *Journal of Intellectual Disability Research,* 51, 702–714. doi:10.1111/j.1365-2788.2007.00960.x

Beck, A. T. (1963). Thinking and depression: Idiosyncratic content and cognitive distortions. *Archives of General Psychiatry, 9,* 324–333.

Beck, A. T. (1976). *Cognitive therapy and the emotional disorders.* New York, NY: International Universities Press.

Beck, A. T. (1984). Cognitive approaches to stress. In R. Woolfolk & P. Lehren (Eds.), *Principles and practice of stress management,* 125–155. New York: Guilford.

Beck, A. T., Steer, R. A., & Brown, G. K. (1996). *Beck Depression Inventory-II.* San Antonio, TX: Psychological Corporation.

Beck, A. T., Steer, R. A., & Carbin, M. G. (1988). Psychometric properties of the Beck Depression Inventory: Twenty-five years of evaluation. *Clinical Psychology Review, 8,* 77–100. doi:10.1016/0272-7358(88)90050-5

Beck, A. T., Ward, C., & Mendelson, M. (1961). Beck depression inventory (BDI). *Archives of General Psychiatry, 4,* 561–571.

Beck, A. T., Weissman, A., Lester, D., & Trexler, L. (1974). The measurement of pessimism: The Hopelessness Scale. *Journal of Consulting and Clinical Psychology, 42,* 861–865. http://doi.org/10.1037/h0037562

Becker, W. C. (1971). *Parents are teachers: A child management program.* Retrieved from http://www.eric.ed.gov/ERICWebPortal/recordDetail?accno=ED047826

Beebe-Frankenberger, M., Lane, K. L., Bocian, K. M., Gresham, F. M., & MacMillan, D. L. (2005). Students with or at risk for problem behavior: Betwixt and between teacher and parent expectations. *Preventing School Failure: Alternative Education for Children and Youth, Winter,* 10–17. doi:10.3200/PSFL.49.2.10-17

Behr, S. K., Murphy, D. L., & Summers, J. A. (1992). *User's manual: Kansas Inventory of Parental Perceptions (KIPP): Measures of perceptions of parents who have children with special needs.* Lawrence, KS: Beach Center on Families and Disability.

Bellack, A. S., Hersen, M., & Turner, S. M. (1976). Generalization effects of social skills training in chronic schizophrenics: An experimental analysis. *Behaviour Research and Therapy, 14,* 391–398. http://doi.org/10.1016/0005-7967(76)90085-1

Ben Chaabane, D. B., Alber-Morgan, S. R., & DeBar, R. M. (2009). The effects of parent-implemented PECS training on improvisation of mands by children with autism. *Journal of Applied Behavior Analysis, 42,* 671–677. doi:10.1901/jaba.2009.42-671

Benn, R., Akiva, T., Arel, S., & Roeser, R. W. (2012). Mindfulness training effects for parents and educators of children with special needs. *Developmental Psychology, 48,* 1476–1487. doi http://dx.doi.org/10.1037/a0027537

Benson, H., Beary, J. F., & Carol, M. P. (1974). The relaxation response. *Psychiatry,* 37, 37–46. doi.:10.1521/00332747.1974.11023785

Bernard, M. E. (1990). *Taking the stress out of teaching.* Melbourne, Australia: Collins Dove.

Bernheimer, L. P., & Weisner, T. S. (2007). "Let me just tell you what i do all day...": The family story at the center of intervention research and practice. *Infants and Young Children, 20,* 192–201. doi:10.1097/01.IYC.0000277751.62819.9b

Bezdek, J., Summers, J. A., & Turnbull, A. (2010). Professionals' attitudes on partnering with families of children and youth with disabilities. *Education and Training in Autism and Developmental Disabilities, 45,* 356–365. Retrieved from http://daddcec.org/Portals/0/CEC/Autism_Disabilities/Research/Publications/Education_Training_Development_Disabilities/Full_Journals/ETDD201009V45n3.pdf#page=39

Biglan, A., Glasgow, R. E., & Singer, G. (1990). The need for a science of larger social units: A contextual approach. *Behavior Therapy, 21,* 195–215. doi:10.1016/S0005-7894(05)80277-1

Binnendyk, L., & Lucyshyn, J. M. (2009). A family-centered positive behavior support approach to the amelioration of food refusal behavior. An empirical case study. *Journal of Positive Behavior Interventions, 11,* 47–62.

Bishop, S. R., Lau, M., Shapiro, S., Carlson, L., Anderson, N. D., Carmody, J., . . . Devins, G. (2004). Mindfulness: A proposed operational definition. *Clinical Psychology: Science and Practice, 11,* 230–241. http://doi.org/10.1093/clipsy.bph077

Blair, K. C., Lee, I.-S., Cho, S.-J., & Dunlap, G. (2011). Positive behavior support through family-school collaboration for young children with autism. *Topics in Early Childhood Special Education, 31*, 22–36. doi:10.1177/0271121410377510

Blanchard, L., Powers, L., Ginsberg, C, Marquis, J., & Singer, G H. S. (1996). *The Coping Efficacy Inventory: Measuring parents perceptions of coping with a child with a disability and family problems.* Unpublished manuscript. University of North Carolina Medical School, Chapel Hill, NC.

Blumberg, S. J., Bramlett, M. D., Kogan, M. D., Schieve, L. A., Jones, J. R., & Lu, M. C. (2013). Changes in prevalence of parent-reported autism spectrum disorder in school-aged US children: 2007 to 2011–2012. *National Health Statistics Reports, 65*, 1–11.

Bolton, P. F., Golding, J., Emond, A., & Steer, C. D. (2012). Autism spectrum disorder and autistic traits in the Avon longitudinal study of parents and children: Precursors and early signs. *Journal of the American Academy of Child and Adolescent Psychiatry, 51*, 249.e25–260.e25. doi:10.1016/j.jaac.2011.12.009

Bor, W., Sanders, M. R., & Markie-Dadds, C. (2002). The effects of the Triple P-Positive Parenting Program on preschool children with co-occurring disruptive behavior and attentional/hyperactive difficulties. *Journal of Abnormal Child Psychology, 30*, 571–587.

Borenstein, M., Hedges, L. V., Higgins, J. P. T., & Rothstein, H. R. (2009). *Introduction to meta analysis.* Chichester, UK: Wiley.

Boyd, B. A. (2002). Examining the relationship between stress and lack of social support in mothers of children with autism. *Focus on Autism and Other Developmental Disabilities, 17*, 208–215.

Boyle, C. A., Boulet, S., Schieve, L. A., Cohen, R. A., Blumberg, S. J., Allsopp, M. Y., ... Kogan, M. D. (2011). Trends in the prevalence of developmental disabilities in US Children 1997–2008. *Pediatrics, 127*, 1034–1042. doi:10.1542/peds.2010-2989.

Braddock, D., Hemp, R., Rizzolo, M. C., Haffer, L., Tanis, E. S., & Wu, J. (2011). *The state of the states in developmental disabilities 2011.* Washington, DC: American Association on Intellectual and Developmental Disabilities.

Braddock, D., Hemp, R., Rizzolo, M. C., Tanis, E. S., Haffer, L., Lulinski, A., & Wu, J. (2013). *The state of the states in developmental disabilities* (9th ed.). Washington, DC: American Association on Intellectual and Developmental Disabilities.

Braddock, D., Hemp, R., Rizzolo, M. C., Tanis, E. S., Haffer, L., & Wu, J. (2015). *The state of the states in intellectual and developmental disabilities: Emerging from the great recession.* Washington, DC: American Association on Intellectual and Developmental Disabilities.

Bradley, V. J., & Moseley, C. (2007). National core indicators: Ten years of collaborative performance measurement. *Intellectual and Developmental Disabilities, 45*, 354–358. http://doi.org/10.1352/0047-6765(2007)45[354:NCITYO]2.0.CO;2

Brantlinger, E. (1991). Home-school partnerships that benefit children with special needs. *Elementary School Journal, 91*, 249–259. Retrieved from http://www.jstor.org/stable/1001711

Brehony, K. A., Benson, B. A., Solomon, L. J., & Luscomb, R. L. (1980). Parents as behavior modifiers: Intervention for three problem behaviors in a severely retarded child. *Journal of Clinical Child and Adolescent Psychology, 9*, 213–216.

Brereton, A., & Tonge, B. (2005). *Pre-schoolers with autism: A parent education and skills training programme.* London, England: Kingsley.

Brestan, E. V., & Eyberg, S. M. (1998). Effective psychosocial treatments of conduct-disordered children and adolescents: 29 years, 82 studies, and 5,272 kids. *Journal of Clinical Child Psychology, 27*, 180–189.

Brewer, E. J., McPherson, M., Magrab, P. R., & Hutchins, V. L. (1989). Family-centered, community-based, coordinated care for children with special health care needs. *Pediatrics, 83*, 1055–1060.

Brightman, R. P., Baker, B. L., Clark, D. B., & Ambrose, S. A. (1982). Effectiveness of alternative parent training formats. *Journal of Behavior Therapy and Experimental Psychiatry, 13*, 113–117.

Brinckerhoff, J. L., & Vincent, L. J. (1986). Increasing parental decision-making at the individualized educational program meeting. *Journal of Early Intervention, 11*(1), 46–58.

Bristol, M. M., Gallagher, J. J., & Holt, K. D. (1993). Maternal depressive symptoms in autism: Response to psychoeducational intervention. *Rehabilitation Psychology, 38*(1), 3.

Bristol, M. M., Gallagher, J. J., & Schopler, E. (1988). Mothers and fathers of young developmentally disabled and nondisabled boys: Adaptation and spousal support. *Developmental Psychology, 24*, 441.

Brotherson, M. J., Cook, C. C., Erwin, E. J., & Weigel, C. J. (2008). Understanding self-determination and families of young children with disabilities in home environments. *Journal of Early Intervention, 31*(1), 22–43. doi:10.1177/1053815108324445

Buchan, L., Clemerson, J., & Davis, H. (1988). Working with families of children with special needs: The parent adviser scheme. *Child: Care, Health and Development, 14*(2), 81–91. http://doi.org/10.1111/j.1365-2214.1988.tb00565.x

Budd, K. S. (1992). *Behavioral feeding assessment parent interview form.* Unpublished manuscript. DePaul University, Chicago.

Buelow, J. M. (2007). An intervention for parents of children with epilepsy and significant learning problems: Lessons learned from a feasibility study. *Journal of the American Psychiatric Nurses Association, 13*, 146–152. doi:10.1177/1078390307303747

Buelow, J. M., Johnson, C. S., Perkins, S. M., Austin, J. K., & Dunn, D. W. (2013). Creating Avenues for Parent Partnership (CAPP): An intervention for parents of children with epilepsy and learning problems. *Epilepsy and Behavior, 27*(1), 64–69. doi:http://dx.doi.org/10.1016/j.yebeh.2012.12.013

Burke, M. M. (2013). Improving parental involvement: Training special education advocates. *Journal of Disability Policy Studies, 23*, 225–234. doi:10.1177/1044207311424910

Buschbacher, P., Fox, L., & Clarke, S. (2004). Recapturing desired family routines: A parent-professional behavioral collaboration. *Research and Practice for Persons with Severe Disabilities, 29*, 25–39.

Butler, A. C., Chapman, J. E., Forman, E. M., & Beck, A. T. (2006). The empirical status of cognitive-behavioral therapy: A review of meta-analyses. *Clinical Psychology Review, 26*(1), 17–31. doi:10.1016/j.cpr.2005.07.003

Call, N. A., Wacker, D. P., Ringdahl, J. E., & Boelter, E. W. (2005). Combined antecedent variables as motivating operations within functional analyses. *Journal of Applied Behavior Analysis, 38*, 385–389. doi:10.1901/jaba.2005.51-04

Carlson, C. R., & Hoyle, R. H. (1993). Efficacy of abbreviated progressive muscle relaxation training: A quantitative review of behavioral medicine research. *Journal of Consulting and Clinical Psychology, 61*, 1059–1067. doi:10.1037/0022-006X.61.6.1059

Carr, E. G., Dunlap, G., Horner, R. H., Koegel, R. L., Turnbull, A. P., Sailor, W., ... Fox, L. (2002). Positive behavior support: Evolution of an applied science. *Journal of Positive Behavior Interventions, 4*, 4–20.

Carr, E. G., & Durand, V. M. (1985). Reducing behavior problems through functional communication training. *Journal of Applied Behavior Analysis, 18*, 111–126.

Carr, E. G., Levin, L., McConnachie, G., Carlson, J. I., Kemp, D. C., & Smith, C. E. (1994). *Communication-based intervention for problem behavior: A user's guide for producing positive change.* Baltimore, MD: Brookes.

Carr, E. G., Levin, L., McConnachie, G., Carlson, J. I., Kemp, D. C., Smith, C. E., & McLaughlin, D. M. (1999). Comprehensive multisituational intervention for problem behavior in the community: Long-term maintenance and social validation. *Journal of Positive Behavior Interventions, 1*, 5–25.

Carter, A. S., Messinger, D. S., Stone, W. L., Celimli, S., Nahmias, A. S., & Yoder, P. (2011). A randomized controlled trial of Hanen's "More Than Words" in toddlers with early autism symptoms. *Journal of Child Psychology and Psychiatry, 52*(7), 741–752. doi:10.1111/j.1469-7610.2011.02395.x

Carter, E. W., Owens, L., Trainor, A. A., Sun, Y., & Swedeen, B. (2009). Self-determination skills and opportunities of adolescents with severe intellectual and developmental disabilities. *American Association on Intellectual and Developmental Disabilities, 114*, 179–192. doi:10.1352/1944-7558-114.3.179

Casenhiser, D. M., Shanker, S. G., & Stieben, J. (2013). Learning through interaction in children with autism: Preliminary data from asocial-communication-based intervention. *Autism, 17*, 220–241. doi:10.1177/1362361311422052

Chadwick, O., Momčilović, N., Rossiter, R., Stumbles, E., & Taylor, E. (2001). A randomized trial of brief individual versus group parent training for behaviour problems in children with severe learning disabilities. *Behavioural and Cognitive Psychotherapy, 29*, 151–167. doi:10.1017/S135246580100203X

Charlop-Christy, M. H., & Carpenter, M. H. (2000). Modified incidental teaching sessions: A procedure for parents to increase spontaneous speech in their children with autism. *Journal of Positive Behavior Interventions, 2*, 98–112. doi:10.1177/109830070000200203

Chen, D., Downing, J. E., & Peckham-Hardin, K. D. (2002). Positive behavior support with families of diverse cultural and linguistic backgrounds: Consderations for culturally-responsive practices. In J. M. Lucyshyn, G. Dunlap, & R. W. Albin (Eds.), *Families in positive behavior support: Addressing problem behavior and family context* (pp. 131–151). Baltimore, MD: Brookes.

Cheremshynski, C., Lucyshyn, J. M., & Olson, D. L. (2013). Implementation of a culturally appropriate positive behavior support plan with a Japanese mother of a child with autism: An experimental and qualitative analysis. *Journal of Positive Behavior Interventions, 15*, 242–253. doi:10.1177/1098300712459904.

Cherlin, A. J. (2010). Demographic trends in the United States: A review of research in the 2000s. *Journal of Marriage and Family, 72*(3), 403–419.

Chiesa, A., & Serretti, A. (2009). Mindfulness-based stress reduction for stress management in healthy people: A review and meta-analysis. *Journal of Alternative and Complementary Medicine, 15*, 593–600. http://doi.org/10.1089/acm.2008.0495

Christenson, S. L. (2004). The family-school partnership: An opportunity to promote the learning competence of all students. *School Psychology Review, 33*, 83–104. Retrieved from http://dx.doi.org/10.1521/scpq.18.4.454.26995

Christopherson, E. R., Arnold, C. M., Hill, D. W., & Quilitch, H. R. (1972). The home point system: Token reinforcement procedures for application by parents of children with behavior problems. *Journal of Applied Behavior Analysis, 5*, 485–497.

Chronis, A. M., Chacko, A., Fabiano, G. A., Wymbs, B. T., & Pelham, W. E. P., Jr. (2004). Enhancements to the behavioral parent training paradigm for families of children with ADHD: Review and future directions. *Clinical Child and Family Psychology Review, 7*(1), 1–27. doi:10.1023/B:CCFP.0000020190.60808.a4

Clarke, S., Dunlap, G., & Vaughn, B. (1999). Family-centered, assessment-based intervention to improve behavior during an early morning routine. *Journal of Positive Behavior Interventions, 1*, 235–241. doi:10.1177/109830079900100406

Cohen, J. (1987). *Statistical power analysis for the behavioral sciences.* Hillside, NJ: Erlbaum.

Coolican, J., Smith, I. M., & Bryson, S. E. (2010). Brief parent training in pivotal response treatment for preschoolers with autism. *Journal of Child Psychology and Psychiatry, 51,* 1321–1330. doi:10.1111/j.1469-7610.2010.02326.x

Cooper, H. M., Hedges, L. V., & Valentine, J. C. (2009). *The handbook of research synthesis and meta-analysis.* New York, NY: Russell Sage Foundation.

Cooper, J. O., Heron, T. E., & Heward, W. L. (2007). *Applied behavior analysis.* Retrieved from http://europepmc.org/articles/PMC1285958/pdf/jaba00099-0113.pdf

Coots, J. (1998). Family resources and parent participation in schooling activities for their children with developmental delays. *Journal of Special Education, 31,* 498–520. doi:10.1177/002246699803100406

Corcoran, K. J. (1981). Experiential empathy: A theory of a felt-level experience. *Journal of Humanistic Psychology, 21*(1), 29–38.

Corrigan, P. W. (1991). Social skills training in adult psychiatric populations: A meta-analysis. *Journal of Behavior Therapy and Experimental Psychiatry, 22,* 203–210. http://doi.org/10.1016/0005-7916(91)90017-Y

Coughlin, M., Sharry, J., Fitzpatrick, C., Guerin, S., & Drumm, M. (2009). A controlled clinical evaluation of the parents plus children's programme: A video-based programme for parents of children aged 6 to 11 with behavioural and developmental problems. *Clinical Child Psychology and Psychiatry, 14,* 541–558.

Crepaz, N., Passin, W. F., Herbst, J. H., Rama, S. M., Malow, R. M., Purcell, D. W., . . . HIV/AIDS Prevention Research Synthesis Team. (2008). Meta-analysis of cognitive-behavioral interventions on HIV-positive persons' mental health and immune functioning. *Health Psychology: Official Journal of the Division of Health Psychology, American Psychological Association,* 27(1), 4–14. doi:10.1037/0278-6133.27.1.4.

Crnic, K. A., & Greenberg, M. T. (1990). Minor parenting stresses with young children. *Child Development, 61,* 1628–1637. doi:10.1111/j.1467-8624.1990.tb02889.x

Crnic, K. A., Greenberg, M. T., Ragozin, A. S., Robinson, N. M., & Basham, R. B. (1983). Effects of stress and social support on mothers and premature and full-term infants. *Child Development, 54,* 209–217. http://doi.org/10.2307/1129878

Crockett, J. L., Fleming, R. K., Doepke, K. J., & Stevens, J. S. (2007). Parent training: Acquisition and generalization of discrete trials teaching skills with parents of children with autism. *Research in Developmental Disabilities, 28*(1), 23–36. doi:10.1016/j.ridd.2005.10.003

Cullen, M., & Wallace, L. (2010). *Stress management and relaxation techniques in education (SMART) training manual.* Unpublished manual, Impact Foundation: Aurora, CO.

Cunconan-Lahr, R., & Brotherson, M. J. (1996). Advocacy in disability policy: Parents and consumers as advocates. *Mental Retardation, 34,* 352–358.

Davis, H., & Rushton, R. (1991). Counselling and supporting parents of children with developmental delay: A research evaluation. *Journal of Intellectual Disability Research, 35,* 89–112. http://doi.org/10.1111/j.1365-2788.1991.tb01039.x

Davis, N. O., & Carter, A. S. (2008). Parenting stress in mothers and fathers of toddlers with autism spectrum disorders: Associations with child characteristics. *Journal of Autism and Developmental Disorders, 38,* 1278–1291.

Davison, K. P., Pennebaker, J. W., & Dickerson, S. S. (2000). Who talks? The social psychology of illness support groups. *American Psychologist, 55,* 205. doi:10.1037/0003-066X.55.2.205

Dawson, G., Rogers, S., Munson, J., Smith, M., Winter, J., Greenson, J., . . . & Varley, J. (2010). Randomized, controlled trial of an intervention for toddlers with autism: the Early Start Denver Model. *Pediatrics, 125*(1), e17–e23.

Dekker, M. C., Koot, H. M., Ende, J. van der, & Verhulst, F. C. (2002). Emotional and behavioral problems in children and adolescents with and without intellectual disability. *Journal of Child Psychology and Psychiatry, 43,* 1087–1098. doi:10.1111/1469-7610.00235

Delaney, E. M., & Kaiser, A. P. (2001). The effects of teaching parents blended communication and behavior support strategies. *Council for Children with Behavioral Disorders, 26,* 93–101.

Derby, K. M., Wacker, D. P., Berg, W., Deraad, A., Ulrich, S., Asmus, J., . . . Stoner, E. A. (1997). The long-term effects of functional communication training in home settings. *Journal of Applied Behavior Analysis, 30,* 507–531.

Developmental Disabilities Assistance and Bill of Rights Act, 42 U.S.C. § 15001 (1994 & Supp., 2000).

Diener, E., Emmons, R. A., Larsen, R. J., & Griffin, S. (1985). The satisfaction with life scale. *Journal of Personality Assessment, 49*(1), 71–75. http://doi.org/10.1207/s15327752jpa4901_13

Dobson, K. S. (2009). *Handbook of cognitive-behavioral therapies* (3rd ed.). New York, NY: Guilford Press.

Drew, A., Baird, G., Baron-Cohen, S., Cox, A., Slonims, V., Wheelwright, S., . . . & Charman, T. (2002). A pilot randomised control trial of a parent training intervention for pre-school children with autism. *European child & adolescent psychiatry, 11*(6), 266–272.

Ducharme, J. M., & Drain, T. L. (2004). Errorless academic compliance training: Improving generalized cooperation with parental requests in children with autism. *Journal of the American Academy of Child and Adolescent Psychiatry, 43,* 163–171. doi:10.1097/00004583-200402000-00011

Ducharme, J. M., Harris, K., Milligan, K., & Pontes, E. (2003). Sequential evaluation of reinforced compliance and graduated request delivery for the treatment of noncompliance in children with developmental disabilities. *Journal of Autism and Developmental Disorders, 33,* 519–526. doi:10.1023/A:1025831528809

Ducharme, J. M., Pontes, E., Guger, S., Crozier, K., Lucas, H., & Popynick, M. (1994). Errorless compliance to parental requests: II. Increasing clinical practicality through abbreviation of treatment parameters. *Behavior Therapy, 25,* 469–487. doi:10.1016/S0005-7894(05)80158-3

Ducharme, J. M., & Popynick, M. (1993). Errorless compliance to parental requests: Treatment effects and generalization. *Behavior Therapy, 24,* 209–226. doi:10.1016/S0005-7894(05)80264-3

Ducharme, J. M., Popynick, M., Pontes, E., & Steele, S. (1996). Errorless compliance to parental requests: III. Group parent training with parent observational data and long-term follow-up. *Behavior Therapy, 27,* 353–372. doi:10.1016/S0005-7894(96)80022-0

Ducharme, J. M., & Worling, D. E. (1994). Behavioral momentum and stimulus fading in the acquisition and maintenance of child compliance in the home. *Journal of Applied Behavior Analysis, 27,* 639–647.

Duda, M. A., Clarke, S., Fox, L., & Dunlap, G. (2008). Implementation of positive behavior support with a sibling set in a home environment. *Journal of Early Intervention, 30,* 213–236.

Dunlap, G., Ester, T., Langhans, S., & Fox, L. (2006). Functional communication training with toddlers in home environments. *Journal of Early Intervention, 28,* 81–96.

Dunst, C. J. (2002). Family-centered practices: Birth through high school. *Journal of Special Education, 36,* 139–147.

Dunst, C. J., Trivette, C. M., & Deal, A. G. (1988). *Enabling and empowering families: Principles and guidelines for practice.* Cambridge, MA: Brookline Books.

Dunst, C. J., Trivette, C. M., Gordon, N. J., & Starnes, A. L. (1993). Family-centered case management practices: Characteristics and consequences. In G. H. Singer & L. L. Powers (Eds.), *Families, disability, and empowerment: Active coping skills and strategies for family interventions* (pp. 89–118). Baltimore, MD: Brookes.

Dunst, C. J., Trivette, C. M., & Hamby, D. W. (2007). Meta-analysis of family-centered helpgiving practices research. *Mental Retardation and Developmental Disabilities, 13,* 370–378. doi:10.1002/mrdd.20176

Durand, V. M. (2001). Future directions for children and adolescents with mental retardation. *Behavior Therapy, 32,* 633–650. doi:10.1016/S0005-7894(01)80013-7

Durand, V. M., & Hieneman, M. (2008). *Helping parents with challenging children positive family intervention facilitator guide.* New York, NY: Oxford University Press.

Durand, V. M., Hieneman, M., Clarke, S., Wang, M., & Rinaldi, M. L. (2013). Positive family intervention for severe challenging behavior: I. A multisite randomized clinical trial. *Journal of Positive Behavior Interventions, 15,* 133–143. doi:10.1177/1098300712458324

Dykens, E. M., Fisher, M. H., Taylor, J. L., Lambert, W., & Miodrag, N. (2014). Reducing distress in mothers of children with autism and other disabilities: A randomized trial. *Pediatrics, 134,* 454–463. doi:10.1542/peds.2013-3164

D'Zurilla, T. J., & Goldfried, M. R. (1971). Problem solving and behavior modification. *Journal of Abnormal Psychology, 78,* 107–126. http://doi.org/10.1037/h0031360

D'Zurilla, T. J., & Nezu, A. M. (2009). Problem solving therapy. In K. S. Dobson (Ed.) *Handbook of cognitive-behavioral therapies* (3rd ed., pp. 197–225). New York, NY: Guilford Press.

Eber, L., Sugai, G., Smith, C. R., & Scott, T. M. (2002). Wraparound and positive behavioral interventions and supports in the schools. *Journal of Emotional and Behavioral Disorders, 10,* 171–180. doi:10.1177/10634266020100030501

Ellis, A. (1970). *The essence of rational psychotherapy: A comprehensive approach to treatment.* New York: Institute for Rational Living.

Ellis, A. (1994). *Reason and emotion in psychotherapy: A comprehensive method of treating human disturbances.* New York, NY: Carol.

Erbas, D. (2010). A collaborative approach to implementing positive behavior support plans for children with problem behaviors: A comparison of consultation versus consultation and feedback approach. *Education and Training in Autism and Developmental Disabilities, 45,* 94–106.

Ergüner-Tekinalp, B., & Akkök, F. (2004). The effects of a coping skills training program on the coping skills, hopelessness, and stress levels of mothers of children with autism. *International Journal for the Advancement of Counselling, 26,* 257–269. http://doi.org/10.1023/B:ADCO.0000035529.92256.0d

Estes, A., Vismara, L., Mercado, C., Fitzpatrick, A., Elder, L., Greenson, J., … Rogers, S. (2014). The impact of parent-delivered intervention on parents of very young children with autism. *Journal of Autism and Developmental Disorders, 44,* 353–365. doi:10.1007/s10803-013-1874-z

Eyberg, S. M., Nelson, M. M., & Boggs, S. R. (2008). Evidence-based psychosocial treatments for children and adolescents with disruptive behavior. *Journal of Clinical Child and Adolescent Psychology, 37,* 215–237.

Farber, B., & Kirk, S. (1959). Effects of a severely mentally retarded child on family integration. *Monographs of the Society for Research in Child Development, 24*(2), 1–112.Feldman, M. A., Condillac, R. A., Tough, S., Hunt, S., & Griffiths, D. (2002). Effectiveness of community positive behavioral intervention for persons with developmental disabilities and severe problem behavior disorders. *Behavior Therapy, 33,* 377–398.

Feldman, M. A., & Werner, S. E. (2002). Collateral effects of behavioral parent training on families of children with developmental disabilities and behavior disorders. *Behavioral Interventions, 17*(2), 75–83. doi:10.1002/bin.111

Fettig, A., Schultz, T. R., & Sreckovic, M. A. (2015). Effects of coaching on the implementation of functional assessment–based parent intervention in reducing challenging behaviors. *Journal of Positive Behavior Interventions, 17*, 170–180.

Field, S., & Hoffman, A. (2002). Lessons learned from implementing the Steps to Self-Determination curriculum. *Remedial and Special Education, 23*(2), 90–98. doi:10.1177/074193250202300205

Fish, W. W. (2008). The IEP meeting: Perceptions of parents of students who receive special education services. *Preventing School Failure: Alternative Education for Children and Youth, 53*(1), 8–14.

Fixsen, D. L., Naoom, S. F., Blasé, K. A., & Friedman, R. M. (2005). *Implementation research: A synthesis of the literature.* Retrieved from http://www.popline.org/node/266329

Floyd, F. J., & Gallagher, E. M. (1997). Parental stress, care demands, and use of support services for school-age children with disabilities and behavior problems. *Family Relations, 46*, 359–371. doi:10.2307/585096

Folkman, S., & Lazarus, R. S. (1980). An analysis of coping in a middle-aged community sample. *Journal of Health and Social Behavior, 21*, 219–239. doi:10.2307/2136617

Forehand, R., Sturgis, E. T., McMahon, R. J., Aguar, D., Green, K., Wells, K. C., & Breiner, J. (1979). Parent behavioral training to modify child noncompliance treatment generalization across time and from home to school. *Behavior Modification, 3*(1), 3–25.

Fox, L., Vaughn, B. J., Wyatte, M. L., & Dunlap, G. (2002). "We can't expect other people to understand": Family perspectives on problem behavior. *Exceptional Children, 68*(4), 437–450. doi:10.1177/001440290206800402

Fransella, F., Bell, R., & Bannister, D. (2004). *A manual for repertory grid technique.* West Sussex, England: Wiley.

Friman, P. C., & Altman, K. (1990). Parent use of DRI on high rate disruptive behavior: Direct and collateral benefits. *Research in Developmental Disabilities, 11*, 249–254.

Friman, P. C., Barnard, J. D., Altman, K., & Wolf, M. M. (1986). Parent and teacher use of DRO and DRI to reduce aggressive behavior. *Analysis and Intervention in Developmental Disabilities, 6*, 319–330.

Fujiura, G. T. (2010). Aging families and the demographics of family financial support of adults with disabilities. *Journal of Disability Policy Studies, 20*, 241–250. doi:10.1177/1044207309350560

Fujiura, G. T., & Yamaki, K. (2000). Trends in demography of childhood poverty and disability. *Exceptional Children, 66*, 187–199.

Gallimore, R., Goldenberg, C. N., & Weisner, T. S. (1993). The social construction and subjective reality of activity settings: Implications for community psychology. *American Journal of Community Psychology, 21*, 537–560. doi:10.1007/BF00942159

Gammon, E. A., & Rose, S. D. (1991). The coping skills training program for parents of children with developmental disabilities: An experimental evaluation. *Research on Social Work Practice, 1*, 244–256. doi:10.1177/104973159100100302

Ganz, M. L. (2007). The lifetime distribution of the incremental societal costs of autism. *Archives of Pediatric and Adolescent Medicine, 161*, 343–349. doi:10.1001/archpedi.161.4.343.

Garriott, P. P., Wandry, D., & Snyder, L. (2001). Teachers as parents, parents as children: What's wrong with this picture? *Preventing School Failure: Alternative Education for Children and Youth, 45*(1), 37–43.

Gillett, J. N., & LeBlanc, L. A. (2007). Parent-implemented natural language paradigm to increase language and play in children with autism. *Research in Autism Spectrum Disorders, 1*, 247–255. doi:10.1016/j.rasd.2006.09.003

Glidden, L. M. (2003). Positive psychology and parenting children with developmental disabilities: Still happy after all these years? *Psychology in Mental Retardation and Developmental Disabilities, 29*(2), 3–4.

Glidden, L. M., Billings, F. J., & Jobe, B. M. (2006). Personality, coping style and well-being of parents rearing children with developmental disabilities. *Journal of Intellectual Disability Research, 50*, 949–962. http://doi.org/10.1111/j.1365-2788.2006.00929.x

Glidden, L. M., & Schoolcraft, S. A. (2003). Depression: Its trajectory and correlates in mothers rearing children with intellectual disability. *Journal of Intellectual Disability Research, 47*, 250–263. doi:10.1046/j.1365-2788.2003.00487.x

Goldberg, D. P., & Hillier, V. F. (1979). A scaled version of the General Health Questionnaire. *Psychological Medicine, 9*, 139–145. doi:10.1017/S0033291700021644

Goldstein, S., & Turnbull, A. P. (1982). Strategies to increase parent participation in IEP conferences. *Exceptional Children, 48*, 360–361.

Graziano, A. M., & Diament, D. M. (1992). Parent behavioral training an examination of the paradigm. *Behavior Modification, 16*(1), 3–38. doi:10.1177/01454455920161001

Greaves, D. (1997). The effect of rational-emotive parent education on the stress of mothers of young children with Down syndrome. *Journal of Rational-Emotive and Cognitive-Behavior Therapy, 15*, 249–267. doi:10.1023/A:1025063425172

Green, J., Charman, T., McConachie, H., Aldred, C., Slonims, V., Howlin, P., ... Pickles, A. (2010). Parent-mediated communication-focused treatment in children with autism (PACT): A randomised controlled trial. *Lancet, 375*, 2152–2160. doi:10.1016/S0140-6736(10)60587-9

Griffin, C., Guerin, S., Sharry, J., & Drumm, M. (2010). A multicentre controlled study of an early intervention parenting programme for young children with behavioural and developmental difficulties. *International Journal of Clinical Health and Psychology, 10*(2). Retrieved from http://search.ebscohost.com/login.aspx?direct=true&profile=ehost&scope=site&authtype=crawler&jrnl=16972600&AN=49186570&h=H8TraD3FixLYvrm%2Fl2iYlcPAORBIe%2B5PdTWoXzeYWAN%2FVbKqNg2PB43Lr7oEoxB%2FK%2FQUHUSmdryBBdZX%2ByLKDg%3D%3D&crl=c

Griffiths, R. (1954). *The abilities of babies: A study in mental measurement.* New York, NY: McGraw-Hill.

Griffiths, R. (1970). *The abilities of young children.* London: Child Development Research Centre.

Guidubaldi, J., & Cleminshaw, H. K. (1985). The development of the Cleminshaw–Guidubaldi Parent Satisfaction Scale. *Journal of Clinical Child Psychology, 14*, 293–298. doi:10.1207/s15374424jccp1404_4

Hagner, D., Kurtz, A., Cloutier, H., Arakelian, C., Brucker, D. L., & May, J. (2012). Outcomes of a family-centered transition process for students with autism spectrum disorders. *Focus on Autism and Other Developmental Disabilities, 27*(1), 42–50. doi:10.1177/1088357611430841

Hand, A., Raghallaigh, C. N., Cuppage, J., Coyle, S., & Sharry, J. (2013). A controlled clinical evaluation of the Parents Plus Children's Programme for parents of children aged 6–12 with mild intellectual disability in a school setting. *Clinical Child Psychology and Psychiatry, 18*, 536–555. doi:10.1177/1359104512460861

Handen, B. L., Parrish, J. M., McClung, T. J., Kerwin, M. E., & Evans, L. D. (1992). Using guided compliance versus time out to promote child compliance: A preliminary comparative analysis in an analogue context. *Research in Developmental Disabilities, 13*, 157–170.

Harris, S. L. (1984). Intervention planning for the family of the autistic child: A multilevel assessment of the family system. *Journal of Marital and Family Therapy, 10*, 157–166. doi:10.1111/j.1752-0606.1984.tb00006.x

Harrold, M., Lutzker, J. R., Campbell, R. V., & Touchette, P. E. (1992). Improving parent-child interactions for families of children with developmental disabilities. *Journal of Behavior Therapy and Experimental Psychiatry, 23*(2), 89–100. doi:10.1016/0005-7916(92)90006-5

Hastings, R. P., Allen, R., McDermott, K., & Still, D. (2002). Factors related to positive perceptions in mothers of children with intellectual disabilities. *Journal of Applied Research in Intellectual Disabilities, 15*, 269–275. doi:10.1046/j.1468-3148.2002.00104.x

Hastings, R. P., & Beck, A. (2004). Practitioner review: Stress intervention for parents of children with intellectual disabilities. *Journal of Child Psychology and Psychiatry, 45*, 1338–1349. doi:10.1111/j.1469-7610.2004.00357.x

Hastings, R. P., Beck, A., & Hill, C. (2005). Positive contributions made by children with an intellectual disability in the family: Mothers' and fathers' perceptions. *Journal of Intellectual Disabilities, 9*, 155–165. doi:10.1177/1744629505053930

Hastings, R. P., Kovshoff, H., Ward, N. J., degli Espinosa, F., Brown, T., & Remington, B. (2005). Systems analysis of stress and positive perceptions in mothers and fathers of pre-school children with autism. *Journal of Autism and Developmental Disorders, 35*, 635–644. doi:10.1007/s10803-005-0007-8

Hastings, R. P., & Taunt, H. M. (2002). Positive perceptions in families of children with developmental disabilities. *American Journal of Mental Retardation: AJMR, 107*, 116–127. doi:10.1352/0895-8017(2002)107<0116:PPIFOC>2.0.CO;2

Hawkins, N. E. & Singer, G. H. S. (1988). *Stress Management Manual.* Unpublished manuscript. Gevirtz Graduate School of Education, University of California Santa Barbara.

Hawkins, R. P., Peterson, R. F., Schweid, E., & Bijou, S. W. (1966). Behavior therapy in the home: Amelioration of problem parent-child relations with the parent in a therapeutic role. *Journal of Experimental Child Psychology, 4*(1), 99–107.

Heiman, T. (2002). Parents of children with disabilities: Resilience, coping, and future expectations. *Journal of Developmental and Physical Disabilities, 14*, 159–171. doi:10.1023/A:1015219514621

Heitzman-Powell, L. S., Buzhardt, J., Rusinko, L. C., & Miller, T. M. (2013). Formative evaluation of an aba outreach training program for parents of children with autism in remote areas. *Focus on Autism and Other Developmental Disabilities, 29*(1), 23N38. doi:10.1177/1088357613504992

Heppner, P., & Petersen, C. H. (1982). The development and implications of a personal problem-solving inventory. *Journal of Counseling Psychology, 29*(1), 66–75. doi:10.1037/0022-0167.29.1.66

Hill, N. E., Castellino, D. R., Lansford, J. E., Nowlin, P., Dodge, K. A., Bates, J. E., & Pettit, G. S. (2004). Parent academic involvement as related to school behavior, achievement, and aspirations: Demographic variations across adolescence. *Child Development, 75*, 1491–1509. doi:10.1111/j.1467-8624.2004.00753.x

Hoffman, A., & Field, S. (1995). Promoting self-determination through effective curriculum development. *Intervention in School and Clinic, 30*, 134–141. doi:10.1177/105345129503000302

Holahan, C. J., Moos, R. H., & Schaefer, J. A. (1996). Coping, stress resistance, and growth: Conceptualizing adaptive functioning. In M. Zeidner & N. S. Endler (Eds.), *Handbook of coping: Theory, research, applications* (pp. 24–43). Oxford, UK: Wiley.

Holroyd, J. (1974). The Questionnaire on Resources and Stress: An instrument to measure family response to a handicapped family member. *Journal of Community Psychology, 2*(1), 92–94. doi:10.1002/1520-6629(197401)2:1<92::AID-JCOP2290020133>3.0.CO;2-A

Hoover-Dempsey, K. V., Walker, J. M. T., Sandler, H. M., Whetsel, D., Green, C. L., Wilkins, A. S., & Closson, K. (2005). Why do parents become involved? Research findings and implications. *Elementary School Journal, 106,* 105–130. doi:10.1086/499194

Horner, R. H., Albin, R. W., Sprague, J. R., & Todd, A. W. (1999). Positive behavior support. In M. E. Snell & F. Brown, (Eds.), *Instruction of students with severe disabilities* (5th Ed., pp. 207–243). Upper Saddle River, NJ: Merrill.

Horner, R. H., Carr E. G., McGee, G., Odom, S., & Wolery, M. (2005). The use of single subject design research to identify evidence-based practice in special education. *Exceptional Children, 71,* 165–179. doi:10.1177/001440290507100203

Horner, R. H., Sugai, G., Smolkowski, K., Eber, L., Nakasato, J., Todd, A. W., & Esperanza, J. (2009). A randomized, wait-list controlled effectiveness trial assessing school-wide positive behavior support in elementary schools. *Journal of Positive Behavior Interventions, 11,* 133–144. doi:10.1177/1098300709332067

Hsieh, H.-H., Wilder, D. A., & Abellon, O. E. (2011). The effects of training on caregiver implementation of incidental teaching. *Journal of Applied Behavior Analysis, 44,* 199–203. doi:10.1901/jaba.2011.44-199

Hudson, A. M. (1982). Training parents of developmentally handicapped children: A component analysis. *Behavior Therapy, 13,* 325–333.

Hudson, A., Cameron, C., & Matthews, J. (2008). The wide-scale implementation of a support program for parents of children with an intellectual disability and difficult behaviour. *Journal of Intellectual and Developmental Disability, 33,* 117–126.

Hudson, A. M., Matthews, J. M., Gavidia-Payne, S. T., Cameron, C. A., Mildon, R. L., Radler, G. A., & Nankervis, K. L. (2003). Evaluation of an intervention system for parents of children with intellectual disability and challenging behaviour. *Journal of Intellectual Disability Research, 47,* 238–249. doi:10.1046/j.1365-2788.2003.00486.x

Hudson, A., Matthews, J., Gavidia-Payne, S., Cameron, C., Nankervis, K., Radler, G., & Mildon, R. (2001). *Report to the Department of Human Services on the development and trialling of Signposts for Building Better Behaviour, a support package for parents of children with an intellectual disability and difficult behaviour.* Melbourne, Australia: RMIT University.

Humm, S. P., Blampied, N. M., & Liberty, K. A. (2005). Effects of parent-administered, home-based, high-probability request sequences on compliance by children with developmental disabilities. *Child and Family Behavior Therapy,* 27(3), 27–45.

Huynen, K. B., Lutzker, J. R., Bigelow, K. M., Touchette, P. E., & Campbell, R. V. (1996). Planned activities training for mothers of children with developmental disabilities community generalization and follow-up. *Behavior Modification, 20,* 406–427. doi:10.1177/01454455960204003

Individuals with Disabilities Education Act (IDEA). (2004). 34 C.F.R. § 300.321. Retrieved from http://idea.ed.gov/explore/view/p/,root,regs,300,D,300%252E321

Ingersoll, B., & Gergans, S. (2007). The effect of a parent-implemented imitation intervention on spontaneous imitation skills in young children with autism. *Research in Developmental Disabilities, 28,* 163–175. doi:10.1016/j.ridd.2006.02.004

Ingersoll, B., & Wainer, A. (2013). Initial efficacy of Project ImPACT: A parent-mediated social communication intervention for young children with ASD. *Journal of Autism and Developmental Disorders, 43,* 2943–2952. doi:10.1007/s10803-013-1840-9

Ireys, H. T., Sills, E. M., Kolodner, K. B., & Walsh, B. B. (1996). A social support intervention for parents of children with juvenile rheumatoid arthritis: Results of a randomized trial. *Journal of Pediatric Psychology, 21*, 633–641. http://doi.org/10.1093/jpepsy/21.5.633

Irvine, A. B., Biglan, A., Smolkowski, K., Metzler, C. W., & Ary, D. V. (1999). The effectiveness of a parenting skills program for parents of middle school students in small communities. *Journal of Consulting and Clinical Psychology, 67*, 811–825.

Jang, J., Dixon, D. R., Tarbox, J., Granpeesheh, D., Kornack, J., & de Nocker, Y. (2012). Randomized trial of an eLearning program for training family members of children with autism in the principles and procedures of applied behavior analysis. *Research in Autism Spectrum Disorders, 6*, 852–856. doi:10.1016/j.rasd.2011.11.004

Jensen, S. A., & Grimes, L. K. (2010, August). Increases in parent attendance to behavioral parent training due to concurrent child treatment groups. In *Child and Youth Care Forum* (Vol. 39, No. 4, pp. 239–251). Springer US.

Jocelyn, L. J., Casiro, O. G., Beattie, D., Bow, J., & Kneisz, J. (1998). Treatment of children with autism: A randomized controlled trial to evaluate a caregiver-based intervention program in community day-care centers. *Journal of Developmental and Behavioral Pediatrics: JDBP, 19*, 326–334.

Joyce, B. R., & Showers, B. (2002). *Student achievement through staff development.* Alexandria, VA: Association for Supervision and Curriculum Development.

Kabat-Zinn, J. (1994). *Wherever you go, there you are: Mindfulness meditation in everyday life.* New York, NY: Hyperion.

Kabat-Zinn, J., & Hanh, T. N. (2009). *Full catastrophe living: Using the wisdom of your body and mind to face stress, pain, and illness.* New York, NY: Random House.

Kaiser, A. P., Hancock, T. B., & Nietfeld, J. P. (2000). The effects of parent-implemented enhanced milieu teaching on the social communication of children who have autism. *Early Education and Development, 11*, 423–446. doi:10.1207/s15566935eed1104_4

Kalyanpur, M., Harry, B., & Skrtic, T. (2000). Equity and advocacy expectations of culturally diverse families' participation in special education. *International Journal of Disability, Development and Education, 47*, 119–136. doi:10.1080/713671106

Kanner, L. (1943). Autistic disturbances of affective contact. *Nervous Child, 2*, 217–250.

Kansas Institute for Positive Behavior Support. (2011). *Positive behavior support online training module.* Lawrence: University of Kansas. Retrieved from http://www.kipbs.org/kmhpbs/index.html

Kashima, K. J., Baker, B. L., & Landen, S. J. (1988). Media-based versus professionally led training for parents of mentally retarded children. *American Journal on Mental Retardation, 93*, 209–217. Retrieved from http://psycnet.apa.org/psycinfo/1989-27126-001

Kashinath, S., Woods, J., & Goldstein, H. (2006). Enhancing generalized teaching strategy use in daily routines by parents of children with autism. *Journal of Speech, Language, and Hearing Research, 49*, 466–485. doi:10.1044/1092-4388(2006/036)

Kazantzis, N., & Deane, F. P. (1999). Psychologists' use of homework assignments in clinical practice. *Professional Psychology: Research and Practice, 30*, 581. doi:http://dx.doi.org/10.1037/0735-7028.30.6.581

Kazantzis, N., Deane, F. P., & Ronan, K. R. (2000). Homework assignments in cognitive and behavioral therapy: A meta-analysis. *Clinical Psychology: Science and Practice, 7*, 189–202. doi:10.1093/clipsy.7.2.189

Kazdin, A. E. (1997). Parent management training: Evidence, outcomes, and issues. *Journal of the American Academy of Child and Adolescent Psychiatry, 36*, 1349–1356.

Kazdin, A. E. (2005). *Parent management training: Treatment for oppositional, aggressive, and antisocial behavior in children and adolescents*. New York, NY: Oxford University Press.

Kazdin, A. E. (2007). Mediators and mechanisms of change in psychotherapy research. *Annual Review of Clinical Psychology, 3*, 1–27. doi:10.1146/annurev.clinpsy.3.022806.091432

Kessler, R. C., Berglund, P. A., Bruce, M. L., Koch, J. R., Laska, E. M., Leaf, P. J., ... Wang, P. S. (2001). The prevalence and correlates of untreated serious mental illness. *Health Services Research, 36*(6 Pt 1), 987–1007.

Kim, N. H., & Park, J. (2012). The effects of the family-involved SDLMI on academic engagement and goal attainment of middle school students with disabilities who exhibit problem behavior. *International Journal of Special Education, 27*, 117–127.

Kim, W.-H., & Turnbull, A. (2004). Transition to adulthood for students with severe intellectual disabilities: Shifting toward person-family interdependent planning. *Research and Practice for Persons with Severe Disabilities, 29*, 53–57. doi:10.1177/088572889902200102

Kirkham, M. A. (1993). Two-year follow-up of skills training with mothers of children with disabilities. *American Journal on Mental Retardation, 97*, 509–520.

Kirkham, M. A., & Schilling, R. F. (1990). Life skills training with mothers of handicapped children. *Journal of Social Service Research, 13*, 67–87. doi:10.1300/J079v13n02_05

Klass, E. T. (1987). Situational approach to assessment of guilt: Development and validation of a self-report measure. *Journal of Psychopathology and Behavioral Assessment, 9*(1), 35–48. doi:10.1007/BF00961630

Koegel, L. K., Steibel, D., & Koegel, R. L. (1998). Reducing aggression in children with autism toward infant or toddler siblings. *Journal of the Association for Persons with Severe Handicaps, 23*, 111–118.

Koegel, R. L., & Kern Koegel, L. (2006). *Pivotal response treatments for autism: Communication, social, and academic development*. Baltimore, MD: Brookes.

Koegel, R. L., Symon, J. B., & Koegel, L. K. (2002). Parent education for families of children with autism living in geographically distant areas. *Journal of Positive Behavior Interventions, 4*, 88–103. doi:10.1177/109830070200400204

Konstantareas, M. M., & Homatidis, S. (1989). Assessing child symptom severity and stress in parents of autistic children. *Journal of Child Psychology and Psychiatry, 30*, 459–470.

Koren, P. E., DeChillo, N., & Friesen, B. J. (1992). Measuring empowerment in families whose children have emotional disabilities: A brief questionnaire. *Rehabilitation Psychology, 37*, 305.

Kozlowski, A. M., Matson, J. L., Horovitz, M., Worley, J. A., & Neal, D. (2011). Parents' first concerns of their child's development in toddlers with autism spectrum disorders. *Developmental Neurorehabilitation, 14*(2), 72–78. doi:10.3109/17518423.2010.539193

Krantz, P. J., MacDuff, M. T., & McClannahan, L. E. (1993). Programming participation in family activities for children with autism: Parents' use of photographic activity schedules. *Journal of Applied Behavior Analysis, 26*, 137–138. doi:10.1901/jaba.1993.26-137

Lafasakis, M., & Sturmey, P. (2007). Training parent implementation of discrete-trial teaching: Effects on generalization of parent teaching and child correct responding. *Journal of Applied Behavior Analysis, 40*, 685–689. doi:10.1901/jaba.2007.685-689

Lalli, J. S., Casey, S. D., & Kates, K. (1997). Noncontingent reinforcement as treatment for severe problem behavior: Some procedural variations. *Journal of Applied Behavior Analysis, 30*, 127–137.

Landesman, S., & Butterfield, E.C. (1987). Normalization and deinstitutionalization of mentally retarded individuals: Controversy and facts. *American Psychologist, 42*, 809–816.

Larson, S. A., Lakin, K. C., Anderson, L. L., Kwak, N., Lee, J. H., & Anderson, D. (2001). Prevalence of mental retardation and developmental disabilities: Estimates from the 1994/1995 National Health Interview Survey Disability Supplements. *American Journal on Mental Retardation, 106,* 231–252.

Laski, K. E., Charlop, M. H., & Schreibman, L. (1988). Training parents to use the natural language paradigm to increase their autistic children's speech. *Journal of Applied Behavior Analysis, 21,* 391–400. doi:10.1901/jaba.1988.21-391

Lazarus R., & Folkman, S. (1984). *Stress, appraisal, and coping.* New York, NY: Springer.

Lee, P., Niew, W., Yang, H., Chen, V. C., & Lin, K. (2012). A meta-analysis of behavioral parent training for children with attention deficit hyperactivity disorder. *Research in Developmental Disabilities, 33,* 2040–2049.

Lerman, D. C., Swiezy, N., Perkins–Parks, S., & Roane, H. S. (2000). Skill acquisition in parents of children with developmental disabilities: Interaction between skill type and instructional format. *Research in Developmental Disabilities, 21,* 183–196. doi:10.1016/S0891-4222(00)00033-0

Levy, R. L., & Feld, A. D. (1999). Increasing patient adherence to gastroenterology treatment and prevention regimens. *American Journal of Gastroenterology, 94,* 1733–1742. doi:10.1111/j.1572-0241.1999.01200.x

Lincoln, T. M., Wilhelm, K., & Nestoriuc, Y. (2007). Effectiveness of psychoeducation for relapse, symptoms, knowledge, adherence and functioning in psychotic disorders: A meta-analysis. *Schizophrenia Research, 96*(1–3), 232–245. doi:10.1016/j.schres.2007.07.022116–127.

Lovaas, O. I. (1977). *The autistic child: Language development through behavior modification.* Irvington.

Lovaas, O. I., Koegel, R. L., Simmons, J. Q., & Long, J. S. (1973). Some generalization and follow-up measures on autistic children in behavior therapy. *Journal of Applied Behavior Analysis, 6,* 131–166.

Lucksted, A., McFarlane, W., Downing, D., & Dixon, L. (2012). Recent developments in family psychoeducation as an evidence-based practice. *Journal of Marital and Family Therapy, 38*(1), 101–121. doi:10.1111/j.17520606.2011.00256.x

Lucyshyn, J. M., & Albin, R. W. (1993). Comprehensive support to families of children with disabilities and behavior problems: Keeping it "friendly." In G. H. S. Singer & L. E. Powers (Eds.), *Families, disability, and empowerment: Active coping skills and strategies for family interventions* (pp. 365–407). Baltimore, MD: Brookes.

Lucyshyn, J. M., Albin, R. W., Horner, R. H., Mann, J. C., Mann, J. A., & Wadsworth, G. (2007). Family implementation of positive behavior support for a child with autism: Longitudinal, single-case, experimental, and descriptive replication and extension. *Journal of Positive Behavior Interventions, 9,* 131–150. doi:10.1177/10983007070090030201.

Lucyshyn, J. M., Albin, R. W., & Nixon, C. D. (1997). Embedding comprehensive behavioral support in family ecology: An experimental, single-case analysis. *Journal of Consulting and Clinical Psychology, 65,* 241–251.

Lucyshyn, J. M., Blumberg E. R., & Kayser, A. T. (2000). Improving the quality of support to families of children with severe behavior problems in the first decade of the new millennium. *Journal of Positive Behavior Interventions, 2,* 113–114.

Lucyshyn, J. M., Dunlap, G., & Albin, R. W. (Eds.). (2002). *Families and positive behavior support: Addressing problem behavior in family contexts.* Baltimore, MD: Brookes.

Lucyshyn, J. M., Fossett, B., Bakeman, R., Cheremshynski, C., Miller, L., Lohrmann, S., & Irvin, L. K. (2015). Transforming parent-child interaction in family routines: Longitudinal analysis with families of children with developmental disabilities. *Journal of Child and Family Studies*. Published online. doi 10.1007/s10826-015-0154-2

Lutzker, J. R., & Campbell, R. (1994). *Ecobehavioral family interventions in developmental disabilities*. Pacific Grove, CA: Brooks/Cole.

Lutzker, J. R., & Steed, S. E. (1998). *Parent training for families of children with developmental disabilities*. Retrieved from http://psycnet.apa.org/psycinfo/1997-36836-009

Lutzker, J. R., Campbell, R. V., Harrold, M., & Huynen, K. (1992). Project Ecosystems: An ecobehavioral approach to families with children with developmental disabilities. *Journal of Developmental and Physical Disabilities, 4*, 1–14.

Maenner, M. J., Rice, C. E., Arneson, C. L., Cunniff, C., Schieve, L. A., Carpenter, L. A., . . . Durkin, M. S. (2014). Potential impact of DSM-5 criteria on autism spectrum disorder prevalence estimates. *JAMA Psychiatry, 71*, 292–300. doi:10.1001/jamapsychiatry.2013.3893

Mahoney, M. J. (1976). *Scientist as subject: The psychological imperative* (Vol. 14). Oxford, UK: Ballinger.

Mancil, G. R. (2006). Functional communication training: A review of the literature related to children with autism. *Education and Training in Developmental Disabilities, 41*, 213–224.

Manzoni, G., Pagnini, F., Castelnuovo, G., & Molinari, E. (2008). Relaxation training for anxiety: A ten-years systematic review with meta-analysis. *BMC Psychiatry, 8*(1), 41. doi:10.1186/1471-244X-8-41

Marckel, J. M., Neef, N. A., & Ferreri, S. J. (2006). A preliminary analysis of teaching improvisation with the Picture Exchange Communication System to children with autism. *Journal of Applied Behavior Analysis, 39*, 109–115. doi:10.1901/jaba.2006.131-04

Marcus, B. A., Swanson, V., & Vollmer, T. R. (2001). Effects of parent training on parent and child behavior using procedures based on functional analyses. *Behavioral Interventions, 16*, 87–104.

Mason, C. Y., McGahee-Kovac, M., Johnson, L., & Stillerman, S. (2002). Implementing student-led IEPs: Student participation and student and teacher reactions. *Career Development for Exceptional Individuals, 25*, 171–192.

Matson, J. L., Dixon, D. R., & Matson, M. L. (2005). Assessing and treating aggression in children and adolescents with developmental disabilities: A 20-year overview. *Educational Psychology, 25*(2-3), 151–181. doi:10.1080/0144341042000301148

Matson, J. L., & Francis, K. L. (1994). Generalizing spontaneous language in developmentally delayed children via a visual cue procedure using caregivers as therapists. *Behavior Modification, 18*, 186–197. doi:10.1177/01454455940182003

Maul, C. A., & Singer, G. H. S. (2009). "Just good different things": specific accommodations families make to positively adapt to their children with developmental disabilities. *Topics in Early Childhood Special Education, 29*(3), 155–170. doi:10.1177/0271121408328516

Maurice, C. E., Green, G. E., & Luce, S. C. (1996). *Behavioral intervention for young children with autism: A manual for parents and professionals*. Pro-ed.

McCubbin, H. I., Joy, C. B., Cauble, A. E., Comeau, J. K., Patterson, J. M., & Needle, R. H. (1980). Family stress and coping: A decade review. *Journal of Marriage and the Family, 42*, 855–871.

McCubbin, H. I., & Patterson, J. M. (1983). The family stress process: The double ABCX model of adjustment and adaptation. *Marriage and Family Review, 6*(1–2), 7–37.

McDonald, M. R., & Budd, K. S. (1983). "Booster shots" following didactic parent training effects of follow-up using graphic feedback and instructions. *Behavior Modification, 7*, 211–223.

McFarlane, W. R., Link, B., Dushay, R., Marchal, J., & Crilly, J. (1995). Psychoeducational multiple family groups: Four-year relapse outcome in schizophrenia. *Family Process, 34*, 127–144. doi:10.1111/j.1545-5300.1995.00127.x

McIntyre, L. L. (2008a). Adapting Webster-Stratton's incredible years parent training for children with developmental delay: Findings from a treatment group only study. *Journal of Intellectual Disability Research, 52,* 1176–1192. doi:10.1111/j.1365-2788.2008.01108.x

McIntyre, L. L. (2008b). Parent training for young children with developmental disabilities: Randomized controlled trial. *American Journal of Mental Retardation, 113,* 356–368. Retrieved from http://www.aaiddjournals.org/aamronline/?request=get-abstract&doi=10.1352%2F2008.113:356-368

McNair, D. M., Lorr, M., & Droppelman, L. F. (1971). Manual for the profile of mood states. *San Diego: Educational and Industrial Testing Services Review, 6*(1–2), 7–37. doi:10.1300/J002v06n01_

Meissner, W. W. (2010). Some notes on the epistemology of empathy. *The Psychoanalytic Quarterly, 79*(2), 421–469. doi:10.1002/j.2167-4086.2010.tb00454.x

Meltzer, L. J., & Mindell, J. A. (2007). Relationship between child sleep disturbances and maternal sleep, mood, and parenting stress: A pilot study. *Journal of Family Psychology, 21*(1), 67.

Mildon, R. L., Moore, D. W., & Dixon, R. S. (2004). Combining noncontingent escape and functional communication training as a treatment for negatively reinforced disruptive behavior. *Journal of Positive Behavior Interventions, 6,* 92–102.

Miner, C. A., & Bates, P. E. (1997). The effect of person centered planning activities on the IEP/Transition planning process. *Education and Training in Developmental Disabilities, 32,* 105–112.

Minke, K. M., & Anderson, K. K. (2005). Family-school collaboration and positive behavior support. *Journal of Positive Behavior Interventions, 7,* 181–185. Retrieved from http://www.monarchcenter.org/pdfs/Minke_2005.pdf

Mitchell, D., Morton, M., & Hornby, G. (2010). Review of the literature on individual education plans: Report to the New Zealand Ministry of Education. *Christchurch: College of Education, University of Canterbury.*

Moes, D. R., & Frea, W. D. (2002). Contextualized behavioral support in early intervention for children with autism and their families. *Journal of Autism and Developmental Disorders, 32,* 519–533.

Moran, D. R., & Whitman, T. L. (1985). The multiple effects of a play-oriented parent training program for mothers of developmentally delayed children. *Analysis and Intervention in Developmental Disabilities, 5*(1), 73–96. doi:10.1016/S0270-4684(85)80007-0

Mueller, T. G., & Carranza, F. (2011). An examination of special education due process hearings. *Journal of Disability Policy Studies, 22,* 131–139. doi:10.1177/1044207311392762

Mueller, T. G., Singer, G. H., & Draper, L. M. (2008). Reducing parental dissatisfaction with special education in two school districts: Implementing conflict prevention and alternative dispute resolution. *Journal of Educational and Psychological Consultation, 18,* 191–233. doi:10.1080/10474410701864339

Muscott, H. S., Mann, E. L., & LeBrun, M. R. (2008). Positive behavioral interventions and supports in New Hampshire effects of large-scale implementation of Schoolwide Positive Behavior Support on student discipline and academic achievement. *Journal of Positive Behavior Interventions, 10,* 190–205. doi:10.1177/1098300708316258

Nachshen, J. S. (2005). Empowerment and families: Building bridges between parents and professionals, theory and research. *Journal of Developmental Disabilities, 11*(1), 67–76. Retrieved from http://www.oadd.org/publications/journal/issues/vol11no1/download/nachshen.pdf

Najdowski, A. C., Wallace, M. D., Doney, J. K., & Ghezzi, P. M. (2003). Parental assessment and treatment of food selectivity in natural settings. *Journal of Applied Behavior Analysis, 36,* 383–386.

National Autism Center (NAC). (2009). *National Standards Project—Addressing the need for evidence-based practice guidelines for autism spectrum disorders.* Retrieved from http://www.nationalautismcenter.org/pdf/NAC%20Standards%20Report.pdf

National Research Council (US) & Committee on Educational Interventions for Children with Autism. (2001). *Educating children with autism.* Washington, DC: National Academy Press. Retrieved from http://site.ebrary.com/id/10032464

Nefdt, N., Koegel, R., Singer, G., & Gerber, M. (2010). The use of a self-directed learning program to provide introductory training in pivotal response treatment to parents of children with autism. *Journal of Positive Behavior Interventions, 12*(1), 23–32. doi:10.1177/1098300709334796

Niemeyer, A. J., & Fox, J. (1990). Reducing aggressive behavior during car riding through parent-implemented DRO and fading procedures. *Education and Treatment of Children, 13*(1), 21–35.

Nixon, C. D., & Singer, G. H. (1993). Group cognitive behavioral treatment for excessive parental self-blame and guilt. *American Journal on Mental Retardation, 97,* 665–672.

Odom, S. L., Boyd, B. A., Hall, L. J., & Hume, K. (2010). Evaluation of comprehensive treatment models for individuals with autism spectrum disorders. *Journal of Autism and Developmental Disorders, 40,* 425–436. doi:10.1007/s10803-009-0825-1

Odom, S. L., Brantlinger, E., Gersten, R., Horner, R., Thompson, B., & Harris, K. (2005). Research in special education: Scientific methods and evidence-based practices. *Exceptional Children, 71,* 137–148.

Offit, P. A. (2008). *Autism's false prophets: Bad science, risky medicine, and the search for a cure.* New York, NY: Columbia University Press.

O'Neill, R. E., Horner, R. H., Albin, R. W., Storey, K., Sprague, J. R., & Newton, J. S. (1997). *Functional assessment of problem behavior: A practical assessment guide.* Pacific Grove, CA: Brooks/Cole.

Oosterling, I., Visser, J., Swinkels, S., Rommelse, N., Donders, R., Woudenberg, T., ... Buitelaar, J. (2010). Randomized controlled trial of the focus parent training for toddlers with autism: 1-year outcome. *Journal of Autism and Developmental Disorders, 40,* 1447–1458. doi:10.1007/s10803-010-1004-0

O'Reilly, M., Lancioni, G., & Taylor, I. (1999). An empirical analysis of two forms of extinction to treat aggression. *Research in Developmental Disabilities, 20,* 315–325.

Parish, S. L., Rose, R. A., Grinstein-Weiss, M., & Richman, E. L. (2008). Material hardship in U.S. families raising children with disabilities. *Exceptional Children, 75*(1), 71–92.

Park, J., Turnbull, A. P., & Turnbull, H. R. (2002). Impacts of poverty on quality of life in families of children with disabilities. *Exceptional Children, 68*(2), 151–170. doi:10.1177/001440290206800201

Patterson, G. R. (1965). An application of conditioning techniques to the control of a hyperactive child. *Case studies in behavior modification* (pp. 370–375). New York, NY: Holt, Rinehart & Winston.

Patterson, G. R., Chamberlain, P., & Reid, J. B. (1982). A comparative evaluation of a parent-training program. *Behavior Therapy, 13,* 638–650. doi:10.1016/S0005-7894(82)80021-X

Patterson, J. M. (1988). Families experiencing stress: I. The family adjustment and adaptation response model: II. Applying the FAAR model to health-related issues for intervention and research. *Family Systems Medicine, 6,* 202–237. doi:10.1037/h0089739

Patterson, J. M. (2002). Integrating family resilience and family stress theory. *Journal of Marriage and Family, 64,* 349–360. doi:10.1111/j.1741-3737.2002.00349.x

Pelham, W. E., Jr., Wheeler, T., & Chronis, A. (1998). Empirically supported psychosocial treatments for attention deficit hyperactivity disorder. *Journal of Clinical Child Psychology, 27,* 190–205.

Peterson, C., Semmel, A., von Baeyer, C., Abramson, L. Y., Metalsky, G. I., & Seligman, M. E. P. (1982). The Attributional Style Questionnaire. *Cognitive Therapy and Research, 6,* 287–299. doi:10.1007/BF01173577

Pfiffner, L., & Kaiser, N. (2010). Behavioral parent training. In M. K. Dulcan (Ed.), *The (AAPI) textbook of child and adolescent psychiatry* (pp. 845–868). Washington, DC: American Psychiatric Publishing. Retrieved from http://www.pn.psychiatryonline.org/content.aspx?bookID=24&sectionID=1315113

Phaneuf, L., & McIntyre, L. L. (2011). The application of a three-tier model of intervention to parent training. *Journal of Positive Behavior Interventions, 13,* 198–207. doi:10.1177/1098300711405337

Phillips, E. L. (1968). Achievement place: Token reinforcement procedures in a home-style rehabilitation setting for "predelinquent" boys. *Journal of Applied Behavior Analysis, 1,* 213–223.

Phillips, R. (1999). Intervention with siblings of children with developmental disabilities from economically disadvantaged families. *Families in Society: The Journal of Contemporary Social Services, 80,* 569–577. doi:10.1606/1044-3894.1781

Pierce, K. L., & Schreibman, L. (1994). Teaching daily living skills to children with autism through pictorial self-management. *Journal of Applied Behavior Analysis, 27,* 471–481. doi:10.1901/jaba.1994.27-471

Plant, K. M., & Sanders, M. R. (2007). Reducing problem behavior during care-giving in families of preschool-aged children with developmental disabilities. *Research in Developmental Disabilities, 28,* 362–385. doi:10.1016/j.ridd.2006.02.009

Powers, L. E., Singer, G. H., Stevens, T., & Sowers, J.-A. (1992). Behavioral parent training in home and community generalization settings. *Education and Training in Mental Retardation,* 27(1), 13–27. Retrieved from http://psycnet.apa.org/psycinfo/1992-28291-001

Powers, L. E., Turner, A., Ellison, R., Matuszewski, J., Wilson, R., Phillips, A., & Rein, C. (2001). A multi-component intervention to promote adolescent self-determination. *Journal of Rehabilitation,* 67(4), 13–19.

Powers, L. E., Turner, A., Westwood, D., Matuszewski, J., Wilson, R., & Phillips, A. (2001). TAKE CHARGE for the future: A controlled field-test of a model to promote student involvement in transition planning. *Career Development for Exceptional Individuals,* 24(1), 89–104. doi:10.1177/088572880102400107

Prieto-Bayard, M., & Baker, B. L. (1986). Parent training for Spanish-speaking families with a retarded child. *Journal of Community Psychology, 14,* 134–143.

Quine, L. (1991). Sleep problems in children with mental handicap. *Journal of Intellectual Disability Research, 35,* 269–290.

Quine, L., & Pahl, J. (1985). Examining the causes of stress in families with severely mentally handicapped children. *British Journal of Social Work, 15,* 501–517.

Quinn, M., Carr, A., Carroll, L., & O'Sullivan, D. (2006). An evaluation of the Parents Plus Programme for pre-school children with conduct problems: A comparison of those with and without developmental disabilities. *Irish Journal of Psychology, 27,* 168–182.

Quinn, M., Carr, A., Carroll, L., & O'Sullivan, D. (2007). Parents Plus Programme 1: Evaluation of its effectiveness for pre-school children with developmental disabilities and behavioural problems. *Journal of Applied Research in Intellectual Disabilities, 20,* 345–359.

Reagon, K. A., & Higbee, T. S. (2009). Parent-implemented script fading to promote play-based verbal initiations in children with autism. *Journal of Applied Behavior Analysis, 42,* 659–664. doi:10.1901/jaba.2009.42-659

Reed, G. K., Ringdahl, J. E., Wacker, D. P., Barretto, A., & Andelman, M. S. (2005). The effects of fixed-time and contingent schedules of negative reinforcement on compliance and aberrant behavior. *Research in Developmental Disabilities, 26,* 281–295.

Reid, M. J., Webster-Stratton, C., & Baydar, N. (2004). Halting the development of conduct problems in Head Start children: The effects of parent training. *Journal of Clinical Child and Adolescent Psychology, 33,* 279–291.

Reid, M. J., Webster-Stratton, C., & Hammond, M. (2007). Enhancing a classroom social competence and problem-solving curriculum by offering parent training to families of moderate- to high-risk elementary school children. *Journal of Clinical Child and Adolescent Psychology, 36,* 605–620. doi:10.1080/15374410701662741

Reinke, W. M., Splett, J. D., Robeson, E. N., & Offutt, C. A. (2009). Combining school and family interventions for the prevention and early intervention of disruptive behavior problems in children: A public health perspective. *Psychology in the Schools, 46*(1), 33–43. doi:10.1002/pits.20352

Reschly, A. L., & Christenson, S. L. (2009). Parents as essential partners for fostering students' learning outcomes. In R. Gilman, E. S. Huebner, & M. J. Furlong (Eds.), *Handbook of positive psychology in schools* (pp. 257–272). New York, NY: Routledge.

Richdale, A., Francis, A., Gavidia-Payne, S., & Cotton, S. (2000). Stress, behaviour, and sleep problems in children with an intellectual disability. *Journal of Intellectual and Developmental Disability, 25,* 147–161.

Richman, N., Stevenson, J., & Graham, P. J. (1982). *Pre-school to school: A behavioural study.* New York, NY: Academic.

Rickards, A. L., Walstab, J. E., Wright-Rossi, R. A., Simpson, J., & Reddihough, D. S. (2007). A randomized, controlled trial of a home-based intervention program for children with autism and developmental delay. *Journal of Developmental and Behavioral Pediatrics, 28,* 308–316. doi:10.1097/DBP.0b013e318032792e

Rickards, A. L., Walstab, J. E., Wright-Rossi, R. A., Simpson, J., & Reddihough, D. S. (2009). One-year follow-up of the outcome of a randomized controlled trial of a home-based intervention programme for children with autism and developmental delay and their families. *Child: Care, Health and Development, 35,* 593–602. doi:10.1111/j.1365-2214.2009.00953.x

Risdal, D., & Singer, G. H. S. (2004). Marital adjustment in parents of children with disabilities: A historical review and meta-analysis. *Research and Practice for Persons with Severe Disabilities, 29,* 95–103.

Roach, M. A., Orsmond, G. I., & Barratt, M. S. (1999). Mothers and fathers of children with Down syndrome: Parental stress and involvement in childcare. *American Journal on Mental Retardation, 104,* 422–436.

Roberts, C., Mazzucchelli, T., Studman, L., & Sanders, M. R. (2006). Behavioral family intervention for children with developmental disabilities and behavioral problems. *Journal of Clinical Child and Adolescent Psychology, 35,* 180–193. doi:10.1207/s15374424jccp3502_2

Roberts, J., Williams, K., Carter, M., Evans, D., Parmenter, T., Silove, N., . . . Warren, A. (2011). A randomised controlled trial of two early intervention programs for young children with autism: Centre-based with parent program and home-based. *Research in Autism Spectrum Disorders, 5,* 1553–1566. doi:10.1016/j.rasd.2011.03.001

Rocha, M. L., Schreibman, L., & Stahmer, A. C. (2007). Effectiveness of training parents to teach joint attention in children with autism. *Journal of Early Intervention, 29,* 154–172. doi:10.1177/105381510702900207

Rogers, S. J., & Dawson, G. (2009). Play and engagement in early autism: The Early Start Denver Model. New York: Guilford.

Rogers, S. J., Estes, A., Lord, C., Vismara, L., Winter, J., Fitzpatrick, A., ... Dawson, G. (2012). Effects of a brief Early Start Denver Model (ESDM)–based parent intervention on toddlers at risk for autism spectrum disorders: A randomized controlled trial. *Journal of the American Academy of Child and Adolescent Psychiatry, 51,* 1052–1065. doi:10.1016/j.jaac.2012.08.003

Rosenthal, R., Rosnow, R. L., & Rubin, D. B. (2000). *Contrasts and effect sizes in behavioral research: A correlational approach.* Cambridge, UK: Cambridge University Press.

Ruble, L. A., Dalrymple, N. J., & McGrew, J. H. (2010). The effects of consultation on individualized education program outcomes for young children with autism: The collaborative model for promoting competence and success. *Journal of Early Intervention, 32,* 286–301. doi:10.1177/1053815110382973

Russell, D., & Matson, J. (1998). Fathers as intervention agents for their children with developmental disabilities. *Child and Family Behavior Therapy, 20*(3), 29–49.

Rutter, M., Tizard, J., & Whitmore, K. (1970). *Education, health and behaviour.* London, UK: Longmans.

Rutter, M., Tizard, J., Yule, W., Graham, P., & Whitmore, K. (1976). Isle of Wight Studies, 1964–1974. *Psychological Medicine, 6,* 313–332. doi:10.1017/S003329170001388X

Ryff, C. D. (2014). Psychological well-being revisited: Advances in science and practice. *Psychotherapy and Psychosomatics, 83*(1), 10–28. doi:10.1159/000353263

Sanders, M. R. (1987). *Child management training.* University of Queensland. Department of Psychology Training Manual.

Sanders, M. R. (1999). Triple P-positive parenting program: Towards an empirically validated multilevel parenting and family support strategy for the prevention of behavior and emotional problems in children. *Clinical Child and Family Psychology Review, 2*(2), 71–90. doi:10.1023/A:1021843613840

Sanders, M. R., & Dadds, M. R. (1982). The effects of planned activities and child management procedures in parent training: An analysis of setting generality. *Behavior Therapy, 13,* 452–461.

Sanders, M. R., & Dadds, M. R. (1993). *Behavioral family intervention.* New York, NY: Prentice Hall.

Sanders, M. R., Markie-Dadds, C., Tully, L. A., & Bor, W. (2000). The triple P-positive parenting program: A comparison of enhanced, standard, and self-directed behavioral family intervention for parents of children with early onset conduct problems. *Journal of Consulting and Clinical Psychology, 68,* 624.

Sanders, M. R., Mazzucchelli, T. G., & Studman, L. J. (2004). Stepping Stones Triple P: The theoretical basis and development of an evidence-based positive parenting program for families with a child who has a disability. *Journal of Intellectual and Developmental Disability, 29,* 265–283.

Sanders, M. R., & Plant, K. (1989). Programming for generalization to high and low risk parenting situations in families with oppositional developmentally disabled preschoolers. *Behavior Modification, 13,* 283–305. doi:10.1177/01454455890133001

Santelli, B., Turnbull, A. P., Marquis, J. G., & Lerner, E. P. (1995). Parent to parent programs: A unique form of mutual support. *Infants and Young Children, 8*(2), 48–57.

Santelli, B., Turnbull, A., Marquis, J., & Lerner, E. (1997). Parent-to-parent programs: A resource for parents and professionals. *Journal of Early Intervention, 21*(1), 73–83.

Santelli, B., Turnbull, A., Sergeant, J., Lerner, E. P., & Marquis, J. G. (1996). Parent to parent programs: Parent preferences for supports. *Infants and Young Children, 9*(1), 53–62.

Schertz, H. H., & Odom, S. L. (2007). Promoting joint attention in toddlers with autism: A parent-mediated developmental model. *Journal of Autism and Developmental Disorders, 37,* 1562–1575. doi:10.1007/s10803-006-0290-z

Schreibman, L. (2000). Intensive behavioral/psychoeducational treatments for autism: Research needs and future directions. *Journal of Autism and Developmental Disorders, 30,* 373–378.

Schultz, C. L., Schultz, N. C., Bruce, E. J., Smyrnios, K. X., Carey, L. B., & Carey, C. L. (1993). Psychoeducational support for parents of children with intellectual disability: An outcome study. *International Journal of Disability, Development and Education, 40,* 205–216. doi:10.1080/0156655930400307

Schultz, N. C., & Schultz, C. L. (1997). *Care for caring parents.* Melbourne, Australia: Australian Council for Educational Research.

Schulz, K. F., Altman, D. G., & Moher, D. (2010). CONSORT 2010 statement: Updated guidelines for reporting parallel group randomised trials. *BMC Medicine, 8*(1), 18. doi:10.1186/1741-7015-8-18

Seiverling, L., Williams, K., Sturmey, P., & Hart, S. (2012). Effects of behavioral skills training on parental treatment of children's food selectivity. *Journal of Applied Behavior Analysis, 45,* 197–203.

Seligman, M. E. P. (2002). Positive psychology, positive prevention, and positive therapy. In C.R. Snyder & S.J. Lopez (Eds.), *Handbood of positive psychology* (pp. 3–12). New York: Oxford University Press.

Seligman, M. E. P., Steen, T. A., Park, N., & Peterson, C. (2006). Positive psychology progress: Empirical validation of interventions. *American Psychologist, 60,* 410–421.

Seltzer, G. B., Begun, A., Mailick Seltzer, M., & Krauss, M. W. (1991). Adults with mental retardation and their aging mothers: Impacts of siblings. *Family Relations, 40,* 310–317.

Seltzer, M. M., Almeida, D. M., Greenberg, J. S., Savla, J., Stawski, R. S., Hong, J., & Taylor, J. L. (2009). Psychosocial and biological markers of daily lives of midlife parents of children with disabilities. *Journal of Health and Social Behavior, 50*(1), 1–15. doi:10.1177/002214650905000101

Seltzer, M. M., Greenberg, J. S., Floyd, F. J., Pettee, Y., & Hong, J. (2001). Life course impacts of parenting a child with a disability. *American Journal of Mental Retardation, 106,* 265–286. doi:10.1352/0895-8017(2001)106<0265:LCIOPA>2.0.CO;2

Serketich, W. J., & Dumas, J. E. (1996). The effectiveness of behavioral parent training to modify antisocial behavior in children: A meta-analysis. *Behavior Therapy, 27,* 171–186. doi:10.1016/S0005-7894(96)80013-X

Sharry, J., & Fitzpatrick, C. (1998). *Parent Plus Programme: A practical and positive video-based course for managing and solving discipline problems in children.* Manual and Videos. Department of Child and Family Psychiatry, Mater Misericordiae Hospital, Dublin.

Sharry, J., Guerin, S., Griffin, C., & Drumm, M. (2005). An evaluation of the Parents Plus Early Years Programme: A video-based early intervention for parents of pre-school children with behavioural and developmental difficulties. *Clinical Child Psychology and Psychiatry, 10,* 319–336.

Sheridan, S. M., Eagle, J. W., Cowan, R. J., & Mickelson, W. (2001). The effects of conjoint behavioral consultation results of a 4-year investigation. *Journal of School Psychology, 39,* 361–385. doi: http://dx.doi.org/10.1016/S0022-4405(01)00079-6

Sheridan, S. M., Meegan, S. P., & Eagle, J. W. (2002). Assessing the social context in initial conjoint behavioral consultation interviews: An exploratory analysis investigating processes and outcomes. *School Psychology Quarterly, 17,* 299–324. doi:10.1521/scpq.17.3.299.20882

Siller, M., Hutman, T., & Sigman, M. (2013). A parent-mediated intervention to increase responsive parental behaviors and child communication in children with ASD: A randomized clinical trial. *Journal of Autism and Developmental Disorders, 43,* 540–555. doi:10.1007/s10803-012-1584-y

Siller, M., Swanson, M., Gerber, A., Hutman, T., & Sigman, M. (2014). A parent-mediated intervention that targets responsive parental behaviors increases attachment behaviors in children with ASD: Results from a randomized clinical trial. *Journal of Autism and Developmental Disorders, 44,* 1720–1732. doi:10.1007/s10803-014-2049-2

Silverman, W. K., Kurtines, W. M., Ginsburg, G. S., Weems, C. F., Rabian, B., & Serafini, L. T. (1999). Contingency management, self-control, and education support in the treatment of childhood phobic disorders: A randomized clinical trial. *Journal of Consulting and Clinical Psychology, 67*, 675.

Simon, B. S. (2001). Family involvement in high school: Predictors and effects. *NASSP Bulletin, 85*(627), 8–19. doi:10.1177/019263650108562702

Singer, G. H. S. (2002). Suggestions for a pragmatic program of research on families and disability. *Journal of Special Education, 36*, 150–156.

Singer, G. H. S. (2006). Meta-analysis of comparative studies of depression in mothers of children with and without developmental disabilities. *American Journal of Mental Retardation, 111*, 155–169. doi:10.1352/0895-8017(2006)111[155:MOCSOD]2.0.CO;2

Singer, G. H. S., Biegel, D. E., & Ethridge, B. L. (2009). Toward a cross disability view of family support for caregiving families. *Journal of Family Social Work, 12*, 97–118. doi:10.1080/10522150902874859

Singer, G. H. S., Biegel, D. E., & Ethridge, B. L. (2010). Trends impacting public policy support for caregiving families. *Journal of Family Social Work, 13*(3), 191–207. doi:10.1080/10522151003773867

Singer, G. H. S., Ethridge, B. L., & Aldana, S. I. (2007). Primary and secondary effects of parenting and stress management interventions for parents of children with developmental disabilities: A meta-analysis. *Mental Retardation and Developmental Education: Disabilities Research Reviews, 13*, 357–369.

Singer, G. H. S., Glang, A., Nixon, C., Cooley, E., Kerns, K. A., Williams, D., & Powers, L. E. (1994). A comparison of two psychosocial interventions for parents of children with acquired brain injury: An exploratory study. *Journal of Head Trauma Rehabilitation, 9*(4), 38–49.

Singer, G. H. S., Goldberg-Hamblin, S. E., Peckham-Hardin, K. D., Barry, L., & Santarelli, G. E. (2002). Towards a synthesis of family support practices and positive behavior support. In J. M. Lucyshyn, G. Dunlap, & R. W. Abidin (Eds.), *Families and positive behavior support: Addressing problem behavior in family contexts* (pp. 155–184). Baltimore, MD: Brookes.

Singer, G. H. S., Hornby, G., Park, J., Wang, M., & Xu, J. (2012). Parent to parent peer support across the Pacific Rim. *Journal of the International Special Needs Education, 15*, 89–106.

Singer, G. H. S., & Irvin, L. K. (Eds.). (1989). *Support for caregiving families: Enabling positive adaptation to disability*. Baltimore, MD: Brookes.

Singer, G. H. S., Irvin, L. K., & Hawkins, N. (1988). Stress management training for parents of children with severe handicaps. *Mental Retardation, 26*, 269–277. Retrieved from http://psycnet.apa.org/psycinfo/1989-12813-001

Singer, G. H. S., Irvin, L. K., Irvine, B., Hawkins, N., & Cooley, E. (1989). Evaluation of community-based support services for families of persons with developmental disabilities. *Journal of the Association for Persons with Severe Handicaps, 14*, 312–323.

Singer, G. H. S., Marquis, J., Powers, L. K., Blanchard, L., Divenere, N., Santelli, B., . . . Sharp, M. (1999). A multi-site evaluation of parent to parent programs for parents of children with disabilities. *Journal of Early Intervention, 22*, 217–229. doi:10.1177/105381519902200305

Singer, G. H., Singer, J., & Horner, R. H. (1987). Using pretask requests to increase the probability of compliance for students with severe disabilities. *Research and Practice for Persons with Severe Disabilities, 12*, 287–291.

Skinner, B. F. (1938). *The behavior of organisms: An experimental analysis*. Retrieved from http://psycnet.apa.org/psycinfo/1939-00056-000

Skinner, B. F. (1953). *Science and human behavior.* New York, NY: Macmillan. Retrieved from http://books.google.com/books?hl=en&lr=&id=Pjjknd1HREIC&oi=fnd&pg=PA1&dq=skinner+1953&ots=iOxhCxH0kF&sig=bVLTV11jmW6zfw9l-sRFRXF9tio

Skouge, J. R., Kelly, M. L., Roberts, K. D., Leake, D. W., & Stodden, R. A. (2007). Technologies for self-determination for youth with developmental disabilities. *Education and Training in Developmental Disabilities, 42,* 475–485. Retrieved from http://daddcec.org/Portals/0/CEC/Autism_Disabilities/Research/Publications/Education_Training_Development_Disabilities/2007v42_Journals/ETDD_200712v42n4p475-482_Technologies_Self-Determination_Youth_With_Developmental.pdf

Smith, D. D., & Salzberg, C. (1994). The shortage of special education faculty: Toward a better understanding. *Teacher Education and Special Education, 17*(1), 52–61. doi:10.1177/088840649401700106

Smith, M. R., & Lerman, D. C. (1999). A preliminary comparison of guided compliance and high-probability instructional sequences as treatment for noncompliance in children with developmental disabilities. *Research in Developmental Disabilities, 20,* 183–195.

Smith, T., Buch, G. A., & Gamby, T. E. (2000). Parent-directed, intensive early intervention for children with pervasive developmental disorder. *Research in Developmental Disabilities, 21,* 297–309. doi:10.1016/S0891-4222(00)00043-3

Snell, M. E., & Brown, F. (2006). Designing and implementing instructional programs. In M. Snell & F. Brown (Eds.), *Instruction of students with severe disabilities* (6th ed., pp. 111–169). Upper Saddle River, NJ: Prentice Hall.

Sofronoff, K., Jahnel, D., & Sanders, M. (2011). Stepping Stones Triple P seminars for parents of a child with a disability: A randomized controlled trial. *Research in Developmental Disabilities, 32,* 2253–2262.

Sofronoff, K., Leslie, A., & Brown, W. (2004). Parent management training and Asperger syndrome: A randomized controlled trial to evaluate a parent based intervention. *Autism, 8,* 301–317. doi:10.1177/1362361304045215

Solomon, M., Ono, M., Timmer, S., & Goodlin-Jones, B. (2008). The effectiveness of parent–child interaction therapy for families of children on the autism spectrum. *Journal of Autism and Developmental Disorders, 38,* 1767–1776. doi:10.1007/s10803-008-0567-5

Sparrow, S. S., Balla, D. A., & Cicchetti, D. V. (1984). *Vineland adaptive behavior scales.* Circle Pines, MN: American Guidance Service.

Spielberger, C. D., Gorsuch, R. L., Lushene, R., Vagg, P. R., & Jacobs, G. A. (1983). *Manual for the State-Trait Anxiety Inventory.* Palo Alto, CA: Consulting Psychologists Press.

Stainton, T., & Besser, H. (1998). The positive impact of children with an intellectual disability on the family. *Journal of Intellectual and Developmental Disability, 23*(1), 57–70.

Steer, R. A., & Beck, A. T. (1997). Beck Anxiety Inventory. In C. P. Zalaquett & R. J. Wood (Eds.), *Evaluating stress: A book of resources* (pp. 23–40). Lanham, MD: Scarecrow.

Stiebel, D. (1999). Promoting augmentative communication during daily routines a parent problem-solving intervention. *Journal of Positive Behavior Interventions, 1,* 159–169. doi:10.1177/109830079900100304

Stores, R., & Stores, G. (2004). Evaluation of brief group administered instruction for parents to prevent or minimize sleep problems in young children with Down syndrome. *Journal of Applied Research in Intellectual Disabilities, 17*(2), 61–70. doi:10.1111/j.1360-2322.2004.00174.x

Stormshak, E. A., Fosco, G. M., & Dishion, T. J. (2010). Implementing interventions with families in schools to increase engagement: The Family Check-Up model. *School Mental Health, 2*(2), 82–92. doi:10.1007/s12310-009-9025-6

Sugavanam, T., Mead, G., Bulley, C., Donaghy, M., & van Wijck, F. (2012). The effects and experiences of goal setting in stroke rehabilitation: A systematic review. *Disability and Rehabilitation, 35*, 177–190. doi:10.3109/09638288.2012.690501

Summers, J., Hoffman, L., Marquis, J., Turnbull, A., Poston, D., & Nelson, L. (2005). Measuring the quality of family-professional partnerships in special education services. *Exceptional Children, 72*(1), 65–81.

Summers, J. A., Marquis, J., Mannan, H., Turnbull, A. P., Fleming, K., Poston, D. J., . . . Kupzyk, K. (2007). Relationship of perceived adequacy of services, family–professional partnerships, and family quality of life in early childhood service programmes. *International Journal of Disability, Development and Education, 54*, 319–338. doi:10.1080/10349120701488848

Swift, C., & Levin, G. (1987). Empowerment: An emerging mental health technology. *Journal of Primary Prevention, 8*(1–2), 71–94.

Symon, J. B. (2005). Expanding interventions for children with autism parents as trainers. *Journal of Positive Behavior Interventions, 7*, 159–173. doi:10.1177/10983007050070030501

Tarbox, J., Wallace, M. D., & Tarbox, R. S. F. (2002). Successful generalized parent training and failed schedule thinning of response blocking for automatically maintained object mouthing. *Behavioral Interventions, 17*, 169–178. doi:10.1002/bin.116

Tavormina, J. B. (1975). Relative effectiveness of behavioral and reflective group counseling with parents of mentally retarded children. *Journal of Consulting and Clinical Psychology, 43*(1), 22.

Taylor, S. E., Klein, L. C., Lewis, B. P., Gruenewald, T. L., Gurung, R. A., & Updegraff, J. A. (2000). Biobehavioral responses to stress in females: Tend-and-befriend, not fight-or-flight. *Psychological Review, 107*, 411–429. .20175doi:10.1177/00224669020360030501

Thackeray, E. J., & Richdale, A. L. (2002). The behavioural treatment of sleep difficulties in children with an intellectual disability. *Behavioral Interventions, 17*, 211–231.

Tiger, J. H., Hanley, G. P., & Bruzek, J. (2008). Functional communication training: A review and practical guide. *Behavior Analysis in Practice, 1*(1), 16–23.

Tonge, B., Brereton, A., Kiomall, M., Mackinnon, A., King, N., & Rinehart, N. (2006). Effects on parental mental health of an education and skills training program for parents of young children with autism: A randomized controlled trial. *Journal of the American Academy of Child and Adolescent Psychiatry, 45*, 561–569. doi:10.1097/01.chi.0000205701.48324.26

Tonge, B., Brereton, A., Kiomall, M., Mackinnon, A., & Rinehart, N. J. (2014). A randomised group comparison controlled trial of "preschoolers with autism": A parent education and skills training intervention for young children with autistic disorder. *Autism, 18*, 166–177. doi:10.1177/1362361312458186

Trach, J., & Shelden, D. (2000). Meeting attendance and transition outcomes as reflected in students' individualized education programs. In D. R. Johnson & E. J. Emanuel (Eds.), *Issues influencing the future of transition programs and services in the United States* (pp. 127–136). Minneapolis, MN: University of Minnesota.

Trainor, A. A. (2002). Self-determination for students with learning disabilities: Is it a universal value? *International Journal of Qualitative Studies in Education, 15*, 711–725. doi:10.1080/0951839022000014394

Trainor, A. A. (2008). Diverse approaches to parent advocacy during special education home-school interactions. *Remedial and Special Education, 31*(1), 34–47. doi:10.1177/0741932508324401

Trent, J. W. (1994). *Inventing the feeble mind: A history of mental retardation in the United States*. Berkeley, CA: University of California Press.

Trivette, C. M., & Dunst, C. J. (1992). Characteristics and influences of role division and social support among mothers of preschool children with disabilities. *Topics in Early Childhood Special Education, 12*, 367–385. doi:10.1177/027112149201200308

Tunali, B., & Power, T. G. (2002). Coping by redefinition: Cognitive appraisals in mothers of children with autism and children without autism. *Journal of Autism and Developmental Disorders, 32*(1), 25–34. doi:10.1023/A:1017999906420

Turnbull, A. P., Blue-Banning, M., Behr, S., & Kerns, G. (1986). Family research and intervention: A value and ethical examination. In P. R. Dokecki & R. M. Zaner (Eds.), *Ethics of dealing with persons with severe handicaps* (pp. 119–140). Baltimore, MD: Brookes.

Turnbull, A. P., Summers, J. A., Turnbull, R., Brotherson, M. J., Winton, P., Roberts, R., . . . Stroup-Rentier, V. (2007). Family supports and services in early intervention: A bold vision. *Journal of Early Intervention, 29*, 187–206. http://doi.org/10.1177/105381510702900301

Van Hasselt, V. B., Sisson, L. A., & Aach, S. R. (1987). Parent training to increase compliance in a young multihandicapped child. *Journal of Behavior Therapy and Experimental Psychiatry, 18*, 275–283.

Van Kuiken, D. (2004). A meta-analysis of the effect of guided imagery practice on outcomes. *Journal of Holistic Nursing: Official Journal of the American Holistic Nurses' Association, 22*, 164–179. doi:10.1177/0898010104266066

Vaughn, B. J., Clarke, S., & Dunlap, G. (1997). Assessment-based intervention for severe behavior problems in a natural family context. *Journal of Applied Behavior Analysis, 30*, 713–716. doi:10.1901/jaba.1997.30-713

Vaughn, B. J., Wilson, D., & Dunlap, G. (2002). Family-centered intervention to resolve problem behaviors in a fast-food restaurant. *Journal of Positive Behavior Interventions, 4*, 38–45.

Vismara, L. A., Colombi, C., & Rogers, S. J. (2009). Can one hour per week of therapy lead to lasting changes in young children with autism? *Autism, 13*(1), 93–115. doi:10.1177/1362361307098516

Vollmer, T. R., Marcus, B. A., & Ringdahl, J. E. (1995). Noncontingent escape as treatment for self-injurious behavior maintained by negative reinforcement. *Journal of Applied Behavior Analysis, 28*(1), 15–26. doi:10.1901/jaba.1995.28-15

Vollmer, T. R., Roane, H. S., Ringdahl, J. E., & Marcus, B. A. (1999). Evaluating treatment challenges with differential reinforcement of alternative behavior. *Journal of Applied Behavior Analysis, 32*(1), 9–23.

Wacker, D. P., Berg, W. K., Harding, J. W., Barretto, A., Rankin, B., & Ganzer, J. (2005). Treatment effectiveness, stimulus generalization, and acceptability to parents of functional communication training. *Educational Psychology, 25*, 233–256. doi:10.1080/0144341042000301184

Wacker, D. P., Berg, W. K., Harding, J. W., Derby, K. M., Asmus, J. M., & Healy, A. (1998). Evaluation and long-term treatment of aberrant behavior displayed by young children with disabilities. *Journal of Developmental and Behavioral Pediatrics, 19*, 260–266.

Wacker, D. P., Lee, J. F., Dalmau, Y. C. P., Kopelman, T. G., Lindgren, S. D., Kuhle, J., . . . Waldron, D. B. (2013). Conducting functional communication training via telehealth to reduce the problem behavior of young children with autism. *Journal of Developmental and Physical Disabilities, 25*(1), 35–48. doi:10.1007/s10882-012-9314-0

Wagner, M., Newman, L., Cameto, R., Levine, P., & Marder, C. (2007). Perceptions and expectations of youth with disabilities. A special topic report of findings from the National Longitudinal Transition Study-2 (NLTS2). NCSER 2007-3006. National Center for Special Education Research. Retrieved from http://files.eric.ed.gov/fulltext/ED498185.pdf

Wang, M., McCart, A., & Turnbull, A. P. (2007). Positive behavior support with Chinese American families: Enhancing cultural competence. *Journal of Positive Behavior Interventions, 9,* 38–51. doi:10.1177/10983007070090010501.

Webster-Stratton, C. (1984). Randomized trial of two parent-training programs for families with conduct-disordered children. *Journal of Consulting and Clinical Psychology, 52*(4), 666–678. doi:10.1037/0022-006X.52.4.666

Webster-Stratton, C. (1997). From parent training to community building. *Families in Society: The Journal of Contemporary Social Services, 78,* 156–171.

Webster-Stratton, C. (1998). Preventing conduct problems in Head Start children: Strengthening parenting competencies. *Journal of Consulting and Clinical Psychology, 66,* 715–730. doi:10.1037/0022-006X.66.5.715

Webster-Stratton, C. (2001). The Incredible Years: Parents, teachers, and children training series. *Residential Treatment for Children and Youth, 18*(3), 31–45. doi:10.1300/J007v18n03_04

Webster-Stratton, C. (2006). *The Incredible Years: A trouble-shooting guide for parents of children ages 3–8 years.* Seattle, WA: Incredible Years Press.

Webster-Stratton, C., & Reid, M. J. (2010). The Incredible Years parents, teachers, and children training series: A multifaceted treatment approach for young children with conduct disorders. In J. Weisz & A. Kazdin (Eds.), *Evidence-based psychotherapies for children and adolescents* (2nd ed.). New York, NY: Guilford.

Webster-Stratton, C., Reid, M. J., & Hammond, M. (2001). Preventing conduct problems, promoting social competence: A parent and teacher training partnership in Head Start. *Journal of Clinical Child and Adolescent Psychology, 30,* 283–302. doi:10.1207/S15374424JCCP3003_2

Webster-Stratton, C., Reid, M. J., & Hammond, M. (2004). Treating children with early-onset conduct problems: Intervention outcomes for parent, child, and teacher training. *Journal of Clinical Child and Adolescent Psychology, 33*(1), 105–124. doi:10.1207/S15374424JCCP3301_11

Webster-Stratton, C., & Taylor, T. (2001). Nipping early risk factors in the bud: Preventing substance abuse, delinquency, and violence in adolescence through interventions targeted at young children (0–8 years). *Prevention Science, 2,* 165–192. doi:10.1023/A:1011510923900

Wechsler, D. (1989). *WPPSI-R manual.* San Antonio, TX: Psychological Corp.

Wehmeyer, M. L. (1997). Student-directed learning and self-determination. In M. Agran (Ed.), *Student directed learning: Teaching self-determination skills* (pp. 28–59). Pacific Grove, CA: Brooks/Cole.

Wehmeyer, M. L. (1999). A functional model of self-determination describing development and implementing instruction. *Focus on Autism and Other Developmental Disabilities, 14*(1), 53–61. doi:10.1177/108835769901400107

Wehmeyer, M. L. (2005). Self-determination and individuals with severe disabilities: Re-examining meanings and misinterpretations. *Research and Practice for Persons with Severe Disabilities, 30,* 113–120. doi:http://dx.doi.org/10.2511/rpsd.30.3.113

Wehmeyer, M. L., & Kelchner, K. (1995). *The Arc's self-determination scale.* Arlington, TX: The Arc National Headquarters.

Wehmeyer, M. L., & Palmer, S. B. (2003). Adult outcomes for students with cognitive disabilities three-years after high school: The impact of self-determination. *Education and Training in Developmental Disabilities, 38,* 131–144.

Wehmeyer, M. L., & Schwartz, M. (1997). Self-determination and positive adult outcomes: A follow-up study of youth with mental retardation or learning disabilities. *Exceptional Children, 63,* 245–256.

Wehmeyer, M. L., & Schwartz, M. (1998). *The relationship between self-determination and quality of life for adults with mental retardation*. Retrieved from http://nytransitions.net/data/a2.pdf

Wehmeyer, M. L., Palmer, S. B., Agran, M., Mithaug, D. E., & Martin, J. E. (2000). Promoting causal agency: The self-determined learning model of instruction. *Exceptional Children, 66*, 439–453.

Wehmeyer, M. L., Palmer, S. B., Shogren, K., Williams-Diehm, K., & Soukup, J. H. (2013). Establishing a causal relationship between intervention to promote self-determination and enhanced student self-determination. *Journal of Special Education, 46*, 195–210. doi:10.1177/0022466910392377

Wehmeyer, M. L., Sands, D. J., Doll, B., & Palmer, S. (1997). The development of self-determination and implications for educational interventions with students with disabilities. *International Journal of Disability, Development and Education, 44*, 305–328. doi:10.1080/0156655970440403

Weiskop, S., Matthews, J., & Richdale, A. (2001). Treatment of sleep problems in a 5-year-old boy with autism using behavioural principles. *Autism, 5*, 209–221.

Werle, M. A., Murphy, T. B., & Budd, K. S. (1993). Treating chronic food refusal in young children: Home-based parent training. *Journal of Applied Behavior Analysis, 26*, 421–433.

Whalen, C., & Schreibman, L. (2003). Joint attention training for children with autism using behavior modification procedures. *Journal of Child Psychology and Psychiatry, 44*, 456–468. doi:10.1111/1469-7610.00135

Whitbread, K. M., Bruder, M. B., Fleming, G., & Park, H. J. (2007). Collaboration in special education: Parent-professional training. *Teaching Exceptional Children, 39*(4), 6–14.

Whittingham, K., Sofronoff, K., & Sheffield, J. K. (2006). Stepping Stones Triple P: A pilot study to evaluate acceptability of the program by parents of a child diagnosed with an autism spectrum disorder. *Research in Developmental Disabilities, 27*, 364–380.

Whittingham, K., Sofronoff, K., Sheffield, J., & Sanders, M. R. (2009). Stepping Stones Triple P: An RCT of a parenting program with parents of a child diagnosed with an autism spectrum disorder. *Journal of Abnormal Child Psychology, 37*, 469–480. doi:10.1007/s10802-008-9285-x

Wiggs, L., & Stores, G. (1996). Severe sleep disturbance and daytime challenging behaviour in children with severe learning disabilities. *Journal of Intellectual Disability Research, 40*, 518–528.

Wiggs, L., & Stores, G. (2001). Behavioural treatment for sleep problems in children with severe intellectual disabilities and daytime challenging behaviour: Effect on mothers and fathers. *British Journal of Health Psychology, 6*, 257.

Wikler, L., Wasow, M., & Hatfield, E. (1981). Chronic sorrow revisited: Parent vs. professional depiction of the adjustment of parents of mentally retarded children. *American Journal of Orthopsychiatry, 51*(1), 63–70.

Witt, W. P., Riley, A. W., & Coiro, M. J. (2003). Childhood functional status, family stressors, and psychosocial adjustment among school-aged children with disabilities in the United States. *Archives of Pediatrics and Adolescent Medicine, 157*, 687–695. doi:10.1001/archpedi.157.7.687

Wolman, J., Campeau, P., Dubois, P., Mithaug, D., & Stolarski, V. (1994). *AIR self-determination scale and user guide*. Palo Alto, CA: American Institute for Research.

Wong, C., Odom, S. L., Hume, K., Cox, A. W., Fetting, A., Kucharczyk, S., & Schultz, T. R. (2013). *Evidence-based practices for children, youth, and young adults with autism spectrum disorder*. The University of North Carolina, Frank Porter Graham Child Development Institute, Autism Evidence-Based Practice Review Group, Chapel Hill, NC.

Wong, V. C. N., & Kwan, Q. K. (2010). Randomized controlled trial for early intervention for autism: A pilot study of the Autism 1-2-3 Project. *Journal of Autism and Developmental Disorders, 40,* 677–688. doi:10.1007/s10803-009-0916-z

Zeidner, M., & Endler, N. S. (1996). *Handbook of coping: Theory, research, and applications.* New York, NY: Wiley.

Zeitlin, A. G. (1986). Mentally retarded adults and their siblings. *American Journal on Mental Retardation, 91,* 217–225.

Zhang, D., Wehmeyer, M. L., & Chen, L.-J. (2005). Parent and teacher engagement in fostering the self-determination of students with disabilities: A comparison between the United States and the Republic of China. *Remedial and Special Education, 26*(1), 55–64. doi:10.1177/07419325050260010701

Zimmerman, M. A. (1995). Psychological empowerment: Issues and illustrations. *American Journal of Community Psychology, 23,* 581–599.

Zirpoli, T. J., Hancox, D., Wieck, C., & Skarnulis, E. R. (1994). Partners in policymaking: Empowering people. *Journal of the Association for Persons with Severe Handicaps, 14,* 163–167.

Zwaigenbaum, L., Bryson, S., Rogers, T., Roberts, W., Brian, J., & Szatmari, P. (2005). Behavioral manifestations of autism in the first year of life. *International Journal of Developmental Neuroscience, 23,* 143–152. doi:10.1016/j.ijdevneu.2004.05.001

INDEX

Note: Page numbers in *italics* indicate tables and charts.